Improved Non-Steroid Anti-Inflammatory Drugs

COX-2 Enzyme Inhibitors

The conference organisers wish to thank

Boehringer Ingelheim

for an educational grant to support this conference

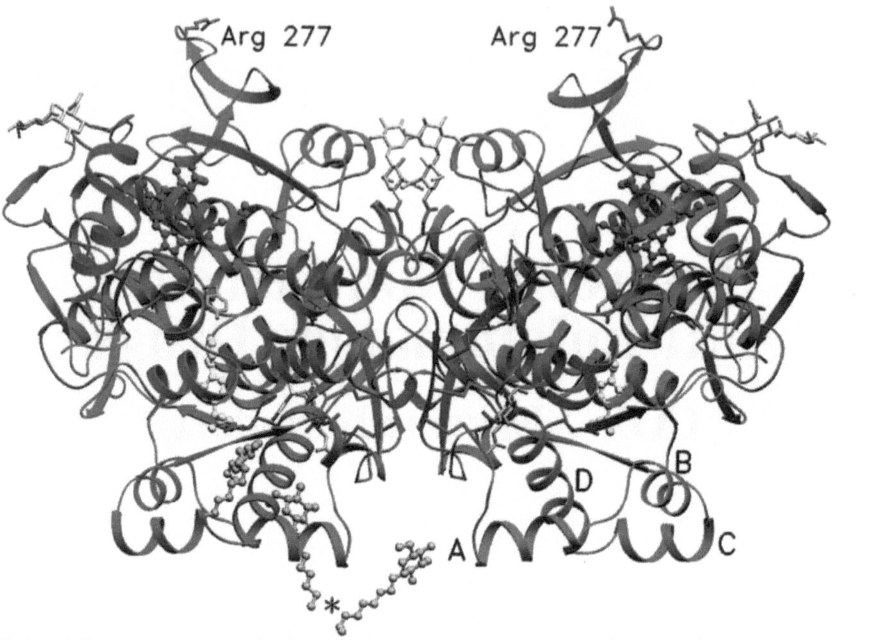

Chapter 2 Figure 1 *A Molescript diagram of the COX-1 dimer derived from the 3.1 Å refined structure. Heme groups are shown in red, Tyr385 in green and flurbiprofen in yellow. The bound detergent molecules are shown in orange where the two near the asterisk are involved in crystal contacts; the other detergent molecule which is in the cyclooxygenase channel also appears in the other monomer. Helices A, B, C, D of the membrane binding domain as well as the site of trypsin cleavage, Arg277, are also labelled*

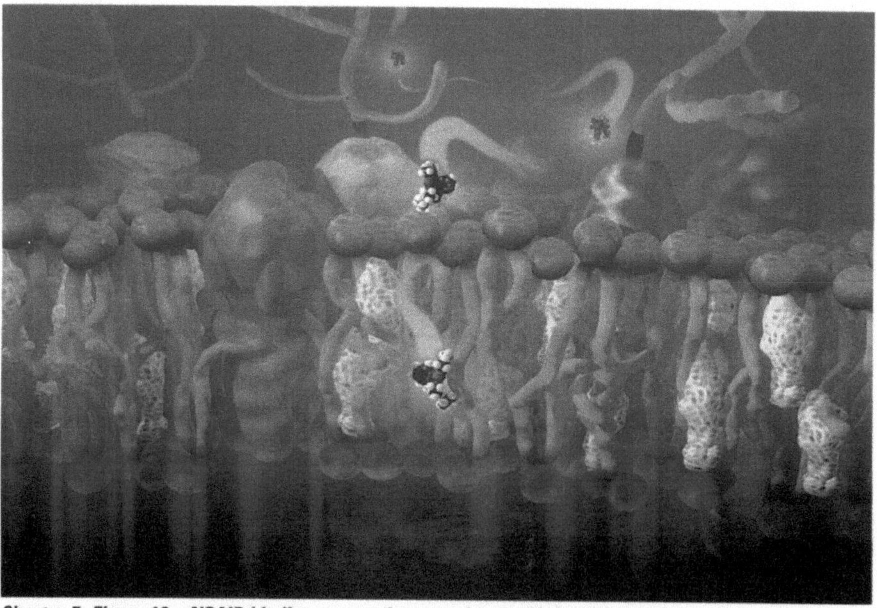

Chapter 5 Figure 10 *NSAID binding approach to membrane. Molecular depiction of the binding of an NSAID to the lipid bilayer structure as a necessary and first step to binding to the COX enzyme.*

Improved Non-Steroid Anti-Inflammatory Drugs
COX-2 Enzyme Inhibitors

Edited by

SIR JOHN VANE, DR JACK BOTTING and DR REGINA BOTTING
The William Harvey Research Institute, Saint Bartholomew's Hospital Medical College, London, United Kingdom

Proceedings of a conference held
on October 10–11, 1995,
at Regent's College, London

KLUWER ACADEMIC PUBLISHERS
DORDRECHT/BOSTON/LONDON

WILLIAM HARVEY
PRESS

Distributors

for the United States and Canada: Kluwer Academic Publishers, PO Box 358, Accord Station, Hingham, MA 02018-0358, USA
for all other countries: Kluwer Academic Publishers Group, Distribution Center, PO Box 322, 3300 AH Dordrecht, The Netherlands

A catalogue record for this book is available from the British Library

ISBN-13:978-94-010-9031-5 e-ISBN-13:978-94-010-9029-2
DOI: 10.1007/978-94-010-9029-2

Published in the United Kingdom by Kluwer Academic Publishers, PO Box 55, Lancaster, UK, and William Harvey Press, Charterhouse Square, London, UK.

Kluwer Academic Publishers BV incorporates the publishing programmes of D. Reidel, Martinus Nijhoff, Dr W. Junk and MTP Press.

Typeset by Lasertext Ltd, Stretford, Manchester.

Contents

List of Contributors

D. Nicholas Bateman
Regional Drugs and Therapeutics Centre, Wolfson Unit, Claremont Place, Newcastle-upon-Tyne NE1 4LP, UK,

Nicolas G. Bazan
Department of Ophthalmology and LSU Neuroscience Center of Excellence, Louisiana State University Medical Center, School of Medicine, 2020 Gravier Street, Suite B, New Orleans LA 70112, USA
Co-authors: Geoffrey Allan and Victor Marcheselli

Phillip Bennett
Royal Postgraduate Medical School, Institute of Obstetrics and Gynaecology, Queen Charlotte's and Chelsea Hospital, Goldhawk Road, London W6 0XG, UK
Co-author: Donna Slater

Leslie J. Crofford
Department of Internal Medicine, Division of Rheumatology, University of Michigan, Ann Arbor, MI 48109, USA

Paul Emery
Rheumatology and Rehabilitation Research Unit, University of Leeds, 36 Clarendon Road, Leeds LS2 9JT UK

Jürgen C. Frölich
Institute of Clinical Pharmacology, Hannover Medical School, 30623 Hannover, Germany
Co-author: Dirk Stichtenoth

R. Michael Garavito
Department of Biochemistry, 522 Biochemistry Building, Michigan State University, East Lansing, MI 48824-1319, USA

Leo G. Herbette
Biomolecular Structure Analysis Center, University of Connecticut Health Center, Farmington, CT 06030, USA
Co-authors: Michelle Vecchiarelli and Günther Trummlitz

Michel Pairet
Department of Biological Research, Boehringer Ingelheim Research Laboratories, Birkendorfer Strasse 65, 88397 Biberach an der Riss, Germany
Co-author: Günther Engelhardt

Carlo Patrono
University of Chieti, 'G D'Annunzio' School of Medicine, Via dei Vestini 31, 66013 Chieti, Italy
Co-authors: Paola Patrignani, Maria Panara, Francesco Cipollone, Giovanna Santini, Maria Sciulli, Maria Rotondo, Roberto Padovano and Maria di Giamberardino

Daniel L. Simmons
Department of Chemistry and Biochemistry, E280 BNSN, Brigham Young University, Provo, UT 84602, USA
Co-authors: Xiaojun Lu, William Bradshaw and Weilin Xie

John R. Vane
The William Harvey Research Institute, St Bartholomew's Hospital Medical College, Charterhouse Square, London EC1M 6BQ, UK
Co-author: Regina M. Botting

Derek Willoughby
Department of Experimental Pathology, St Bartholomew's Hospital Medical College, William Harvey Research Institute, London EC1M 6BQ, UK
Co-authors: Annette Tomlinson, Derek Gilroy and Dean Willis

Preface

In 1971, Vane proposed that the mechanism of action of the aspirin-like drugs was through their inhibition of prostaglandin biosynthesis. Since then, there has been intense interest in the interaction between this diverse group of inhibitors and the enzyme known as cyclooxygenase (COX). It exists in two isoforms, COX-1 and COX-2 (discovered some 5 years ago). Over the last two decades several new drugs have reached the market based on COX-1 enzyme screens. Elucidation of the three-dimensional structure of COX-1 has provided a new understanding for the actions of COX inhibitors. The constitutive isoform of COX, COX-1 has clear physiological functions. Its activation leads, for instance, to the production of prostacyclin which when released by the endothelium is anti-thrombogenic and anti-atherosclerotic, and in the gastric mucosa is cyto-protective. COX-1 also generates prostaglandins in the kidney, where they help to maintain blood flow and promote natriuresis. The inducible isoform, COX-2, was discovered through its activity being increased in a number of cells by pro-inflammatory stimuli. A year or so later, COX-2 was identified as a distinct isoform encoded by a different gene from COX-1. COX-2 is induced by inflammatory stimuli and by cytokines in migratory and other cells. Thus the anti-inflammatory actions of non-steroid anti-inflammatory drugs (NSAIDs) may be due to the inhibition of COX-2, whereas the unwanted side-effects such as irritation of the stomach lining and toxic effects on the kidney are due to inhibition of the constitutive enzyme, COX-1. This hypothesis has led to intense research to establish, *inter alia*, the relative activities of the currently used NSAIDs against COX-1 and COX-2, the sites of expression of COX-2 and the therapeutic activity and toxicity profile of new, highly selective COX-2 inhibitors.

The following chapters, written by leaders in the field, review the current status of this research. In the next few years, we can expect improved therapy of inflammatory disease, arising from further knowledge of the pathophysiological significance of the COX enzymes.

John R. Vane

1 Overview – mechanisms of action of anti-inflammatory drugs

J.R. VANE and R.M. BOTTING

Inflammation is the response of living tissues to injury. It involves a complex battery of enzyme activation, mediator release, extravasation of fluid, cell migration, tissue breakdown and repair. This overview will concentrate on the actions of anti-inflammatory drugs, with special reference to the prostaglandin system. This system is activated by phospholipase A_2, which liberates arachidonic acid, the substrate for cyclooxygenase (COX or PGH_2 synthase). This leads to an increased production of prostaglandins (Figure 1). Prostaglandin E_2 is the predominant eicosanoid detected in inflammatory conditions in man ranging from experimental acute oedema and sunburn through to chronic arthritis. Because inflammation is one of the few conditions in which PGE_2 is a major product of COX it is possible that the process of inflammation directs the enzymic pathway towards this product. A second enzyme, 5-lipoxygenase converts arachidonic acid to the leukotrienes[1], which are important mediators of asthma, but this aspect will not be discussed here.

Prostaglandin E_2 accounts for the characteristic vasodilatation and erythema (redness) seen in acute inflammation[2]. Vasodilatation increases the flow of blood through inflamed tissues and this augments the extravasation of fluid (oedema) caused by agents which increase vascular permeability such as bradykinin and histamine[3]. Prostaglandin E_2 also acts synergistically with other mediators to produce inflammatory pain: although it has no direct pain-producing activity, PGE_2 sensitizes receptors on afferent nerve endings to the actions of bradykinin and histamine[4]. PGE_2 is also a potent pyretic agent and its production, stimulated by the release of interleukin-1 (IL-1), in bacterial and viral infections contributes to the associated fever[5].

Many other COX products have been detected in inflammatory lesions. These include $PGF_{2\alpha}$, PGD_2, prostacyclin (as 6-keto-$PGF_{1\alpha}$) and thromboxane A_2 (TXA_2; as TXB_2), but these are usually present at less than a quarter of the concentrations of PGE_2. Prostacyclin is probably the most important of these products in terms of inflammatory signs, for it is also a potent vasodilator and is a more potent hyperalgesic agent than PGE_2. It is likely, therefore, that both PGE_2 and prostacyclin contribute to the development of inflammatory erythema and pain[6].

There was a new dawn in inflammatory research when Needleman and his colleagues found that COX activity was substantially increased by bacterial endotoxin in human monocytes in vitro[7] and in mouse peritoneal macrophages

Figure 1 The arachidonic acid cascade

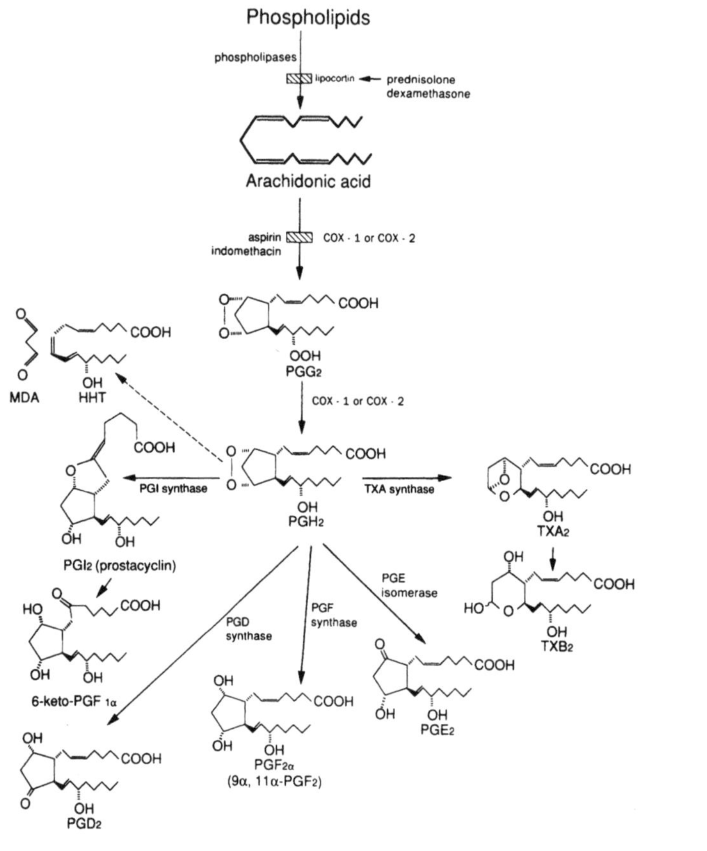

in vivo[8]. This increase was associated with de novo synthesis of new COX protein and was prevented by dexamethasone. A year or so later, an inducible synthase was identified as a distinct isoform of cyclooxygenase (COX-2) encoded by a different gene from the constitutive enzyme (COX-1; see below).

CYCLOOXYGENASE-1

Cyclooxygenase (COX) activity has long been studied in preparations from ram seminal vesicles and a homogeneous, enzymatically active prostaglandin endoperoxide synthase (PGHS) was isolated in 1976[9]. This membrane-bound haemo- and glycoprotein with a molecular weight of 71 kDa is found in greatest amounts in the endoplasmic reticulum of prostanoid-forming cells[10]. It both cyclizes arachidonic acid and adds the 15-hydroperoxy group to form prostaglandin (PG) G_2. The hydroperoxy group of PGG_2 is reduced to the hydroxy group of PGH_2 by a peroxidase (in the same enzyme protein) that utilizes a wide variety of compounds to provide the requisite pair of electrons (Figure 1). The hydroperoxides also drive the cyclooxygenase reaction by maintaining a 'hydroperoxide tone'[11].

Picot, Loll and Garavito[12] gave a strong boost to the field of COX research by determining the three-dimensional structure of COX-1. The enzyme is in a monotopic arrangement with respect to the cell membrane (that is, it integrates into only a single leaflet of the lipid bilayer). This bifunctional enzyme comprises three independent folding units: an epidermal growth factor-like domain, a membrane-binding motif and an enzymatic domain. The sites for peroxidase and cyclooxygenase activity are adjacent but spatially distinct. Three of the helices of the structure form an entrance channel to the active site and their insertion into the membrane could allow arachidonic acid to gain access from the interior of the bilayer.

The COX active site is a long, hydrophobic channel and Picot et al.[12] presented arguments that some of the aspirin-like drugs such as flurbiprofen inhibit COX-1 by excluding arachidonate from the upper portion of the channel. Tyrosine (Tyr) 385 and serine (Ser) 530 are at the apex of the long active site. Aspirin irreversibly inhibits COX-1 by acetylation of Ser530, thereby excluding access for arachidonic acid to Tyr385 by steric hindrance[13]. The acetyl-serine side chain can rotate in the slightly larger channel of COX-2, thus allowing limited access of substrate to the active site. Loll and his colleagues[14] postulated that the salicylate moiety of aspirin or salicylic acid binds with weak affinity to a second binding site below Ser530 (probably to the carboxylate binding site, arginine (Arg) 120). A comparable affinity of the two salicylate molecules for this site would explain the antagonistic effect of salicylic acid on aspirin activity in some systems. Because of the weak affinity for its binding site, salicylic acid would be easily displaced by excess of substrate and would therefore have low intrinsic cyclooxygenase inhibitory activity[14]. The S(–) stereoisomer of flurbiprofen interacts, through its carboxylase, with Arg120, thereby placing the second phenyl ring within van der Waals contact of Tyr385. Other subsites for drug binding may exist in the channel to explain the interactions of anti-inflammatory drugs such as indomethacin or ibuprofen.

COX-1 is constitutively expressed in most tissues, and performs a 'housekeeping' function to synthesize prostaglandins which regulate normal cell activity (Figure 1). The prostaglandins produced are, thus, protective to the organism. The concentration of the enzyme remains largely stable, but small, 2- to 4-fold increases can occur in response to stimulation with hormones or growth factors[15,16].

CYCLOOXYGENASE-2

The cloning of COX-1 from sheep seminal vesicles[17–19] provided useful probes for the study of the relationship between prostaglandin production and COX mRNA induction. Many of these studies revealed a lack of correlation between COX activity and the induction of COX mRNA. For example, the levels of 2.8 kb COX-1 mRNA in epithelial cells of sheep trachea stimulated with growth factors did not reflect the increase in enzyme activity. However, a second mRNA (4.0 kb) recognized by the COX-1 cDNA probes and formed from a separate gene increased in parallel with prostaglandin production[20]. Needleman and his colleagues[7,21] also reported that dexamethasone inhibited only the inducible COX activity in human IL-1-treated dermal fibroblasts and in human lipopolysaccharide (LPS)-stimulated monocytes. Basal levels of COX were not affected by dexamethasone.

The presence of the gene encoding for a second COX enzyme was discovered serendipitously by Xie et al.[22] while characterizing 'immediate early' genes switched on by expression of the *v-src* oncogene in chicken embryo fibroblasts[22,23]. This new COX isoenzyme was also induced by serum, tetradecanoyl phorbol acetate (TPA) or forskolin in established murine fibroblast cell lines[24,25]. The chicken and mouse COX-2 gene, at 8.3 kb, is similar to the COX-2 gene of human, but smaller than the 22 kb human COX-1 gene. The amino acid sequence of its cDNA shows only a 60% homology with the sequence of the constitutive enzyme, with the size of the mRNA for COX-2 approximating 4.5 kb and that for COX-1 being 2.8 kb[26]. At the amino acid level, the protein sizes of COX-1 and COX-2 enzymes from different sources are approximately 80–90% identical (for review see Ref. 27). However, both enzymes have a molecular weight of 70 kDa and similar active sites for the attachment of arachidonic acid or non-steroid anti-inflammatory drugs (NSAIDs), although the active site of COX-2 is larger than that of COX-1 and can accept a wider range of structures as substrates. Thus, whereas both enzymes oxygenate dihomo-γ-linolenic acid almost equally well, α-linolenic, linoleic and eicosapentaenoic acids are better substrates for COX-2 than for COX-1[28]. Both enzymes have similar K_m and V_{max} values for metabolism of arachidonic acid[29]. Although aspirin is highly selective for COX-1 and produces inhibition by acetylating Ser530, large doses will acetylate Ser516 on COX-2[30]. This acetylated enzyme, however, can still metabolize arachidonic acid to 15-R-HETE. The synthesis of 15-R-HETE therefore provides an additional means of distinguishing between the two isoforms of COX[29]. The finding that aspirin-acetylated COX-2 can accommodate arachidonic acid in its active site, whereas aspirin-acetylated COX-1 cannot, confirms that the active site of COX-2 must be wider than that of COX-1.

Little or no COX-2 is found in resting cells but its expression can be increased dramatically after exposure of fibroblasts, vascular smooth muscle or endothelial cells to growth factors, phorbol esters or cytokines and by LPS in monocytes/macrophages. In chronic inflammation, levels of COX-2 protein also increase in

***Figure 2** Relationship between the pathways leading to the generation of prostaglandins by COX-1 or COX-2. Activation of COX-1 promotes release of eicosanoids involved in physiological processes (e.g. thromboxane A_2, prostacyclin, prostaglandin E_2). Inhibition by NSAIDs of COX-1 results in the side effects (e.g. gastrointestinal irritation, damage). However, the protective effect of aspirin in heart attacks and strokes is also due to inhibition of COX-1 in platelets. Inhibition of COX-2 reduces inflammation. Most currently available NSAIDs are more potent inhibitors of COX-1 than COX-2. NSAIDs that preferentially inhibit COX-2 reduce inflammation with less inhibition of the production of physiologically active eicosanoids so potentially reducing the risk of side effects*

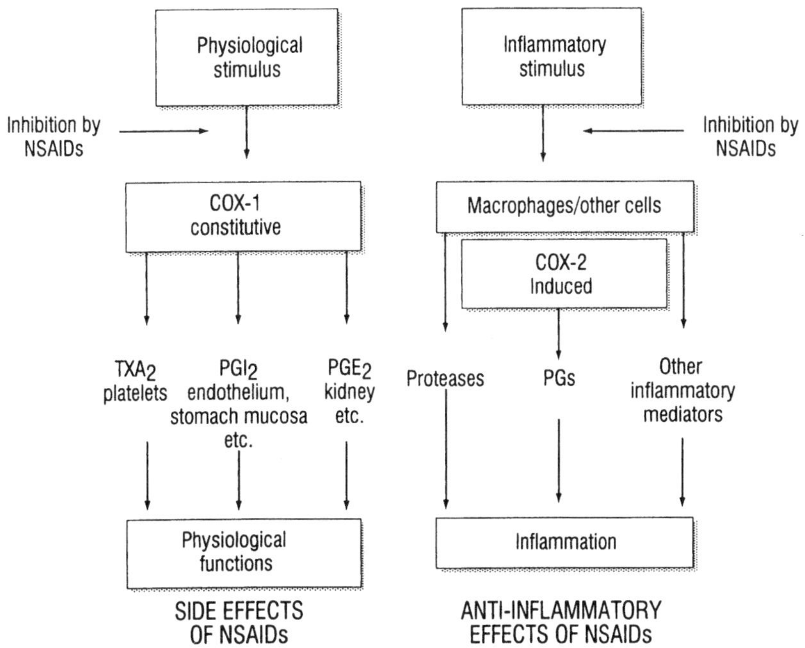

parallel with the over-elaboration of prostaglandins in many cells and tissues. The COX-2 gene may be one of a family of primary response genes, which also includes the gene for inducible nitric oxide synthase (iNOS), induced during inflammation and cell growth (Figure 2).

In cultured Swiss 3T3 cells induced with TPA or in RAW 264.7 macrophages stimulated with LPS, the prostaglandins which accumulate in the culture medium are derived exclusively from endogenous arachidonic acid metabolized by COX-2. Although these cells contain both isoenzymes, their prostaglandin production can be completely inhibited by antisense oligonucleotides to the inducible enzyme. Thus, when expression of COX-2 is increased in these cells, the stores of endogenous substrate (arachidonic acid) seem to be utilized only by COX-2[31].

However, other cells containing only COX-2 still convert exogenous arachidonic acid[32].

The physiological and pathological functions of COX-2 will be better understood when animals lacking a COX-2 gene are bred. Preliminary work with COX-2 null mice has shown abnormal kidney development, cardiac fibrosis and failure of ovulation leading to infertility in females[33].

THE MECHANISM OF ACTION OF STEROIDS IN INFLAMMATION

Corticosteroids inhibit the activity of phospholipase A_2, which reduces the release of arachidonic acid. Thus, corticosteroids ultimately inhibit the formation of prostaglandins, thromboxane and the leukotrienes. Anti-inflammatory steroids inhibit phospholipase A_2 indirectly by the release of an inhibitory protein, identified as lipocortin-1[34] (also known as annexin 1; for review see Ref. 35). The recombinant form of lipocortin-1 has a molecular weight of 37 kDa. This protein is a member of a superfamily of proteins characterized by their ability to bind calcium and anionic phospholipids[36]. Recombinant lipocortin-1 prevents the release of eicosanoids from lungs[37] and is a potent anti-inflammatory agent[38] which inhibits phospholipase-induced oedema in the rat paw. However, not all types of cells produce lipocortin-1 in response to glucocorticoids[39]. It is interesting that inhibition of gene expression of inducible NOS by dexamethasone is mediated by lipocortin, but the expression of COX-2 is inhibited by dexamethasone in some other way[40].

The inhibition by glucocorticoids of the expression of COX-2 is an additional aspect of their anti-inflammatory action. They combine with and activate cytoplasmic glucocorticoid receptors which regulate the transcription of some primary response genes including those expressing inducible cyclooxygenase (COX-2). Thus dexamethasone, through a mechanism different from lipocortin release, inhibits lipopolysaccharide-induced COX-2 gene expression in human monocytes[7] and rat alveolar macrophages[41] as well as inhibiting cytokine-induced COX-2 expression in rat mesangial cells[42].

MECHANISM OF ACTION OF NON-STEROID ANTI-INFLAMMATORY AGENTS

In 1971 we demonstrated that aspirin and indomethacin inhibit the COX enzyme of guinea pig lung homogenates, human platelets and dog spleen in vivo[43–45], thus preventing the synthesis of all prostanoids. This inhibition of prostaglandin production was proposed as the mechanism of action of the NSAIDs[43]. The inhibition by aspirin is due to the irreversible acetylation of the cyclooxygenase component of prostaglandin endoperoxide synthase, leaving the peroxidase activity of the enzyme unaffected[46]. In contrast to this irreversible action of aspirin, other NSAIDs such as indomethacin or ibuprofen produce reversible cyclooxygenase inhibition by competing with the substrate, arachidonic acid, for the active site of the enzyme[47].

The inhibition of prostaglandin synthesis explains all the actions of aspirin-like drugs. They prevent the pathological over-production of prostaglandins by COX-2 which contribute to the inflammatory process (therapeutic effects) and prevent the physiological formation of prostanoids by COX-1 (side effects). For instance, the ulcerogenic activity of aspirin arises from the inhibition of prostacyclin production. Prostacyclin has an important cytoprotective function in the gastric mucosa[48]. Administration of various prostaglandins reverses or prevents experimental gastric ulcers[49] and some of the recently developed prostaglandin derivatives are now available for clinical use. In addition, the inhibition of COX by NSAIDs correlates with their capacity to erode the gastric mucosa (see later).

The inhibition of prostaglandin synthesis by NSAIDs has been demonstrated in a wide variety of cell types and tissues, ranging from whole animals and man to microsomal enzyme preparations. For instance, the concentration of PGE_2 is about 20 ng/ml in the synovial fluid of patients with rheumatoid arthritis. This decreases to zero in patients taking aspirin; a good demonstration of the effect of this drug on prostaglandin synthesis clinically[50]. Several classes of inhibitors have been identified[51] and at least 12 major chemical series are known to affect prostaglandin production directly[52].

High concentrations of sodium salicylate and aspirin inhibit the activation of the transcription factor, nuclear factor-κB (NF-κB) which is instrumental in stimulating the genes for inflammatory mediators such as IL-1, interferon (IFN)-β and tumour necrosis factor (TNF)-α[53]. However, these concentrations may not be achieved therapeutically.

Selective inhibition of COX-2

In anti-inflammatory doses, different NSAIDs cause side effects such as irritation of the stomach to different extents. This was difficult to explain when only one COX was known. Bateman[54] published a comparison of epidemiological data on the side effects of the NSAIDs. In three different studies ibuprofen had the fewest side effects in humans, whereas indomethacin and piroxicam had the most (Table 1). For instance, piroxicam in our whole cell preparations (see below) has an IC_{50} of 0.00242 μmol/l against COX-1 and 0.604 μmol/l against COX-2 (Table 2)[32]. This higher potency against COX-1 than COX-2 can be expressed as a ratio of the IC_{50} for each enzyme: the COX-2/COX-1 ratio for piroxicam is therefore 250. When the epidemiological results are compared to such COX-2/COX-1 ratios, it is evident that high COX-2/COX-1 ratios correlate with severe side effects (Tables 1 and 2).

The release of prostaglandins following inflammatory stimuli is well established. However, the mechanism by which the increased synthesis of prostaglandins is achieved in inflammation (through induction of COX-2) has

***Table 1** Odds ratio for bleeding and perforation (Garcia Rodriguez) or acute gastrointestinal bleeding (Langman), and CSM rank order of adverse reports of gut toxicity expressed per million prescriptions in the first 5 years of marketing. For comparison with the human data, ratios of IC_{50} values for inhibition of COX-2 or COX-1 in intact cells are also provided*

				Ratio COX-2/COX-1 in intact cells	
NSAIDs	*CSM reports*	*Bleeding and perforation*	*Acute gastrointestinal bleeding*	*Vane* (Ref. 32)	*Engelhardt* (Ref. 76)
Ibuprofen	1	2.9	2	15	–
Diclofenac	2	3.9	4.2	0.7	2.2
Naproxen	5	3.1	9.1	0.6	–
Ketoprofen	6	5.4	23.7	–	–
Indomethacin	–	6.3	11.3	60	30
Piroxicam	11	18	13.7	250	33
Azapropazone	12	23.4	31.5	–	–

Human data obtained from Ref. 54.

***Table 2** IC_{50} values (μmol/l) of NSAIDs on COX-2 or COX-1 activity in intact cells*

NSAID	*COX-2*	*COX-1*	*Ratio*	
Tolfenamic acid	0.0191 ± 0.00725	0.00115 ± 0.00267	16.7	(n = 12)
Flurbiprofen	0.102 ± 0.041	0.082 ± 0.041	1.3	(n = 9)
Meloxicam	0.171 ± 0.142	0.214 ± 0.0855	0.8	(n = 18)
Piroxicam	0.604 ± 0.242	0.00242 ± 0.000604	250	(n = 12)
Diclofenac	1.1 ± 0.472	1.57 ± 0.66	0.7	(n = 9)
Indomethacin	1.68 ± 0.223	0.0279 ± 0.0028	60	(n = 12)
Naproxen	5.65 ± 9.57	9.56 ± 4.26	0.6	(n = 12)
Carprofen	10.9 ± 6.28	10.9 ± 1.5	1	(n = 9)
Tolmetin	27.2 ± 4.75	0.156 ± 0.0117	175	(n = 9)
Ibuprofen	72.8 ± 25.9	4.85 ± 0.34	15	(n = 9)
Sulindac	112 ± 65.5	1.12 ± 0.787	100	(n = 9)
Acetaminophen	133 ± 79.5	17.9 ± 13.3	7.4	(n = 9)
Aspirin	278 ± 55.6	1.67 ± 1.11	166	(n = 12)
Sodium salicylate	725 ± 117	254 ± 81.4	2.8	(n = 9)

The NSAIDs are arranged in their order of potency in μmol/l against COX-2. Note that amongst the most potent, meloxicam has the lowest activity ratio (i.e. has less effect on COX-1). Whole cell cultures of J774.2 macrophages treated with *E. coli* lipopolysaccharide were used as a source of COX-2 enzyme, and whole cell cultures of bovine aortic endothelial cells were used as a source of COX-1. (Data obtained from Refs 32, 117.)

only recently become understood. The other factors which were unexplained until the discovery of COX-2 include the differences between the anti-inflammatory action of aspirin and salicylate, and the mechanism of action of acetaminophen (paracetamol).

Salicylate is an order of magnitude less active than aspirin on the crude cyclooxygenase enzyme prepared from lung tissue[43], yet rheumatologists[55] report that salicylate is as potent as aspirin in suppressing arthritis. This observation in patients is supported by the work of Higgs et al.[56], which showed that a crude COX preparation from an inflamed site in the rat had almost the same sensitivity to aspirin as to salicylate. We now know that salicylate has at least half the potency of aspirin in inhibiting COX-2 in certain cell lines (see Table 2). This suggests a relatively low activity of salicylate against the COX-1 in lung homogenates. The profile fits well with the lack of gastric irritation by salicylate[57] and the lack of activity of salicylate on platelets (COX-1)[58].

Acetaminophen is antipyretic and analgesic but has little anti-inflammatory activity. Furthermore, it has only weak activity against most cyclooxygenase preparations, although it is considerably more active in diminishing prostaglandin synthesis in the brain[59]. Perhaps the brain enzyme represents a third isoform of cyclooxygenase, COX-3, which has yet to be characterized.

Even though aspirin should not now be the drug of choice for chronic inflammatory conditions such as rheumatism and arthritis because of its potent inhibitory action on COX-1, it will remain the drug of choice in reducing the number of secondary and primary heart attacks and strokes in high-risk patients, which is an anti-COX-1 effect in platelets[60,61]. A low-dose aspirin regimen of 75 mg/day has been recommended while doses of up to 325 mg/day may be administered in acute emergencies.

Time-dependent inhibition of COX-1 and COX-2

Aspirin inactivates COX enzymes by acetylating the serine 530 on COX-1 or the serine 516 on COX-2. Other COX inhibitors such as indomethacin, flurbiprofen, ibuprofen or piroxicam compete with the substrate, arachidonic acid, for the active sites on the enzymes. When added to the isolated human enzymes without preincubation, these NSAIDs instantaneously inhibited both COX-1 and COX-2, being 3–75 times more potent as inhibitors of COX-1 than of COX-2[62]. After 30 min incubation of the enzyme with the inhibitor, however, indomethacin and flurbiprofen became much more potent inhibitors of both enzymes and lost their selectivity for COX-1. Ibuprofen and piroxicam showed no such time-dependent inhibition, but retained their initial ratios of activity against COX-1/COX-2. After washing indomethacin or flurbiprofen off the enzyme it was not possible to recover full COX-1 activity, whereas COX-2 activity recovered completely. It is likely that after combining with the active site of the enzyme by competition with the substrate, some NSAIDs (including indomethacin and flurbiprofen) induce a secondary time-dependent inhibition of COX-1 activity which is only partially reversible. This possibility is reinforced by the fact that indomethacin binding protects COX-1 enzyme from cleavage by trypsin, indicating that the enzyme has undergone a structural change (Table 3)[63].

Table 3 ***Time dependency of ED_{50} values (μM) for inhibition of COX in different human assays by some non-steroid anti-inflammatory drugs. The COX-2/COX-1 ratio is different for time-dependent inhibitors according to length of preincubation***

	Instantaneous microsomal enzyme (Ref. 62)			*20 min pre-incub microsomal enzyme* (Ref. 75)			*WHRI* 30 min pre-incub HUVEC/A549*		
	COX-1	*COX-2*	*Ratio*	*COX-1*	*COX-2*	*Ratio*	*COX-1*	*COX-2*	*Ratio*
Indomethacin (time-dependent)	13.5	>1000	>74	0.0	0.35	3.5	–	–	–
Ibuprofen (not time-dependent)	4.0	12.5	3.1	14	80	5.7	0.5	0.4	0.9
Meloxicam	–	–	–	36.6	0.49	0.013	0.15	0.05	0.3

*Unpublished results from the William Harvey Research Institute.

Compounds with the general formula of aryl methyl sulphonyls and aryl methyl sulphonamides (such as DuP 697 or NS-398) have equal potency for inhibiting COX-1 or COX-2 enzymes immediately after mixing with the enzyme, but their potency for COX-2 increases selectively with preincubation of 10 min or more[64]. Moreover, while removal of the NSAID by dialysis completely restores the activity of COX-1, COX-2 remains inactive. Thus, these selective COX-2 inhibitors initially bind to the active site competitively and subsequently cause slowly developing irreversible structural changes in the COX-2 but not the COX-1 enzyme (Table 3).

The affinities of NSAIDs for human recombinant COX-2 enzyme measured after incubation with arachidonic acid in vitro for different time intervals, did not reflect their anti-inflammatory activity in vivo[65]. Mitchell et al.[32] had already proposed that a more profitable approach for detecting potential COX-2-inhibitory activity is to measure prostaglandin formation in intact cells. If prostaglandins formed from endogenous arachidonic acid were also measured, this would more closely resemble the normal, physiological state of the cell where NSAIDs such as salicylate with a weak affinity for the COX-2 enzyme would compete with relatively low concentrations of substrate for the active site on the enzyme[65].

Tests for selective COX-2 inhibitors

Selective inhibition of COX-2 should provide anti-inflammatory drugs which will not harm the stomach. With this in mind, we and others have developed models to test the activity of NSAIDs for inhibitory actions against COX-1 and COX-2. As well as using purified enzymes, we have developed whole cell systems because penetration of cell membranes is an important aspect of the activity of NSAIDs[32]. We have also incubated the inhibitor with the cells for 30 min to allow time-dependent inhibition.

Purified enzymes and isolated cells

Cultured bovine aortic endothelial cells serve as a source of COX-1 enzyme and J774.2 macrophages (which have little or no COX-1) stimulated with LPS are the means of testing for anti-COX-2 activity[32]. In both instances prostaglandin release from the cells is measured. We have also used purified enzyme preparations from Cayman Chemicals. Comparing the activity of the known NSAIDs in these two cell types and on the purified enzymes with their ED_{50} in the original experiment carried out by Vane[43] on guinea-pig lung homogenates, it becomes clear that in 1971 the drugs were tested for their activity against COX-1 (see Table 4). It is also clear from comparing the IC_{50} on broken cells in Table 4 with the purified enzymes that there is good agreement for the activity of the NSAIDs in several different species (guinea pig, sheep, cow or mouse).

A series of NSAIDs have also been tested for their relative activities against

***Table 4** IC_{50} values (μg/ml) for inhibition of COX from guinea-pig lungs by non-steroid anti-inflammatory drugs (NSAIDs) compared with those obtained using purified COX-1 and COX-2, cultured cell homogenates and whole cultured cells*

	ED_{50} (Ref. 43)	Purified enzyme (Ref. 32)	Broken cells (Ref. 32)	Whole cells (Ref. 32)
		COX-1/COX-2	COX-1/COX-2	COX-1/COX-2
Aspirin	6.3	5/210	8/200	0.3/50
Indomethacin	0.27	0.1/5	0.01/0.4	0.01/0.6
Salicylate	95	Inactive	In/>1 mg/ml	35/100
Ibuprofen		1/46	3/160	1/15

Pure COX-1 was isolated from ovine seminal vesicles and pure COX-2 from ovine placenta. Cell homogenates and whole cell cultures of J774.2 macrophages treated with *E. coli* lipopolysaccharide were used as a source of COX-2 enzyme, while homogenates and whole cell cultures of bovine aortic endothelial cells were used as a source of COX-1.

COX-1 and COX-2 in the whole cells and tables of activity ratios have been constructed[32]. Piroxicam (250 times more active against COX-1 than COX-2), tolmetin (175 times more active), aspirin (166 times more active) and indomethacin (60 times more active) show as the inhibitors with the worst COX-2/COX-1 ratios (Tables 2 and 4). These drugs are also well known for their propensity to cause gastric bleeding. Compounds with lower activity ratios should have fewer side effects and less irritant action on the stomach. Meloxicam is approaching the market and is one of the new potent NSAIDs with the best activity ratio for COX-2/COX-1. It also has minimal damaging effects on the gastrointestinal tract[66].

Clearly, the well known NSAIDs such as piroxicam, aspirin and indomethacin (Table 2) are much more potent inhibitors of the constitutive COX-1 than of the inflammatory COX-2, which explains their tendency to cause gastric damage. Drugs which have the highest potency against COX-2 and a better activity ratio against COX-2/COX-1 will have potent anti-inflammatory activity with fewer side effects on the stomach and kidney.

Human enzymes

Comparisons were made in a number of studies of the inhibition of human COX-1 and COX-2 by NSAIDS. The affinities of 14 NSAIDs were determined for human COX-1 and COX-2 in microsomal suspensions of transfected cos-1 cells[62]. Measuring instantaneous inhibition, all these were more potent inhibitors of COX-1 than of COX-2 with COX-2/COX-1 ratios of the same order as those estimated by Mitchell et al.[32] in non-human cultured cells. Thus, ibuprofen, flurbiprofen and sulindac had ratios of 3.1, 6.4 and 39.0 compared with our values of 15, 1.3 and 100 (Table 2).

Klein et al.[67] used human washed platelets as a source of COX-1 and

IL-1-stimulated rat mesangial cells which almost exclusively expressed COX-2. After 15 min incubation with different NSAIDs in these two model systems, COX-2/COX-1 ratios for indomethacin, diclofenac and the selective COX-2 inhibitor CGP28238 were 5.9, 0.07 and 0.0002. Under these experimental conditions, the COX-2/COX-1 ratios have rather low values and might not be comparable to other estimates.

In another model for assessing COX inhibitors in vitro and ex vivo[68], COX-1 and COX-2 activities were measured in human blood. Heparinized human whole blood was incubated with LPS and NSAIDs for 4 or 24 h. The PGE_2 levels in separated plasma and COX-2 protein in blood monocytes increased in parallel. This LPS-induced PGE_2 production was inhibited by dexamethasone. Whole blood TXB_2 levels provided a measure of maximally stimulated COX-1 activity of platelets, by endogenously formed thrombin. Platelets were incubated with the COX inhibitor for the 1 h the blood was allowed to clot.

Using this experimental system, indomethacin was, surprisingly, twice as potent in inhibiting COX-2 as COX-1, whereas *S*-indobufen was 20 times more potent on COX-1 than on COX-2. The metabolite of nabumetone, 6-methoxy-2-naphthyl acetic acid (6MNA), inhibited the two isoenzymes to the same degree. The results on indomethacin were in contrast to our own estimates and those reported by other laboratories[29,43]. Perhaps the unexpected COX-2/COX-1 ratio of indomethacin reflects the disparity between the two methods of measuring COX activity in the COX-1 and COX-2 systems. In any event it is clear that, for the comparison of the effects of many different NSAIDs on COX-1 and COX-2, a single method should be used in order to avoid differences due to factors such as time of incubation and enzymes obtained from different species and cell types.

Some selective inhibitors of COX-2

The discovery of COX-2 has stimulated several laboratories to search for selective inhibitors of this enzyme.

Nimesulide

Nimesulide was patented in 1974 in Belgium and the USA and is currently sold in several European countries for the relief of pain associated with inflammatory conditions. It has an unusual pharmacological profile compared with other NSAIDs in that it barely inhibited the bovine seminal vesicle microsomal cyclooxygenase with 1/1000 of the activity of indomethacin[69], while reducing the inflammation of rat adjuvant arthritis and carrageenin paw oedema at similar doses to indomethacin, diclofenac or piroxicam. It only produces gastrointestinal effects at oral doses of > 100 mg/kg, which constitutes 500 times the ED_{40} for inhibition of adjuvant arthritis[70]. In limited clinical trials for its use in acute and chronic inflammation in humans between 1981 and 1984, it was more effective than placebo or had comparable anti-inflammatory activity to established NSAIDs[71-73]. Epidemiological data suggested that, in long term therapeutic use at anti-inflammatory doses (100 mg twice daily), it caused no more serious gastrointestinal symptoms than placebo[74]. This unusual profile became understandable when nimesulide was shown to be a selective COX-2 inhibitor. Our cell systems gave a COX-2/COX-1 ratio of 0.1 which shows definite selectivity for the inhibition of the COX-2 rather than the COX-1 enzyme. (Chemical structures of COX-2-selective NSAIDs are shown in Figure 3.)

Meloxicam

Meloxicam is a selective COX-2 inhibitor with a COX-2/COX-1 ratio of about 0.01 on human recombinant enzymes[75] and about 0.33 in guinea pig peritoneal macrophages[76]. The drug was a potent inhibitor of adjuvant arthritis in rats at doses which only weakly affected the synthesis of prostaglandins in the gastric mucosa and kidneys[66]. In our hands meloxicam also has a ratio in favour of COX-2 (Table 2). Meloxicam is now registered in many countries worldwide.

1,2-Diarylcyclopentene derivatives

Needleman and his group at Monsanto/Searle[77] have made inhibitors which are some 1000-fold more potent against COX-2 than against COX-1. Their prototype, SC 58125, emerged as an effective anti-inflammatory agent in various models of chronic inflammation such as carrageenin-induced oedema of the rat paw, the rat carrageenin-injected air-pouch[78] and rat adjuvant-induced arthritis. Its in vitro selectivity was tested against COX-1 in platelets and against COX-2 in IL-1-stimulated fibroblasts. The IC_{50} was 0.09 μM for COX-2 and >100 μM for COX-1, making it 1400-fold more selective for COX-2[79]. Even at greater than anti-inflammatory doses, SC 58125 did not inhibit PGE_2 synthesis in the stomach or cause gastric ulceration. Under similar experimental conditions, aspirin caused a 55% incidence of stomach ulcers and fenoprofen caused a 15% incidence. No changes in generation of renal prostaglandins were observed at high doses of SC 58125.

DuP 697 was reported some years ago to be a potent anti-inflammatory drug in the rat adjuvant-induced arthritis model[80], with an ED_{50} of 0.18 mg/kg. It did not cause stomach ulcers or alter renal blood flow at doses of up to 400 mg/kg.

L-475,337

Recent reports have described the selective and orally active COX-2 inhibitor L-475,337. In whole cell assays, this compound inhibited COX-2 with an IC_{50} of 20 nM, but it was inactive on COX-1 even at doses of 10 μM (COX-2/COX-1 ratio of 1/500). It reduced carrageenin-induced rat paw oedema with an ED_{50} of

Figure 3 Chemical structures of some more selective COX-2 inhibitors

Meloxicam | Boehringer-Ingelheim

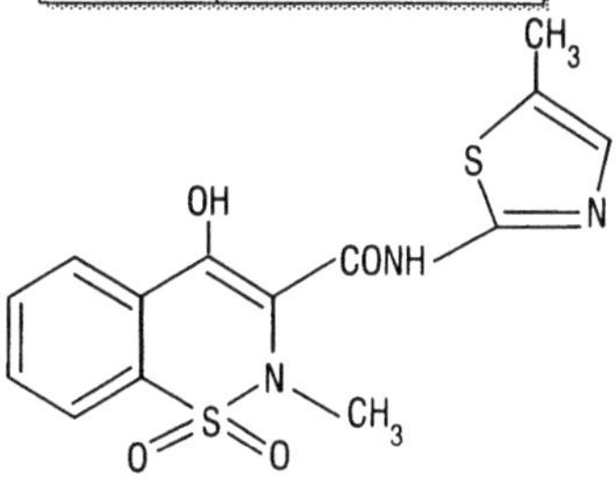

DuP 697 | Dupont Co.

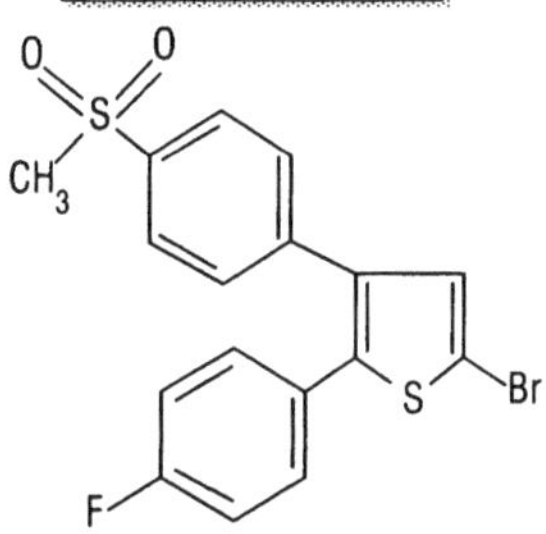

NS-398 | Taisho Pharmaceutical Co.

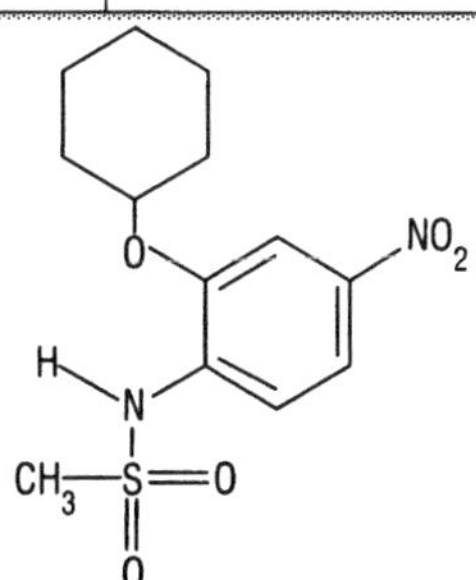

CGP 28238 | Ciba-Geigy Corp.

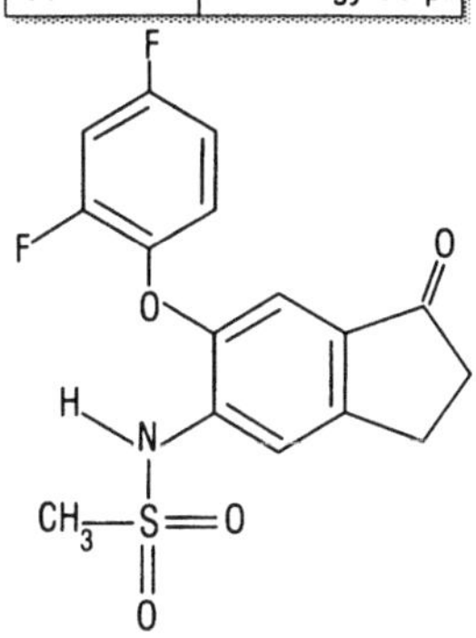

SC 58125 | Searle, Monsanto Co.

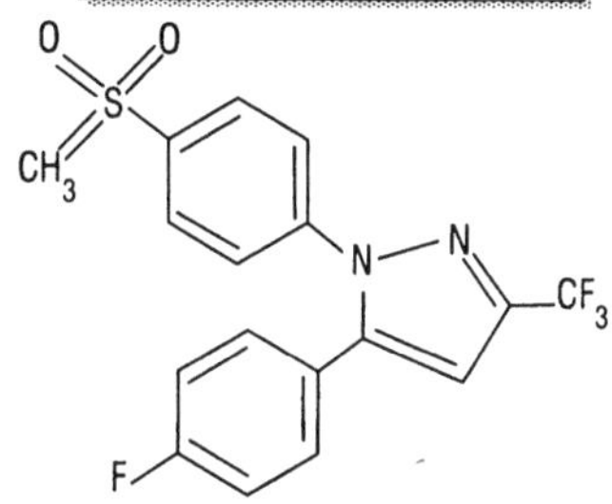

L-745,337 | Merck Frosst

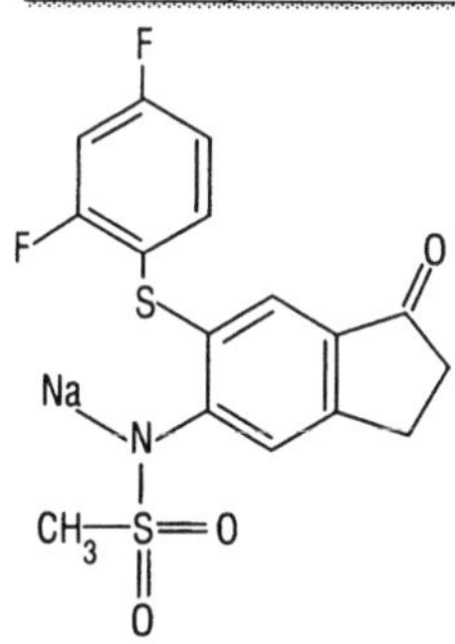

NIMESULIDE
(Aulin, Flogovital, Mesulid Nimed, Sulidene)

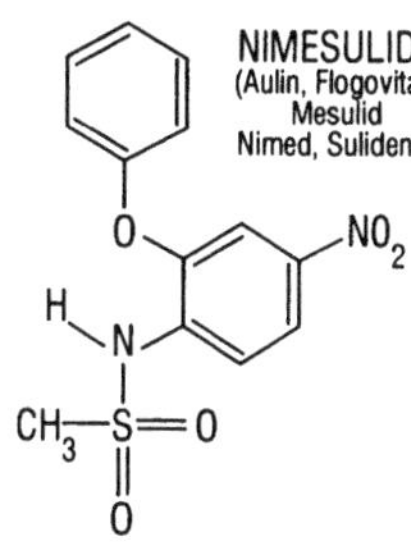

2 mg/kg[81]. Oral doses of L-475,337 reduced carrageenin hyperalgesia in the rat paw with ED_{50} values similar to those of piroxicam and indomethacin (0.37, 0.51 and 1.47 mg/kg respectively). It did not cause stomach lesions at doses of up to 30 mg/kg, whereas the ED_{50} for the ulcerogenic actions of piroxicam and indomethacin was 14 mg/kg[82]. No gastrointestinal bleeding was detected in a ^{51}Cr excretion assay in monkeys at doses of 10 mg/kg given twice daily for 5 days. Indomethacin and flurbiprofen had a significant effect in this test when given at 5 mg/kg for one day[81]. Furthermore, no obvious stomach lesions were found in rats at doses which reduced PGE_2 levels in the inflammatory exudate from the pleural cavity.

CGP 28238

CGP 28238, also known as flosulide (but not on the market), has been described as a highly potent NSAID which does not inhibit COX prepared from sheep seminal vesicles[83]. It is now clear that flosulide is a highly potent, selective inhibitor of COX-2 with an IC_{50} of 15 nM in IL-1-stimulated mesangial cells. At least 1000-fold higher concentrations were required for 50% inhibition of COX-1 in human washed platelets[66]. Early reports commented on the low gastrotoxicity of this compound[84]. Assessment of gastric damage in squirrel monkeys by measuring ^{51}Cr excretion in faeces showed that the two COX-2-selective NSAIDs, flosulide and DuP 697, were considerably less toxic to the stomach than other standard NSAIDs[85].

NS-398

An impressive selectivity for COX-2 was also shown for NS-398, made by Taisho in Japan[86]. This compound inhibited the COX-2 of sheep placenta with a potency equal to that of indomethacin (IC_{50} for NS-398 $= 3.8 \times 10^{-6}$ M), but even at concentrations of 10^{-4} M, NS-398 had no effect on COX-1 of ram seminal vesicles[87]. In analgesic and anti-inflammatory tests in rats, NS-398 (0.3–5 mg/kg, p.o.) was almost as potent as indomethacin, whereas no significant gastric lesions were seen even when 1000 mg/kg was given as a single oral dose[88]. A precise assessment of the COX-2/COX-1 ratio for this compound has not yet been published.

The most selective COX-2 inhibitors are still in the experimental stage. Nimesulide is out of patent, but meloxicam has been registered in many countries. Clearly, anti-inflammatory agents will be far less toxic by the year 2000.

INTERACTIONS BETWEEN THE NITRIC OXIDE SYNTHASE AND COX PATHWAYS

Nitric oxide is an important vasodilator and anti-aggregating mediator made by endothelial cells. The constitutive enzyme which makes it is found in endothelial cells (eNOS) and like COX-2, another less controlled enzyme, inducible nitric oxide synthase (iNOS), is induced by inflammatory mediators and LPS. Patients with rheumatoid arthritis have increased levels of nitrite (formed from nitric oxide) in their serum and synovial fluid. In both diseases synovial fluid nitrite is higher than serum nitrite suggesting that nitric oxide is synthesized by the synovium[89]. Lung samples from patients with different lung diseases formed more nitric oxide than tissues from normal lungs. The increased NOS activity was, however, probably due to constitutive NOS[90]. Thus, like the prostaglandin system, the constitutive NOS is protective whereas iNOS leads to excess NO which is damaging.

Actions of nitric oxide on the COX system

Small amounts of endogenous or exogenous nitric oxide (NO) stimulate COX-1 and COX-2 activity without inducing formation of new protein, whereas inhibition of prostaglandin formation by large amounts of NO has also been demonstrated. The interactions have been studied in cultured cells, perfused organs and in vivo with, sometimes, apparently conflicting results.

Mouse cultured macrophage cells (RAW264.7 and J774.2) can be stimulated with LPS for 12–18 h so that the levels of COX-2 and iNOS enzymes increase markedly, as does their production of prostaglandins and NO. Additional treatment of RAW264.7 cells with inhibitors of NOS such as methyl arginine (MeArg) reduced formation of both NO and prostanoids suggesting that endogenous NO was stimulating the activity of COX[91]. However, treating LPS-induced J774.2 macrophages with MeArg reduced endogenous NO production but enhanced expression of COX-2 protein and release of prostaglandins[92]. Thus, in different cell types NO can either stimulate COX activity or inhibit expression of COX-2.

It is interesting that in our model of chronic inflammation, the murine granulomatous air pouch[93], the levels of COX and NOS in the skin and granulomatous tissues varied throughout the inflammatory process. During both the acute stages (0–24h) and the chronic phase (3–21 days), when levels of iNOS were high, prostaglandin production fell; conversely, during times of high prostaglandin formation NO synthesis was reduced (Figures 4 and 5). Thus, the modulatory actions of NO on COX-2 activity may contribute to the dissociation of activities seen in this model of chronic inflammation[94]. Other reported interactions between the COX and NOS systems are summarized in Table 5.

In inflamed organs endogenous NO generally stimulates prostaglandin production. For example, stimulation of COX by endogenous NO has now been shown in the chronically inflamed kidney of the rabbit. A ureter-obstructed hydronephrotic kidney removed from the animal and perfused ex vivo released PGE_2 in response to an injection of bradykinin. This release of PGE_2 was reduced by inhibition of NOS with MeArg or aminoguanidine, dexamethasone or

***Figure 4** Cyclooxygenase-2 and inducible nitric oxide synthase (iNOS) activity in a model of chronic inflammation during the acute stage. Cyclooxygenase activity was measured by the formation of PGE_2 (□) in normal skin (time 0) and at 6, 12, and 24 h after injection of an irritant. The iNOS activity (■) was measured in the skin samples by the formation of L-citrulline in the absence of calcium. Data represent the mean ± SEM of 14 determinations from seven separate animals*

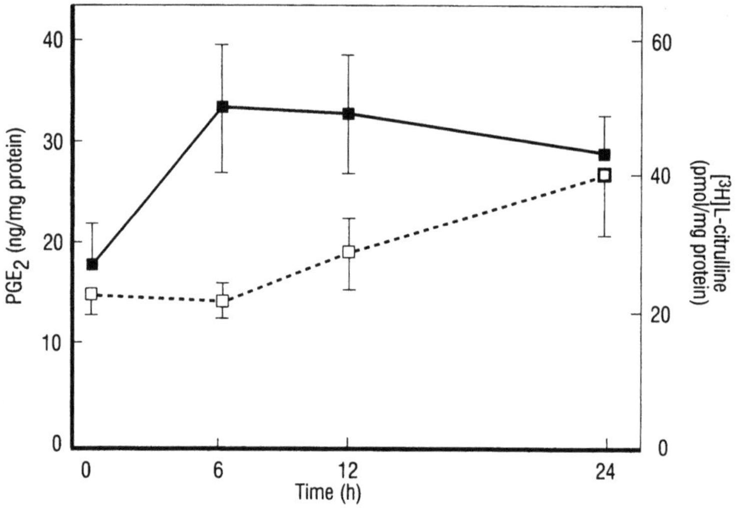

cycloheximide, showing that the prostaglandin was synthesized by induced COX-2 which was driven by endogenous NO. In the contralateral normal kidney perfused ex vivo, bradykinin stimulated the release of nitrite and PGE_2, a response which was also blocked by MeArg. However, dexamethasone or cycloheximide had no effect. In the normal kidney, therefore, NO produced by the constitutive NOS enhanced the activation of COX-1 with bradykinin. Thus, endogenous NO made by either iNOS in the inflamed kidney or constitutive NOS in the normal kidney activates COX-2 or COX-1 enzymes to enhance the release of prostaglandins[95].

Further evidence for a stimulatory action of NO on COX activity was supplied by Sautebin and Di Rosa[96] in lungs removed from LPS-treated rats. Homogenates or chopped lungs from these rats produced increased amounts of 6-keto-$PGF_{1\alpha}$ after incubation with L-arginine and reduced amounts when L-nitroarginine or MeArg was added to the incubation mixture[96]. This is likely to be an enhancement by endogenous NO of COX enzyme activity since NOS inhibitors added to chopped lungs in vitro were also effective. During acute pancreatitis induced with sodium taurocholate in rats, production of prostaglandins was increased. Inhibition of NOS with nitro-arginine reversed the increases in 6-keto-

***Figure 5** Cyclooxygenase-2 and inducible nitric oxide synthase (iNOS) activity in a model of chronic inflammation during the chronic and resolving stages. Cyclooxygenase and iNOS activities were measured in granulomatous tissue at different times after injection of an irritant. Cyclooxygenase activity was measured by the formation of PGE2 (□) at 3, 5, 14, and 21 days. The iNOS activity (■) was measured in the granulomatous tissue by the formation of L-citrulline in the absence of calcium. Data represent the mean ± SEM of 20 determinations from 10 separate animals*

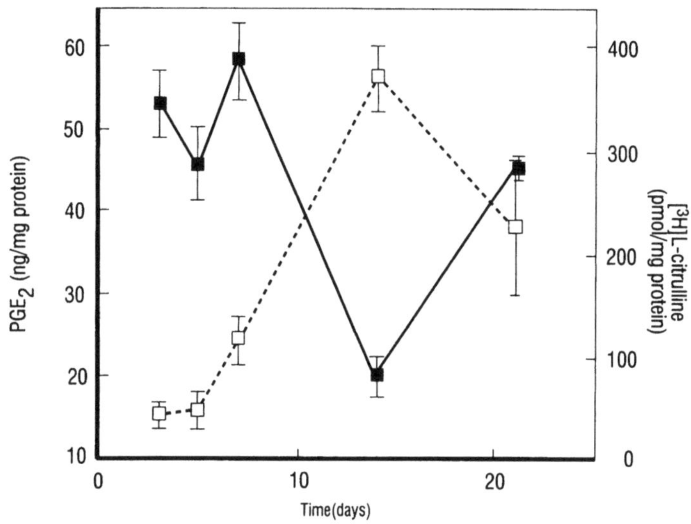

$PGF_{1\alpha}$ and TXB_2 levels indicating that endothelial and platelet prostaglandin generation was NO-dependent[97].

Similarly, in uteri removed from female rats treated with oestrogen, the NO donor sodium nitroprusside stimulated release of prostaglandins and thromboxane, whereas methyl arginine or haemoglobin reduced release. Again, an effect on enzyme activity rather than enzyme expression is probable since the incubation period with inhibitors was only 60 min[98]. Cultured T67 human astrocytoma cells induced with HIV coating gp120 glycoprotein, released increased amounts of nitrite and PGE_2 into the cell supernatants. The increased production of both mediators was antagonized by nitro-arginine but not by methylene blue indicating that stimulation of COX by NO did not involve increases in cGMP levels[99].

An examination of the possible mechanisms by which NO may interact with COX concluded that it is unlikely to combine with the ferric haem in prostaglandin synthase (PGHS). Under aerobic conditions NO has only a weak affinity for the ferric haem in PGHS, reacting more strongly with the ferrous

Table 5 Interactions between the nitric oxide synthase and COX pathways in various biological systems

Systems	*References*
Stimulation of COX by NO	
RAW264.7 macrophages	Salvemini et al.[91]
Human fetal fibroblasts	
Murine rCOX-1, rCOX-2	
Rabbit hydronephrotic kidney	Salvemini et al.[95]
Rabbit normal kidney	
Rat aorta VSMC	Inoue et al.[108]
Isolated islets of Langerhans	Corbett et al.[109]
Rat lung homogenate	Sautebin et al.[96]
Human T67 astrocytoma cells	Mollace et al.[99]
Articular chondrocytes	Stadler et al.[110]
Bovine coronary endothelial cells	Davidge et al.[111]
Inhibition of COX by NO	
J774.2 macrophages	Swierkosz et al.[92]
Articular chondrocytes	Stadler et al.[110]
Rat Kupffer cells	Stadler et al.[112]
Rat peritoneal macrophage	Habib et al.[113]
Human saphenous vein	Barker et al.[114]
No effect of NO on COX activity	
Ovine PGHS-1	Tsai et al.[100]
Activation of NOS by PGs	
Rat peritoneal macrophage	Habib et al.[113]
Rabbit eye	Astin et al.[102]
Rabbit cornea	Ziche et al.[115]
Inhibition of NOS by PGs	
Human saphenous vein	Barker et al.[116]
No effect of PGs on NOS	
Rabbit hydronephrotic kidney	Salvemini et al.[95]
Rabbit normal kidney	

haem of PGHS under anaerobic conditions[100]. However, there is evidence that formation of nitrosothiols is important for enhancement of COX-1 activity by NO. These produce changes in the enzyme structure of COX-1 which result in increased catalytic efficiency[101].

Effect of prostaglandins and cAMP on NOS activity

Products of the COX pathway also influence generation of nitric oxide. Prostaglandin $F_{2\alpha}$ caused hyperaemia of the surface structures of the eye in the conscious rabbit by activating cNOS, since MeArg prevented the increase in blood flow. Only constitutive enzymes appear to be involved in this reaction[102].

However, in primary cultures of mesangial cells from rats, modulation of iNOS expression required incubation with IL-1β for 12h. Curiously, in these cells, endogenous prostaglandins inhibited iNOS expression and nitrite production whereas exogenous carba prostacyclin enhanced IL-1β-induced iNOS mRNA levels and generation of nitrite. Forskolin, which activates adenylate cyclase and raises cAMP levels, mimicked the effect of carba prostacyclin[103].

A number of publications have described the effects of raising cAMP levels on the accumulation of NO in various cells and tissues. Forskolin, other cAMP-elevating agents or dibutyryl-cAMP increased NOS mRNA as well as formation of nitrite. This action synergized with the inducing action of IL-1β on NOS gene expression which was, however, mediated by a different mechanism. In cultured vascular smooth muscle cells from rat thoracic aorta, 8-bromo-cAMP stimulated NO production and increased steady state levels of iNOS mRNA[104], whereas dibutyryl cAMP markedly enhanced IL-1β-stimulated release of NO. Dibutyryl cAMP had no effect on NO synthesis when added alone, but increased iNOS protein and mRNA over that induced by IL-1β only. Cholera toxin, isoprenaline and phosphodiesterase inhibitors mimicked the actions of these cAMP analogues[105].

Inoue et al.[106] found that the COX-2 gene is also regulated by cAMP. In cultured U937 human monocytic cells (expressing COX-2) stimulated with TPA, deletion or destruction of the cAMP response element markedly reduced the promoter activity of the COX-2 gene.

CONCLUSIONS

Even before the identification of the COX-2 enzyme, industrial screening programmes, using models of chronic inflammation in conjunction with models of gastric damage, discovered anti-inflammatory drugs which we now know are selective COX-2 inhibitors with low toxicity for the stomach and kidneys. Needleman postulated the existence of a second COX isoenzyme[7] before its characterization and cloning by Xie et al.[22]. With the firm knowledge of the properties of this enzyme, a wide variety of biological assays was devised to test the selectivity of existing NSAIDs for the two isoforms of COX and to develop more selective COX-2 inhibitors. Some of these highly selective COX-2 inhibitors, which show over 1000-fold greater activity against COX-2 than for COX-1, are now available. Being only weak blockers of COX-1 they also have much less toxicity for the stomach and kidneys. Interestingly, several of the selective COX-2 inhibitors incorporate a sulphonamide moiety (see Figure 3).

It is important to remember that the ratio of the inhibitor activity (IC_{50}) of a drug for COX-1 to its inhibitory activity for COX-2 can vary according to time of incubation and whether tests are performed on pure enzymes, cell homogenates, intact cells or with the types of cells used[107]. Substrate concentration may also be important. Thus, several different values for the same compound may be quoted depending on the biological system used for the tests. Accurate comparisons of the selectivity of these new drugs will only be possible when a standard test is designated for measuring inhibitory potency for the two isoenzymes. Although human cloned COX-1 and COX-2 are very useful for developing structure/activity relationships, these enzyme preparations are not ideal for predicting in vivo activity, since they ignore the effects of cell membranes and intracellular concentrations.

Notwithstanding the impressive recent experimental results with selective COX-2 inhibitors, these drugs may not turn out to be as potent as steroids, even though the lack of side effects will allow the use of higher doses. This is because prostaglandins are not the only mediators involved in chronic inflammation.

Acknowledgements

The William Harvey Research Institute is supported by grants from the ONO Pharmaceutical Company, Schwarz Parma Limited and the Servier International Research Institute.

References

1. Murphy RC, Hammarström S, Samuelsson B. Leukotriene C: a slow-reacting substance from murine mastocytoma cells. Proc Natl Acad Sci USA. 1979;76:4275–9.
2. Solomon LM, Juhlin L, Kirchenbaum MB. Prostaglandins on cutaneous vasculature. J Invest Dermatol. 1968;51:280–2.
3. Williams TJ, Peck MJ. Role of prostaglandin-mediated vasodilatation in inflammation. Nature. 1977;270:530–2.
4. Ferreira SH. Prostaglandins, aspirin-like drugs and analgesia. Nature. 1972;240:200–3.
5. Saxena PN, Begg MMA, Singhal KC, Ahmad M. Prostaglandin-like activity in the cerebrospinal fluid of febrile patients. Indian J Med Res. 1979;79:495–8.
6. Higgs EA, Moncada S, Vane JR. Inflammatory effects of prostacyclin (PGI_2) and 6-oxo-$PGF_{1\alpha}$ in the rat paw. Prostaglandins. 1978;16:153–62.
7. Fu J-Y, Masferrer JL, Seibert K, Raz A, Needleman P. The induction and suppression of prostaglandin H_2 synthase (cyclooxygenase) in human monocytes. J Biol Chem. 1990;265: 16737–40.
8. Masferrer JL, Zweifel BS, Seibert K, Needleman P. Selective regulation of cellular cyclooxygenase by dexamethasone and endotoxin in mice. J Clin Invest. 1990;86:1375–9.
9. Hemler M, Lands WEM, Smith WL. Purification of the cyclo-oxygenase that forms prostaglandins. Demonstration of the two forms of iron in the holoenzyme. J Biol Chem. 1976; 251:5575–9.
10. Miyamoto T, Ogino N, Yamamoto S, Hayaishi O. Purification of prostaglandin endoperoxide synthetase from bovine vesicular gland microsomes. J Biol Chem. 1976;251:2629–36.
11. Kulmacz RJ, Pendleton RB, Lands WEM. Interaction between peroxidase and cyclooxygenase activities in prostaglandin-endoperoxide synthase. Interpretation of reaction kinetics. J Biol Chem. 1994;269:5527–36.
12. Picot D, Loll PJ, Garavito RM. The X-ray crystal structure of the membrane protein prostaglandin H_2 synthase-1. Nature. 1994;367:243–9.
13. Roth GJ, Stanford N, Majerus PW. Acetylation of prostaglandin synthetase by aspirin. Proc Natl Acad Sci USA. 1975;2:3073–6.
14. Loll PJ, Picot D, Garavito RM. The structural basis of aspirin activity inferred from the crystal structure of inactivated prostaglandin H_2 synthase. Nature Struct Biol. 1995;2:637–43.

15. DeWitt D. Prostaglandin endoperoxide synthase: Regulation of enzyme expression. Biochim Biophys Acta. 1991;1083:121–34.
16. Wu KK, Sanduja R, Tsai A-L, Ferhanoglu B, Loose-Mitchell DS. Aspirin inhibits interleukin-1-induced prostaglandin H synthase expression in cultured endothelial cells. Proc Natl Acad Sci USA. 1991;88:2384–7.
17. DeWitt DL, Smith WL. Primary structure of prostaglandin G/H synthase from sheep vesicular gland determined from the complementary DNA sequence. Proc Natl Acad Sci USA. 1988; 85:1412–6.
18. Merlie JP, Fagan D, Mudd J, Needleman P. Isolation and characterisation of the complementary DNA for sheep seminal vesicle prostaglandin endoperoxide synthase (cyclooxygenase). J Biol Chem. 1988;263:3550–3.
19. Yokoyama C, Takai T, Tanabe T. Primary structure of sheep prostaglandin endoperoxide synthase deduced from cDNA sequence. FEBS Lett. 1988;231:347–51.
20. Rosen GD, Birkenmeier TM, Raz A, Holtzman MJ. Identification of a cyclooxygenase-related gene and its potential role in prostaglandin formation. Biochem Biophys Res Commun. 1989; 164:1358–65.
21. Raz A, Wyche A, Needleman P. Temporal and pharmacological division of fibroblast cyclooxygenase expression into transcriptional and translational phases. Proc Natl Acad Sci USA. 1989;86:1657–61.
22. Xie W, Chipman JG, Robertson DL, Erikson RL, Simmons DL. Expression of a mitogen-responsive gene encoding prostaglandin synthase is regulated by mRNA splicing. Proc Natl Acad Sci USA. 1991;88:2692–6.
23. Simmons DL, Levy DB, Yannoni Y, Erikson RL. Identification of a phorbol ester-repressible *v-src* inducible gene. Proc Natl Acad Sci USA. 1989;86:1178–82.
24. Kujubu DA, Fletcher BS, Varnum BC, Lim RW, Herschman HR. TIS10, a phorbol ester tumor promoter-inducible mRNA from Swiss 3T3 cells, encodes a novel prostaglandin synthase/ cyclooxygenase homologue. J Biol Chem. 1991;266:12866–72.
25. Simmons DL, Xie W, Chipman J, Evett G. Multiple cyclooxygenases: Cloning of a mitogen-inducible form. In: Bailey M, editor. Prostaglandin, Leukotrienes, Lipoxins and PAF. London: Plenum Press; 1992:67–78.
26. O'Banion MK, Winn VD, Young DA. cDNA cloning and functional activity of a glucocorticoid-regulated inflammatory cyclooxygenase. Proc Natl Acad Sci USA. 1992;89:4888–92.
27. Xie W, Robertson DL, Simmons DL. Mitogen-inducible prostaglandin G/H synthase: a new target for nonsteroidal antiinflammatory drugs. Drug Dev Res. 1992;25:249–65.
28. Laneuville O, Breuer DK, Xu N et al. Fatty acid substrate specificities of human prostaglandin-endoperoxide H synthase-1 and -2. Formation of 12-hydroxy-(9Z,13E/Z,15Z)-octadecatrienoic acids from α-linolenic acid. J Biol Chem. 1995;270:19330–6.
29. Meade EA, Smith WL, DeWitt DL. Differential inhibition of prostaglandin endoperoxide synthase (cyclooxygenase) isozymes by aspirin and other nonsteroidal anti-inflammatory drugs. J Biol Chem. 1993;268:6610–4.
30. Wennogle LP, Liang H, Quintavalla JC et al. Comparison of recombinant cyclooxygenase-2 to native isoforms: aspirin labelling of the active site. FEBS Lett. 1995;371:315–20.
31. Reddy ST, Herschman HR. Ligand-induced prostaglandin synthesis requires expression of the TIS10/PGS-2 prostaglandin synthase gene in murine fibroblasts and macrophages. J Biol Chem. 1994;269:15473–15480.
32. Mitchell JA, Akarasereenont P, Thiemermann C, Flower RJ, Vane JR. Selectivity of nonsteroidal antiinflammatory drugs as inhibitors of constitutive and inducible cyclooxygenase. Proc Natl Acad Sci USA. 1993;90:11693–7.
33. Dinchuk JE, Focht R, Car B et al. Cyclooxygenase 2 null mice have reduced viability due to abnormal kidney development and exhibit cardiac fibrosis and female infertility. Inflamm Res. 1995;44(Suppl 3):S271.
34. Wallner BP, Mattaliano RJ, Hession C et al. Cloning and expression of human lipocortin, a phospholipase A_2 inhibitor with potent anti-inflammatory activity. Nature. 1986;320:77–81.
35. Flower RJ, Rothwell NJ. Lipocortin-1: cellular mechanisms and clinical relevance. Trends Pharmacol Sci. 1994;15:71–6.
36. Geisow MJ, Walker JH, Boustead C, Taylor W. Localisation and structure of novel calcium-regulated phospholipid-binding proteins. Biochem Soc Trans. 1987;15:800–2.

37. Cirino G, Flower RJ. Human recombinant lipocortin 1 inhibits prostacyclin production by human umbilical artery in vitro. Prostaglandins. 1987;34:59–62.
38. Cirino G, Peers SH, Flower RJ, Browning JL, Pepinsky RB. Human recombinant lipocortin 1 has acute local anti-inflammatory properties in the rat paw edema test. Proc Natl Acad Sci USA. 1989;86:3428–32.
39. Barnes PJ, Adcock I. Anti-inflammatory actions of steroids: molecular mechanisms. Trends Pharmacol Sci. 1993;14:436–41.
40. Wu C-C, Croxtall JD, Perretti M et al. Lipocortin 1 mediates the inhibition by dexamethasone of the induction by endotoxin of nitric oxide synthase in the rat. Proc Natl Acad Sci USA. 1995;92: 3473–7.
41. Lee SH, Soyoola E, Chanmugam P et al. Selective expression of mitogen-inducible cyclo-oxygenase in macrophages stimulated with lipopolysaccharide. J Biol Chem. 1992;267:25934–8.
42. Coyne DW, Nickols M, Bertrand W, Morrison AR. Regulation of mesangial cell cyclooxygenase synthesis by cytokines and glucocorticoids. Am J Physiol. 1992;263:F97–102.
43. Vane JR. Inhibition of prostaglandin synthesis as a mechanism of action for the aspirin-like drugs. Nature. 1971;231:232–5.
44. Smith JH, Willis AL. Aspirin selectively inhibits prostaglandin production in human platelets. Nature. 1971;231:235–7.
45. Ferreira SH, Moncada S, Vane JR. Indomethacin and aspirin abolish prostaglandin release from spleen. Nature. 1971;231:237–9.
46. Van der Ouderaa FJ, Buytenhek M, Nugteren DH, van Dorp DA. Acetylation of prostaglandin endoperoxide synthetase with acetylsalicylic acid. Eur J Biochem. 1980;109:1–8.
47. Vane JR, Flower RJ, Botting RM. History of aspirin and its mechanism of action. Stroke. 1990;(Suppl. IV):12–23.
48. Miller TA. Protective effects of prostaglandins against gastric mucosal damage: current knowledge and proposed mechanisms. Am J Physiol. 1983;245:G601–23.
49. Robert A, Hanchar AJ, Lancaster C, Nezamis JE. Prostacyclin inhibits enteropooling and diarrhea. In: Vane JR, Bergström S, editors. Prostacyclin. New York: Raven Press; 1979:147–58.
50. Higgs GA, Vane JR, Hart FD, Wojtulewski JA. Effects of anti-inflammatory drugs on prostaglandins in rheumatoid arthritis. In: Robinson HJ, Vane JR, editors. Prostaglandin Synthetase Inhibitors. New York: Raven Press; 1974:165–73.
51. Flower RJ. Drugs which inhibit prostaglandin biosynthesis. Pharm Rev. 1974;26:33–67.
52. Shen TY. Prostaglandin synthetase inhibitors. In Vane JR, Ferreira SH, editors. Antiinflammatory Drugs. Berlin: Springer-Verlag; 1979:305–47.
53. Kopp E, Ghosh S. Inhibition of NF-κB by sodium salicylate and aspirin. Science. 1994;265:956–9.
54. Bateman DN. NSAIDs: time to re-evaluate gut toxicity. Lancet. 1994;343:1051–2.
55. Preston SJ, Arnold MH, Beller EM, Brooks PM, Buchanan WW. Comparative analgesic and anti-inflammatory properties of sodium salicylate and acetylsalicylic acid (aspirin) in rheumatoid arthritis. Br J Clin Pharmacol. 1989;27:607–11.
56. Higgs GA, Salmon JA, Henderson B, Vane JR. Pharmacokinetics of aspirin and salicylate in relation to inhibition of arachidonate cyclo-oxygenase and anti-inflammatory activity. Proc Natl Acad Sci USA. 1987;84:1417–20.
57. Whittle BJR, Higgs GA, Eakins KE, Moncada S, Vane JR. Selective inhibition of prostaglandin production in inflammatory exudates and gastric mucosa. Nature. 1980;284:271–3.
58. Vargaftig BB. Salicylic acid fails to inhibit generation of thromboxane A_2 activity in platelets after in vivo administration to the rat. J Pharm Pharmacol. 1978;30:101–4.
59. Flower RJ, Vane JR. Inhibition of prostaglandin synthetase in brain explains the antipyretic activity of paracetamol (4-acetamidophenol). Nature. 1972;240:410–1.
60. Antiplatelet Trialists' Collaboration. Collaborative overview of randomised trials of antiplatelet therapy-I: Prevention of death, myocardial infarction, and stroke by prolonged antiplatelet therapy in various categories of patients. Br Med J. 1994;308:81–106.
61. Funk CD, Funk LB, Kennedy ME, Pong AS, Fitzgerald GA. Human platelet/erythroleukemia cell prostaglandin G/H synthase: cDNA cloning, expression and gene chromosomal assignment. FASEB J. 1991;5:2304–12.
62. Laneuville O, Breuer DK, DeWitt DL, Hla T, Funk CD, Smith WL. Differential inhibition of human prostaglandin endoperoxide H synthases-1 and -2 by nonsteroidal anti-inflammatory drugs. J Pharmacol Exp Ther. 1994;271:927–34.

63. Kulmacz RJ. Topography of prostaglandin H synthase. Antiinflammatory agents and the protease-sensitive arginine 253 region. J Biol Chem. 1989;264:14136–44.
64. Copeland RA, Williams JM, Giannaras J et al. Mechanism of selective inhibition of the inducible isoform of prostaglandin G/H synthase. Proc Natl Acad Sci USA. 1994;91:11202–6.
65. Smith WL, Lecomte M, Laneuville O, Breuer DK, DeWitt DL. Differential inhibition of human prostaglandin endoperoxide H synthases-1 and -2 by aspirin and other nonsteroidal anti-inflammatory drugs. Eur J Med Chem. 1995;30(S):S417–27.
66. Engelhardt G, Homma D, Schlegel K, Utzmann R, Schnitzler C. Anti-inflammatory, analgesic, antipyretic and related properties of meloxicam, a new non-steroidal anti-inflammatory agent with favourable gastrointestinal tolerance. Inflamm Res. 1995;44:423–33.
67. Klein T, Nüsing RM, Pfeilschifter J, Ullrich V. Selective inhibition of cyclooxygenase 2. Biochem Pharmacol. 1994;48:1605–10.
68. Patrignani P, Panara MR, Greco A et al. Biochemical and pharmacological characterization of the cyclooxygenase activity of human blood prostaglandin endoperoxide synthases. J Pharmacol Exp Ther. 1994;271:1705–12.
69. Böttcher I, Schweizer A, Glatt M, Werner H. A sulphonamidoindanone CGP 28237 (ZK 34228), a novel non-steroidal anti-inflammatory agent without gastrointestinal ulcerogenicity in rats. Drugs Exp Clin Res. 1987;13:237–45.
70. Carr DP, Henn R, Green JR, Böttcher I. Comparison of the systemic inhibition of thromboxane synthesis, anti-inflammatory activity and gastro-intestinal toxicity of non-steroidal anti-inflammatory drugs in the rat. Agents Actions. 1986;19:374–5.
71. Weissenbach R. Clinical trials with nimesulide, a new non-steroid anti-inflammatory agent, in rheumatic pathology. J Int Med Res. 1981;9:349–52.
72. Pais JM, Rosteiro FM. Nimesulide in the short-term treatment of inflammatory process of dental tissues: a double-blind controlled trial against oxyphenbutazone. J Int Med Res. 1983;11:149–54.
73. Emami Nouri E. Nimesulide for treatment of acute inflammation of the upper respiratory tract. Clin Ther. 1984;6:142–50.
74. Fusetti G, Magni E, Armandola MC. Tolerability of nimesulide. Epidemiological data. Drugs. 1993;46(Suppl 1):277–80.
75. Churchill L, Graham AG, Shih C-K, Pauletti D, Farina PR, Grob PM. Selective inhibition of human cyclooxygenase-2 by meloxicam. Inflammopharmacology. 1996; (in press).
76. Engelhardt G. Meloxicam. A potent inhibitor of COX-2. 9th International Conference on Prostaglandins and Related Compounds. Florence (Italy), 6–10 June, 1994.
77. Needleman P. In search of a better NSAID. 9th International Conference on Prostaglandins and Related Compounds. Florence (Italy), 6–10 June, 1994.
78. Seibert K, Zhang Y, Leahy K et al. Pharmacological and biochemical demonstration of the role of cyclooxygenase 2 in inflammation and pain. Proc Natl Acad Sci USA. 1994;91:12013–7.
79. Reitz DB, Li JJ, Norton MB et al. Selective cyclooxygenase inhibitors: novel 1,2-diarylcyclopentenes are potent and orally active COX-2 inhibitors. J Med Chem. 1994;37:3878–81.
80. Gans KR, Galbraith W, Roman RJ et al. Anti-inflammatory and safety profile of DuP 697, a novel orally effective prostaglandin synthesis inhibitor. J Pharmacol Exp Ther. 1990;254:180–7.
81. Chan C-C, Boyce S, Brideau C et al. Pharmacology of a selective cyclooxygenase-2 inhibitor, L-745,337: a novel nonsteroidal anti-inflammatory agent with an ulcerogenic sparing effect in rat and nonhuman primate stomach. J Pharmacol Exp Ther. 1995;274:1531–7.
82. Boyce S, Chan C-C, Gordon R et al. L-745,337: A selective inhibitor of cyclooxygenase-2 elicits antinociception but not gastric ulceration in rats. Neuropharmacology. 1994;33:1609–11.
83. Hirschelmann R, Hentschel M Geissler J, Rickinger O. CGP 28238, a new potent nonsteroidal anti-inflammatory agent: its relation to arachidonic acid metabolism. Agents Actions. 1991;32:54–5.
84. Weisenberg-Boettcher I, Schweizer A, Green JR, Mueller K, Maerki F, Pfeilschifter J. The pharmacological profile of CGP 28238, a novel highly potent anti-inflammatory compound. Drugs Exp Clin Res. 1989;15:501–9.
85. Tagari P, Panneton M, Rasori R. Assessment of NSAID gastroenteropathy in primates. Can J Physiol Pharmacol. 1994;72(Suppl 1):267.
86. Parnham MJ. Inflammation '93. Drug News Perspect. 1994;6:737–42.
87. Futaki N, Takahashi S, Yokoyama M, Arai S, Higuchi S, Otomo S. NS-398, a new anti-inflammatory agent, selectively inhibits prostaglandin G/H synthase/cyclooxygenase (COX-2) activity in vitro. Prostaglandins. 1994;47:55–9.

88. Futaki N, Arai I, Hamasaka Y, Takahashi S, Higuchi S, Otomo S. Selective inhibition of NS-398 on prostanoid production in inflamed tissue in rat carrageenan-air-pouch inflammation. J Pharm Pharmacol. 1993;45:753–5.
89. Farrell AJ, Blake DR, Palmer RMJ, Moncada S. Increased concentrations of nitrite in synovial fluid and serum samples suggest increased nitric oxide synthesis in rheumatic diseases. Ann Rheum Dis. 1992;51:1219–22.
90. Belvisi M, Barnes PJ, Larkin S, Yacoub M, Tadjkarimi S, William TJ, Mitchell JA. Nitric oxide activity is elevated in inflammatory lung disease in humans. Eur J Pharmacol. 1995;283:255–8.
91. Salvemini D, Misko TP, Masferrer JL, Seibert K, Currie MG, Needleman P. Nitric oxide activates cyclooxygenase enzymes. Proc Natl Acad Sci USA. 1993;90:7240–4.
92. Swierkosz TA, Mitchell JA, Warner TD, Botting RM, Vane JR. Co-induction of nitric oxide synthase and cyclooxygenase: interactions between nitric oxide and prostanoids. Br J Pharmacol. 1995;114:1335–42.
93. Appleton I, Tomlinson A, Colville-Nash P, Willoughby DA. Temporal and spatial immunolocalization of cytokines in murine chronic granulomatous tissue. Implications for their role in tissue development and repair processes. Lab Invest. 1993;69:405–14.
94. Vane JR, Mitchell JA, Appleton I, Tomlinson A, Bishop-Bailey D, Croxtall J, Willoughby DA. Inducible isoforms of cyclooxygenase and nitric oxide synthase in inflammation. Proc Natl Acad Sci USA. 1994;91:2046–50.
95. Salvemini D, Seibert K, Masferrer JL, Misko TP, Currie MG, Needleman P. Endogenous nitric oxide enhances prostaglandin production in a model of renal inflammation. J Clin Invest. 1994;93:1940–7.
96. Sautebin L, Di Rosa M. Nitric oxide modulates prostacyclin biosynthesis in the lung of endotoxin-treated rats. Eur J Pharmacol. 1994;262:193–6.
97. Closa D, Hotter G, Prats N, Bulbena O, Roselló-Catafau J, Fernández-Cruz L, Gelpí E. Prostanoid generation in early stages of acute pancreatitis: a role for nitric oxide. Inflammation. 1994;18:469–80.
98. Franchi AM, Chaud M, Rettori V, Suburo A, McCann SM, Gimeno M. Role of nitric oxide in eicosanoid synthesis and uterine motility in estrogen-treated rat uteri. Proc Natl Acad Sci USA. 1994;91:539–43.
99. Mollace V, Colasanti M, Rodino P, Lauro GM, Nistico G. HIV coating gp 120 glycoprotein-dependent prostaglandin E_2 release by human cultured astrocytoma cells is regulated by nitric oxide formation. Biochem Biophys Res Commun. 1994;203:87–92.
100. Tsai A-L, Wei C, Kulmacz RJ. Interaction between nitric oxide and prostaglandin H synthase. Arch Biochem Biophys. 1994;313:367–72.
101. Hajjar DP, Lander HM, Pearce SFA, Upmacis RK, Pomerantz KB. Nitric oxide enhances prostaglandin-H synthase activity by a heme-independent mechanism: evidence implicating nitrosothiols. J Am Chem Soc. 1995;117:3340–6.
102. Astin M, Stjernschantz J, Selén G. Role of nitric oxide in $PGF_{2\alpha}$-induced ocular hyperemia. Exp Eye Res. 1994;59:401–7.
103. Tetsuka T, Daphna-Iken D, Srivastava SK, Baier LD, DuMaine J, Morrison AR. Cross-talk between cyclooxygenase and nitric oxide pathways: Prostaglandin E_2 negatively modulates induction of nitric oxide synthase by interleukin 1. Proc Natl Acad Sci USA. 1994;91:12168–72.
104. Ima T, Hirata Y, Kanno K, Marumo F. Induction of nitric oxide synthase by cyclic AMP in rat vascular smooth muscle cells. J Clin Invest. 1994;93:543–9.
105. Hirokawa K, O'Shaughnessy K, Moore K, Ramrakha P, Wilkins MR. Induction of nitric oxide synthase in cultured vascular smooth muscle cells: the role of cyclic AMP. Br J Pharmacol. 1994;112:396–402.
106. Inoue H, Nanayama T, Hara S, Yokoyama C, Tanabe T. The cyclic AMP response element plays an essential role in the expression of the human prostaglandin-endoperoxide synthase 2 gene in differentiated U937 monocytic cells. FEBS Lett. 1994;350:51–4.
107. Battistini B, Botting R, Bakhle YS. COX-1 and COX-2: toward the development of more selective non-steroid anti-inflammatory drugs. Drug News Perspect. 1994;8:501–12.
108. Inoue T, Fukuo K, Morimoo S, Koh E, Ogihara T. Nitric oxide mediates interleukin-1-induced prostaglandin E_2 production by vascular smooth muscle cells. Biochem Biophys Res Commun. 1993;194:420–4.
109. Corbett JA, Kwon G, Turk J, McDaniel ML. IL-1β induces the co-expression of both nitric

oxide synthase and cyclooxygenase by islets of Langerhands: activation of cyclooxygenase by nitric oxide. Biochemistry. 1993;32:13767–70.
110. Stadler J, Stefanovic-Racic M, Billiar TR et al. Articular chondrocytes synthesize nitric oxide in response to cytokines and lipopolysaccharide. J Immunol. 1991;147:3915–20.
111. Davidge ST, Baker PN, McLaughlin MK, Roberts JM. Nitric oxide produced by endothelial cells increases production of eicosanoids through activation of prostaglandin H synthase. Circ Res. 1995;77:274–83.
112. Stadler J, Harbrecht BC, DiSilvio M, Curran RD, Jordan ML, Simmons RL, Billiar TR. Endogenous nitric oxide inhibits the synthesis of cyclooxygenase products and interleukin-6 by rat Kuppfer cells. J Leukocyte Biol. 1993;53:165–72.
113. Habib A, Bernard C, Tedgui A, Maclouf J. Evidence of cross-talks between inducible nitric oxide synthase and cyclooxygenase II in rat peritoneal macrophages. Abstracts of the 9th International Conference on Prostaglandins and Related Compounds, Florence (Italy), June 6–10 1994; 57.
114. Barker JE, Anderson J, Treasure T, Piper PJ. Role of endothelium in the mediation of angiotensin II-stimulated contraction and prostacyclin release in the human saphenous vein. Br J Pharmacol. 1994;111(Suppl):106P.
115. Ziche M, Morbidelli L, Parenti A, Ledda F. Nitric oxide modulates angiogenesis elicited by prostaglandin E_1 in rabbit cornea. Abstracts of the 9th International Conference on Prostaglandins and Related Compounds, Florence (Italy), June 6–10 1994; 11.
116. Barker JE, Anderson J, Treasure T, Piper PJ. Effects of prostaglandins on stimulated release of nitric oxide by angiotensin II from human saphenous vein. Br J Pharmacol. 1994;112(Suppl): 446P.
117. Akarasereenont P, Mitchell JA, Thiemermann C, Vane JR. Relative potency of nonsteroid anti-inflammatory drugs as inhibitors of cyclooxygenase-1 or cyclooxygenase-2. Br J Pharmacol. 1994;122(Suppl):183P.

2 The three-dimensional structure of cyclooxygenases

R.M. GARAVITO

Prostaglandin H_2 synthase (PGHS; EC 1.14.99.1; cyclooxygenase or COX) catalyses the two-step conversion of arachidonic acid to prostaglandin G_2 and thence to prostaglandin H_2, the first committed steps in the biosynthesis of prostaglandins[1,2]. While COX catalyses both steps of this catalytic process (known as the cyclooxygenase and peroxidase steps, respectively), the reactions are carried out in two spatially distinct active sites[2]. At least two isoforms of the enzyme, COX-1 and COX-2, are expressed in mammalian tissues[1,3]. The COX activity is specifically inhibited by the class of compounds known as non-steroid anti-inflammatory drugs (NSAIDs), which includes the commercially and pharmacologically important agents aspirin, ibuprofen, naproxen and indomethacin[4]. NSAIDs have been the common way to treat certain symptoms of inflammatory[5] and cardiovascular diseases[6]. Moreover, a role for aspirin as an anticancer prophylaxis is now quite established[7–9] although the precise molecular basis for this effect is still unclear.

As the emerging opinion[3,10,11] is that COX-2 is the enzyme involved in the short-term responses to inflammatory events, drug therapy aimed at reducing inflammation should be targeted at COX-2. Most NSAIDs currently in clinical use, however, are known to inhibit both isoforms of COX with little selectivity, and many NSAIDs elicit ulcerogenic and other undesirable side effects that are probably due to COX-1 inhibition in the stomach[3,12]. Information about the structural basis of NSAID binding by COX-1 and COX-2 may therefore prove valuable in the process of designing novel isoform-specific inhibitors[4]. We have determined the X-ray crystal structures of four complexes of NSAIDs with ovine COX-1: flurbiprofen[13], a brominated analogue of aspirin[14], iodosuprofen and iodoindomethacin (Loll et al., manuscript submitted). In this report, I will summarize the results of the crystallographic studies and discuss the implications of ligand binding for COX-2.

PROPERTIES OF THE CYCLOOXYGENASE ISOFORMS

For the X-ray crystallographic and many of the early biochemical studies, COX-1 was obtained from ram seminal vesicles but COX-1 from other species, including human, has been fairly well characterized[1]. Ovine COX-1 has a M_{app} of 70 kDa including glycosylation (about 3.5% by weight) which correlates well with molecular weight calculations using the amino acid sequence. The monomer polypeptide has 600 amino acids (including a 24 residue signal sequence) and is N-linked glycosylated at three sites[15]. When extracted from microsomal membranes, the enzyme appears as dimer in 0.1% Tween-20. COX-1 binds 1 mol of high-spin ferric haem per mole monomer.

COX-1 has the cyclooxygenase (bisdioxygenase) and peroxidase activities within the same polypeptide[1]. The catalytic mechanisms of both reactions are fairly well characterized[1,16]: the cyclooxygenase reaction involves a free radical mechanism utilizing a bound radical generated during the peroxidase reaction. A tyrosine radical has been observed during the catalysis[17–19] but it is not clear yet that it is an obligatory intermediate. Few COX inhibitors have been explicitly developed against the peroxidase activity. Many, such as paracetamol (Tylenol) are radical scavengers, and others have a quite broad spectrum of inhibition towards COX and lipoxygenases (e.g. BW755C); others are quite toxic (e.g. cyanide).

COX-2 seems to be catalytically indistinguishable from COX-1 with respect to its general structure, biochemistry and mechanism of prostaglandin biosynthesis[4]. COX-2 is induced in certain cells and tissues after exposure to a variety of cytokines[20–23]. The cDNA sequences of this 'inducible' COX gene and N-terminal analyses of the gene products suggest that subtle, but significant amino acid differences occur between COX-1 and COX-2 (around 60% identities); COX-2 sequences for several species have greater degrees of amino acid identities[1]. Hence, the isoforms of COX should have a high degree of structural homology[4].

NSAIDs generally compete with the COX substrate, arachidonic acid, in a competitive, reversible manner, as is seen with the drug ibuprofen (Advil). However, several classes of NSAIDs irreversibly inhibit COX activity. Aspirin acetylates Ser 530 and prevents access of the substrate to the active site[14]; other NSAIDs such as flurbiprofen, indomethacin or meclofenamate cause an irreversible, time-dependent inhibition of COX, perhaps by a non-covalent structural alteration of the enzyme–ligand complex which creates a tighter complex[4]. In either case, the peroxidase activity is generally unaffected. NSAIDs, as a whole, do not display a high level of structural similarity to the substrate arachidonate nor, in many cases, to each other[1,3]. Even in structurally isosteric classes of NSAIDs (e.g. ibuprofen, flurbiprofen and suprofen), why some members are reversible, competitive inhibitors and others are irreversible, time-dependent inhibitors is still not known.

Clear kinetic differences are observed between the two COX isozymes with regard to the peroxidase activity[20] and cyclooxygenase activity[10,21]. There are also distinct COX isozyme differences in NSAID action[10,21–27]. This isoform effect is rather pronounced with aspirin: aspirin acetylation completely blocks the activity of COX-1, but aspirin-acetylated COX-2 is still capable of oxygenating arachidonic acid, producing 15(R)-hydroperoxy-eicosatrienoic acid (15(R)-HPETE) instead of prostaglandin G_2[21,28,29]. 15-HPETE can be converted to 15(R)-hydroxy-eicosatrienoic acid (15(R)-HETE or 15-epi-lipoxin) by the COX peroxidase. Thus aspirin blockade of COX-1 and COX-2 could have wider physiological effects than just stopping the biosynthesis of prostaglandins[1,3], particularly with regard to the roles of the COX isozyme in cancer[8,9]. Moreover, the serine acetylation in COX-2 must alter the substrate position for catalysis instead of blocking binding as in COX-1, suggesting that the active site topographies of COX-1 and COX-2 are subtly, but distinctly different.

THE X-RAY CRYSTAL STRUCTURE OF OVINE COX-1

We have determined the crystal structure of the ovine COX-1 isoenzyme co-crystallized with the NSAID flurbiprofen at 3.5 Å resolution[13]. The resolution was extended to 3.1 Å resolution[30] and refined using simulated annealing protocols implemented with the program XPLOR v. 3.1 (D. Picot, P.J. Loll, and R.M. Garavito, manuscript in preparation). At the current stage of refinement, the crystallographic R-factor is 19.2% (free R-factor=22.4%) for 39540 X-ray reflections and 9190 non-H atoms; RMSD bond distance is 0.014 Å and RMSD bond angle is 1.89°. A total of 551 amino acid residues (out of 576 possible) are observed in the $(2F_o - F_c)$ electron density map as well as the haem prosthetic group, the inhibitor flurbiprofen, two N-acetylglucosamine moieties at each of the three glycosylation sites (Asn68, Asn144, and Asn410), and four tightly-bound detergent molecules (Figure 1*). The COX monomer is comprised of three folding domains[2,13]: (1) an N-terminal epidermal growth factor (EGF)-like module, with three intradomain disulphide bridges, Cys36–Cys47, Cys41–Cys57 and Cys59–Cys69, and one interdomain disulphide bridge (Cys37–Cys159); (2) a membrane-binding motif, a spiral of four amphipathic helices (Figure 1); and (3) a globular catalytic domain containing the peroxidase and cyclooxygenase active sites. Of the 13 cysteines, the X-ray structure suggests that 10 are involved in disulphide bridges, including Cys569 and Cys575.

The tertiary structure of the catalytic domain bears striking homology to other mammalian peroxidases[2,13,31], particularly myeloperoxidase (MPO), although the overall sequence homology is only about 20%. The peroxidase active site is located at the cleft between two lobes created by bundles of helices in the catalytic domain. The features of the COX haem binding pocket are quite similar to those of MPO; however, the active site is more open, exposing a larger portion of the haem to the solvent. This correlates well with the need of the COX peroxidase active site to accommodate larger hydroperoxide substrates such as PGG_2.

The active centre of COX is located at the end of a long and narrow hydrophobic channel (8×25 Å long), whose axis runs parallel to the molecular two-fold axis. The apex of the channel is separated from the edge of the haem by Tyr385. A tyrosyl free radical is thought to be generated by the peroxidase reaction and has been proposed to activate the substrate in the cyclooxygenase

*See frontispiece

Figure 2 Views of (a) flurbiprofen (Flu), (b) salicylate (SA) after acetylation with bromo-aspirin, (c) iodosuprofen (Isp), and (d) iodoindomethacin (In) bound in the upper, catalytic region of the COX channel; in (b) Ser530 is acetylated (see text). Note the similarity of binding modes between quite different NSAIDs

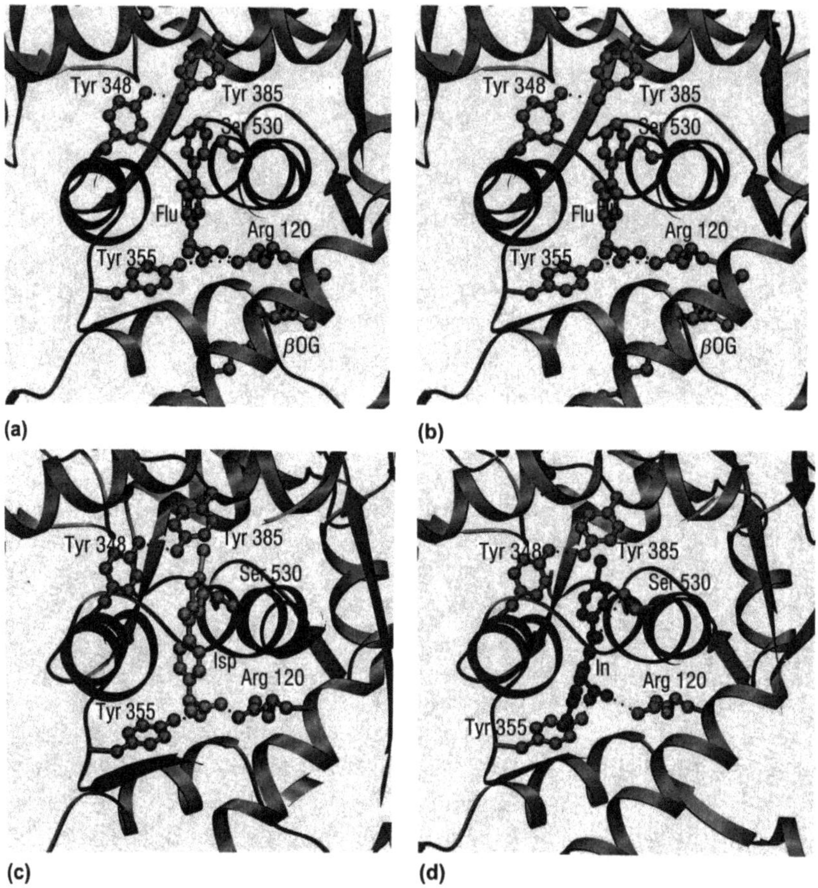

reaction[17,32]. Several lines of evidence suggests that this radical resides on Tyr385. The COX crystals were grown in the presence of the NSAID flurbiprofen and the drug apparently occupies the cyclooxygenase channel between Arg120 and Tyr385 (Figure 2a) where the carboxylate moiety of the drug ligands to Arg120. This arginine is therefore the obvious candidate to ligand the carboxylic group of the substrate arachidonic acid; the rest of the channel is very hydrophobic. Ser530, which is acetylated by aspirin, is located in the upper portion of the channel, within 6 Å of Tyr385.

The globular structure of COX-1 suggests that almost all of the protein should reside on the lumen side of the endoplasmic reticular membrane. The disulphide bridges and the three glycosylation sites also suggest a lumenal localization of the catalytic domain. Finally, the three first helices of the structure and the aminoterminal portion of the fourth helix create a distinct hydrophobic surface facing the exterior of the protein. In the dimer, these surfaces are on the same face of the molecule and the helix axes would lie nearly parallel to the plane of the membrane[33]. To interact with the bilayer, the hydrophobic side chains of this helical surface would penetrate into one leaflet of the bilayer in a manner suggested for amphipathic peptides. As the hydrophobic surface made by these helices would not span the bilayer, we therefore proposed that COX is a monotopic membrane protein[33]. The 3.1 Å refined structure supports this hypothesis: we have found four tightly bound detergent molecules (Figure 1). One β-octyl glucoside (β-OG) detergent molecule is located in each cyclooxygenase channel of the dimer with the alkyl tail pointing into the hydrophobic channel (see Figures 1 and 2a). Two other molecules of β-OG are found at crystal contact sites between the membrane binding domains; their position and orientation support the notion that each membrane binding domain is covered by an extensive detergent shell.

THE SITE(S) OF DRUG INTERACTION

Many factors have prevented us from obtaining strongly diffracting crystals of many COX–drug complexes and, thus, have limited the achievable resolution of the X-ray data. In the cases where the attainable resolution is limited, we have chosen to employ drug analogues which contain electron-dense bromine or iodine atoms, reasoning that the strong scattering power of the halogen atom would allow its unambiguous location in even a low resolution electron density map.

Bromoaspirin

To probe the structure of aspirin-inactivated COX-1, we synthesized the analogue 2-bromo-acetoxy-benzoic acid (bromoaspirin) and soaked it into holo-enzyme crystals. Data were collected and processed as recently described[14] and structure refinement began with the 3.1 Å refined structure of the PGHS–flurbiprofen complex from which the flurbiprofen molecule, carbohydrate and bound detergent had been removed. After structure refinement, the current model for the monomer consists of residues 33–583 of COX-1, one bound haem, the bromoacetyl adduct, salicylate, one bound detergent and four asparagine-linked N-acetyl-glucosamine molecules. The structure of the polypeptide chain in the bromoaspirin crystals is essentially identical to that seen in the flurbiprofen complex[14]. No evidence is seen for significant differences in side chain positions, even in the vicinity of Ser530.

Aspirin is the only NSAID known to inactivate COX-1 through covalent modification, selectively acetylating Ser530[1]. Ser530, which lies along the wall of this channel near Tyr385 (Figure 2b) is evidently not directly involved in catalysis: while acetylation of Ser530 inactivates the enzyme, mutation of this residue to an alanine has no effect on cyclooxygenase activity save to render the enzyme insensitive to aspirin[34]. The structural basis of COX inhibition by aspirin is as follows: the bromoacetyl group on Ser530 extends outward into the channel directly below Tyr385 (Figure 2b); any substrate diffusing up the channel would be prevented from interacting with Tyr385 by the steric hindrance introduced by this adduct.

An $F_o - F_c$ electron density map calculated after completion of the structure refinement strongly suggests that the bromoacetyl–Ser530 side chain has a minor conformer: while the principal conformer protrudes directly into the channel below Tyr385, the minor conformer is folded back into an alcove leading off from the channel[14]. The presence of two conformers at the aspirin acetylation site may be pharmacologically relevant, giving the distinctly different activity aspirin has on the COX isoforms (see above). This effect is unlikely to be due to gross differences in the environment around Ser530, since the amino acids lining the cyclooxygenase site are almost completely conserved between the two isoforms[4]. Our results suggest that the effect may be caused by a change in the preferred rotameric state of the acetylated serine side chain between COX-1 and -2; such an inversion in the ratio of rotamer populations might be caused by subtle differences in side chain conformation and cavity size between the two isoforms.

As COX creates radical species that can be characterized[17,19,35], the question arose as to whether electron paramagnetic resonance (EPR) and electron nuclear double resonance (ENDOR) spectroscopies could provide enough structural information to define the conformation of a ligand and the relative orientation and position on the enzyme. Many NSAIDs can be readily prepared with fluorine and the resonance features of a ^{19}F-substituent can be directly determined and a very reliable distance between the fluorine nucleus and free electron can be measured[36]. In collaboration with Professor M. W. Makinen (The University of Chicago), we prepared monofluoro-acetylsalicylate and have followed the effect of acetylation on the EPR spectrum of the Tyr385 radical species. In COX-1, acetylation by monofluoro-acetylsalicylate does not perturb the EPR spectrum; in mouse COX-2, acetylation alters the EPR signal significantly (S. Stork et al., unpublished observations). Thus, the environment experienced by the tyrosyl radical is different between the two fluoro-acetylated isoforms and provides confirmatory results for our proposals derived from crystallographic observations in bromoacetylated COX-1[14]. We are in the midst of determining whether more detailed structural information about the isoform differences can be obtained from ENDOR measurements.

The transfer of an acetyl group from aspirin to COX generates salicylic acid (SA) as the leaving group. We observed electron density in the active site channel below the acetylation site (Figure 2b) consistent in size and shape with SA. The

SA molecule appears to bind in a manner similar to that observed for flurbiprofen, with its carboxylic acid moiety forming a salt bridge with Arg120 and approaching to within hydrogen bonding distance of the hydroxyl group of Tyr355; the aromatic ring of SA binds in approximately the same position of the channel as the fluorinated ring of flurbiprofen. The mechanism of action for aspirin might then have two steps: aspirin would bind initially at the SA site, at least weakly. Once bound at this site, it then diffuses 5 Å up along the channel until the hydroxyl of Ser530 attacks the acetyl carbon and effects trans-acetylation. Although the salicylate/aspirin binding site is not found at a remote position, as has been suggested by others[37–39], our observation of SA binding is consistent with a large body of pharmacological data on salicylate/aspirin activity[40,41]. The weak COX inhibition by SA is explained by such a site, blocking as it does access to the upper part of the channel where Ser530 is found. Moreover, the antagonistic effect of SA on aspirin activity[40,41] can also be explained by direct competition between aspirin and salicylic acid for the same binding site. Finally, the weak binding of aspirin at this site and the lack of water in the COX channel may explain aspirin's strong and astonishing selectivity for acetylation of this residue.

Iodosuprofen

The starting protein model used in the refinement of the COX-1/iodosuprofen structure (Loll et al., manuscript submitted) was derived by removing all inhibitor, carbohydrate, and detergent molecules from the 3.1 Å refined COX–flurbiprofen structure (Picot et al., manuscript in preparation); individual refined B-values for each atom were retained without further refinement. The refinement converged to a R-value stabilized of 0.189 (free R=0.231), for reflections between 8 and 3.5 Å Luzzati analysis gives an estimate of the rms coordinate error for the COX-1/iodosuprofen complex structure of 0.3 Å. The rms difference in Cα positions between the flurbiprofen and iodosuprofen structures is 0.19 Å. The good R-values obtained throughout the iodosuprofen refinement, particularly in the early stages, suggest that the protein structures in the flurbiprofen and iodosuprofen complexes are indeed very similar.

Iodosuprofen binds to COX-1 at the top of the cyclooxygenase channel (Figure 2c); flurbiprofen has already been found to bind in this site (Figure 2a) and it is not surprising that suprofen would occupy the same site, given its structural similarity to flurbiprofen. As seen with flurbiprofen, side chains lining the channel below the inhibitor, including Tyr355 and Arg120, surround the inhibitor and render it quite inaccessible to solvent. The carboxylic acid moiety of iodosuprofen forms a salt bridge with Arg120 (Figure 2c) and one carboxylic acid oxygen of iodosuprofen evidently forms a hydrogen bond with Tyr355. A hydrogen bond also appears to be formed between the carbonyl oxygen of the inhibitor's ketone moiety and the side chain hydroxyl of Ser530. The iodine atom of the inhibitor lies in a small pocket at the top of the channel and is in close contact with various hydrophobic side chains, including the face of Tyr385. In addition, the iodine may interact with the backbone carbonyl oxygen of Leu384 (Loll et al., manuscript submitted), suggesting that the iodine and oxygen atoms may be engaged in an interaction of the Lewis acid–Lewis base type.

The alpha methyl group of the inhibitor's propionic acid is tucked into a small hydrophobic cleft lined by leucine and valine residues, as was observed in the COX-1/flurbiprofen complex[13]. The basis of the enzyme's stereoselectivity for the *S* stereoisomer of the drug is clear from the structure: the *R* stereoisomer would place the alpha methyl in unfavourably close contact with Tyr355. The region of the channel around Tyr355/Arg120 is quite narrow, forming a constriction that is responsible for enclosing the drugs flurbiprofen, salicylate and iodosuprofen within the channel. One obvious conclusion is that the channel needs to open to allow access to the catalytic center of the COX active site. Hence, the dynamic behaviour of the channel may play a critical role in determining the accessibility of drugs to the upper portion of the channel.

Iodoindomethacin

The refinement of the COX-1/iodoindomethacin structure (Loll et al., manuscript submitted) began with the same starting model as above. Before any refinement, this model yielded an R-value of 0.37 for all data between 8 and 4.5 Å. Rigid body refinement and refinement of an overall anisotropic ΔB reduced the R value to 0.282 (free R=0.285). Despite the low resolution (4.5 Å), a F_o-F_c map calculated at this stage clearly revealed strong electron density for the iodine atom and the iodoindomethacin molecule was placed, fixing the iodine at the site of high electron density and building the remainder of the molecule by hand. After a series of refinement steps, the model had an R-value=0.254 (free R=0.264) for data between 8 and 4.5 Å. The lower resolution available for the COX-1/iodoindomethacin structure makes it difficult to evaluate the accuracy of the model and the refinement protocols. However, the reasonable R-values obtained argue that the model derived from the COX-1/flurbiprofen complex fits the iodoindomethacin data well.

As in the case of COX/iodosuprofen complex, the iodine atom on iodo-indomethacin is observed to bind at the top of the cyclooxygenase channel, packing directly against the aromatic ring of Tyr385 (Figure 2d). Placement of the iodine atom in the initial F_o-F_c map was unambiguous; the distance between the iodine positions in the two structures is 0.6 Å. Although electron density was observed for the light atoms of the iodoindomethacin molecule, the resolution of the data does not allow for their unambiguous fitting into density. However, it was possible to manually build in the light atoms of the iodoindomethacin molecule using the following constraints: (1) using the X-ray crystal structure of the inhibitor[42] for the initial stereochemistry; (2) keeping the iodine position fixed; and (3) assuming that the protein structure is the same as that found in the PGHS–flurbiprofen complex. There are only five bonds in the inhibitor about which free rotation should be possible, and so the conformation space available to the inhibitor is not large. Moreover, the steric constraints contributed by the protein side chains lining the channel severely limited the positions that these atoms could occupy, and very few possible binding modes were identified (Loll et al., manuscript submitted). A 'highly probable' binding model satisfied the following criteria: partial charge neutralization of the carboxylic acid moiety of the inhibitor by Arg120; reasonable values for the torsion angles of the inhibitor; best agreement with the density in the $F_o - F_c$ map; and minimal apparent steric clashes with the protein. After additional refinement, the resulting model is chemically reasonable and appears to agree well with the diffraction data; it should, however, be stressed that other binding modes (or combinations of binding modes) may exist which are consistent with the observed iodine position and which we cannot rigorously rule out at this point.

The model for iodoindomethacin binding is shown in Figure 2d. The iodophenyl group of the inhibitor lies in a hydrophobic pocket at the top of the channel while the carbonyl bridge between the phenyl and indole rings sits further down the channel; a potential hydrogen bond could be made the carbonyl bridge and the γ-hydroxyl of Ser530. The acetic acid moiety would ligand the side chains of Arg120 and Tyr355, much like the carboxylate groups of flurbiprofen[13], iodosuprofen (Figure 2c), and salicylic acid[14] in their respective complexes with PGHS.

DRUG BINDING: SUMMARY

NSAIDs display an unusually large degree of structural diversity and include classes of compounds such as the salicylates, the aryl acetic and propionic acids, the fenamates, the pyrazoles, and the oxicams. While compounds falling within any given class bear obvious resemblance to one another, compounds from different classes may bear little or no resemblance to one another. This suggests that there may exist distinct inhibitor binding sites or subsites on the enzyme which are used by the different inhibitor types. Alternatively, these inhibitors may employ different features of a common site for binding. To date, structures have been determined for COX-1 complexed with inhibitors belonging to three distinct NSAID classes: bromoaspirin[14], iodoindomethacin, an aryl acetic acid, and flurbiprofen[13] and iodosuprofen, both aryl propionic acids. These compounds have common structural features; all contain aromatic rings and carboxylic acid functionalities, for example. However, they differ widely in size and shape, and inhibit COX by at least two distinct mechanisms: bromoaspirin inhibits the cyclooxygenase via acetylation of a serine residue, while the others do not covalently modify the enzyme. Despite the structural and mechanistic differences between these various inhibitors, they all share a common site of action. The

NSAIDs studied all bind at the top of the COX channel in close proximity to the putative catalytic residue Tyr385 (Figures 2 and 3). Their binding therefore blocks access of substrate to the active site cavity that lies at the end of this channel. The blockage is achieved in different ways by different compounds. For example, the acetyl group introduced by bromoaspirin lies at the very top of the channel, just below Tyr385; it does not fill the channel, but evidently occupies enough volume to prevent the substrate from contacting Tyr385. Flurbiprofen, iodosuprofen and iodoindomethacin are substantially larger than this acetyl group, and would fill the entire channel from Tyr385 downwards for a distance of roughly 12–14 Å (Figure 3).

Certain structural details of ligand binding are common between the different compounds. First, Ser530 can apparently hydrogen bond to carbonyls on the drugs. Second, the carboxylic acid moieties of flurbiprofen, iodosuprofen, and iodoindomethacin all form salt bridges with Arg120, and iodosuprofen and iodoindomethacin appear to form hydrogen bonds to the hydroxyl of Tyr355. Salicylic acid, the leaving group generated by acetylation of Ser530 by bromoaspirin and itself a weak cyclooxygenase inhibitor, is also observed to bind in a similar manner with its carboxylic acid group also positioned between Arg120 and Tyr355. Since Arg120 and its salt bridge partner Glu524 are the only charged residues in the otherwise hydrophobic channel interior, and since a carboxylic acid moiety is found in many otherwise structurally dissimilar NSAIDs, it seems likely that this carboxylate–arginine interaction is a common feature of many COX–NSAID complexes. This observation also suggests that the substrate arachidonic acid would bind with its carboxylic acid group liganding to Arg120 and Tyr355.

All of the inhibitors for which structures are available are irreversible or pseudo-irreversible. Bromoaspirin covalently modifies COX and is thus irreversible. Flurbiprofen, iodosuprofen, and iodoindomethacin do not covalently modify the enzyme, but belong to the slow tight-binding class of inhibitors, and hence inhibit pseudo-irreversibly. These compounds exhibit time-dependent inhibition; that is, as the inhibitor is incubated with the enzyme, the inhibition increases with time. This type of binding is believed to involve a two-step mechanism: the initial, rapid formation of the enzyme inhibitor complex EI, followed by a slow conformational change to the more stable form EI*[43]. The similarity between the COX structures in the bromoaspirin, iodosuprofen and flurbiprofen crystals suggests that, if these NSAID binding gives rise to conformational changes, then the magnitude of the change is smaller than can be detected at the current level of resolution. Moreover, the flurbiprofen and iodosuprofen complexes were determined from crystals produced by co-crystallization and, thus, their structures presumably reflect the EI* form.

The iodoindomethacin structure was determined from a crystal of the enzyme–flurbiprofen complex that was soaked in iodoindomethacin to displace the flurbiprofen (Loll et al., manuscript submitted). Although this is a low resolution

Figure 3 ***A stereo view of the residues that form the COX channel. Flurbiprofen (gray) ligands (dotted lines) Tyr355 and Arg120, the residues that mark the location of the channel constriction. Residues Leu357 and Ile523 (both dark gray) are the only residues lining the upper portion of the channel which change in human COX-2 (see Table 1). Thr106 (dark gray), at the junction between helices C and D of the membrane binding motif, is the location where a residue insertion occurs in the human COX-2 sequence***

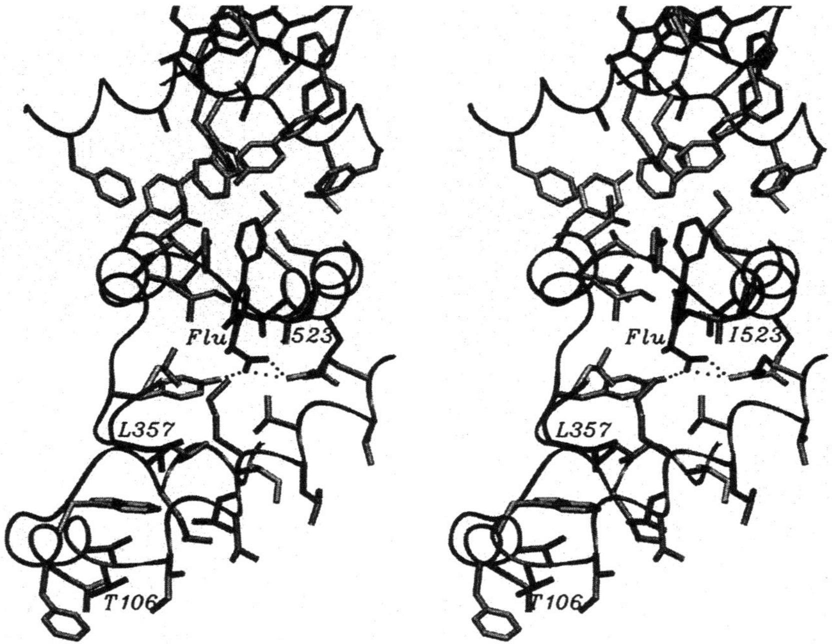

structure, we see no evidence for significant conformational differences in the enzyme between the flurbiprofen and iodoindomethacin complexes. Nonetheless, evaluating the behaviour of drugs that are isosteric with indomethacin as well as the possible conformation heterogeneity of indomethacin[42] suggest that drug stereochemistry may play a variety of roles in the binding process and that there may be multiple binding conformations in COX-1, creating a heterogeneous population of structures (Loll et al., manuscript submitted). This hypothesis might explain the observation that iodoindomethacin, indomethacin, and several other drugs can disorder ovine COX-1 crystals during soaking as well as creating disordered crystals during co-crystallization (P.J. Loll and R.M. Garavito, unpublished observations).

IMPLICATIONS FOR THE DESIGN OF COX-2 SELECTIVE NSAIDs

Sequence comparisons between COX-1 and COX-2 from a variety of species[1] reinforce the idea that the two isoforms are structurally homologous[4]. Using standard modelling algorithms such as ProMod[44], we have built a consensus model of human COX-1 (B. Perman and R.M. Garavito, unpublished results). In the initial stages of modelling, the Ca positions of the 'unrefined' COX-2 structure deviated from the ovine X-ray structure with a RMSD of 0.2 Å. Although the RMSD rose to 0.3 Å after restrained energy minimization of the COX-2, the superposition of the COX-1/COX-2 tertiary structures is excellent (B. Perman and R.M. Garavito, unpublished observations).

Within the COX catalytic centre, the structures of the two isoforms are strikingly similar, an unsurprising observation given the lack of sequence differences in this region (Table 1). From the level of the channel constriction at Tyr355/Arg120 up to Tyr385, only two sequence differences between the isoforms are observed in the residues that line the channel (Figure 3 and Table 1): Leu357 and Ile523 in ovine COX-1 change to Phe and Val, respectively. While these changes will subtly change the topography of the COX catalytic centre, it remains to be seen whether these changes alone can explain the observed isoform selectivity of the newer generation of NSAIDs[3,22,24,25,45,46].

More dramatic sequence variations occur at the mouth of the COX channel in the membrane binding motif (Table 1). The only residue insertion within the main body of the enzyme between COX-1 (-^{103}VNA<u>T</u>FI^{108}-) occurs at the junction between helices C and D in the membrane-binding motif (Table 1 and Figure 3). As mentioned above, all of the inhibitor complexes with COX-1 lead to the inescapable conclusion that the COX channel, particularly at the site of the constriction, must open up to allow the ligand access to the COX catalytic centre. The sequence changes in this region may directly affect the dynamic behaviour of channel opening and closing during ligand binding as the membrane binding motif contributes some of the residues which create the channel constriction (Figure 3). The precise nature of the conformational changes associated with

Table 1 COX channel residues[a]

Membrane Binding Motif	Helix 2	Helix 6-loop
I89V	F198	V344
L921	A202	I345
L93	F205	**Y348**
L99F	T206	V349
W100	F209	L352
F102V	F210	**Y355**
V103		L357F
T106I	**Helix 8 transition**	L359
-106'P[c]	F381	
F107	L384	
I108L	**Y385**	**Helix 17**
T111A	W387	F518
L112I		M522
M113		I523V
L115Y		A527
V116		**S530**
V119S		L531
R120[b]		

[a]Listed residues contribute directly to the COX channel topography. The residues are given as ovine COX-1 residue and number followed by the residue type in human COX-2, if different.
[b]Bold residues are involved in catalysis or ligand binding.
[c]Boxed residues highlight possibly significant differences between ovine COX-1 and human COX-2 (see text). The COX-2 insertion is labelled -106'P.

inhibitor binding will have profound implications for the design of next-generation inhibitors of COX-1 and COX-2; hence, further work is required to clearly delineate the structural and dynamic aspects of NSAID binding. The structures of the uninhibited COX-1 enzyme and the COX-2 enzyme, which both remain to be determined, may elucidate the physical nature of these conformational changes.

Acknowledgements

This work, primarily done at The University of Chicago, was supported by the PHS/NIH program project grant HL-30121 and, in part, by the American Heart Association of Metropolitan Chicago. I would like to thank my co-workers, Drs D. Picot, P.J. Loll, S. Stork, and B. Perman for allowing me to comment on some unpublished aspects of their work.

References

1. Smith WL, Marnett LJ. Prostaglandin endoperoxide synthases. In: Sigal H, Sigel A eds. Metal Ions in Biological Systems. New York: Marcel Dekker; 1994:163–99.
2. Garavito RM, Picot D, Loll PJ. Prostaglandin H synthase. Curr Opin Struct Biol. 1994;4: 529–35.

3. Munroe D, Lau C. Turning down the heat: new routes to inhibition of inflammatory signaling by prostaglandin H2 synthases. Chem Biol. 1995;2:343–50.
4. Loll PJ, Garavito RM. The isoforms of cyclooxygenase: structure and function. Exp Opin Invest Drugs. 1994;3:1171–80.
5. Abramson S. Therapy with and mechanisms of nonsteroidal anti-inflammatory drugs. Curr Opin Rheumatol. 1991;3:336–40.
6. Makheja A. Atherosclerosis: the eicosanoid connection. Mol Cell Biochem. 1992;111:137–42.
7. Giovannucci E, Egan K, Hunter D et al. Aspirin and the risk of colorectal cancer in women. N Engl J Med. 1995;333:609–14.
8. Marnett L. Aspirin and the potential role of prostaglandins in colon cancer. Cancer Res. 1992; 52:5575–89.
9. Marcus A. Aspirin as a prophylaxis against colorectal cancer. N Engl J Med. 1995;333:636–8.
10. Meade AA, Smith WL, DeWitt DL. Differential inhibition of prostaglandin endoperoxide synthase (cyclooxygenase) isozymes by aspirin and other non-steroidal antiinflammatory drugs. J Biol Chem. 1993;268:6610–4.
11. Vane J. Towards a better aspirin. Nature (London). 1994;367:215–6.
12. Rainsford K. Current concepts of the mechanism of side effects of nonsteroidal antiinflammatory drugs as a basis for establishing research priorities: an experimentalist's view. J Rheumatol. 1988;17(Suppl.):63–70.
13. Picot D, Loll PJ, Garavito RM. The X-ray crystal structure of the membrane protein prostaglandin H_2 synthase-1. Nature (Lond.). 1994;367:243–9.
14. Loll P, Picot D, Garavito R. The structural basis of aspirin activity inferred from the crystal structure of inactivated prostaglandin H_2 synthase. Nat Struct Biol. 1995;2:637–43.
15. Otto J, Dewitt D, Smith W. N-glycosylation of prostaglandin endoperoxide synthases-1 and 2 and their orientations in the endoplasmic reticulum. J Biol Chem. 1993;268:18234–42.
16. Marnett L, Maddipati K. Prostaglandin H synthase. In: Everse J, Everse KE, Grisham MB, eds. Peroxidases in Chemistry and Biology. Boca Raton: CRC Press; 1991:293–334.
17. Smith WL, Eling TE, Kulmacz RJ, Marnett LJ, Tsai A. Tyrosyl radicals and their role in hydroperoxide-dependent activation and inactivation of prostaglandin endoperoxide synthase. Biochemistry. 1992;31:3–7.
18. Dietz R, Nastainczyk W, Ruf H. Higher oxidation states of prostaglandin H synthase. Rapid electronic spectroscopy detected two spectral intermediates during the peroxidase reaction with prostaglandin G2. Eur J Biochem. 1988;171:321–8.
19. Karthein R, Dietz R, Nastainczyk W, Ruf HH. Higher oxidation states of prostaglandin H synthase. An EPR study of a transient tyrosyl radical in the enzyme during the peroxidase reaction. Eur J Biochem. 1988;171:313–20.
20. Sirois J, Richards J. Purification and characterization of a novel, distinct isoform of prostaglandin endoperoxide synthase induced by human chorionic gonadotropin in granulosa cells of rat preovulatory follicles. J Biol Chem. 1992;267:6382–8.
21. Holtzman MJ, Turk J, Shornick LP. Identification of a pharmacologically distinct prostaglandin H synthase in cultured epithelial cells. J Biol Chem. 1992;267:21438–45.
22. Mitchell JA, Akarasereenont P, Thiemermann C, Flower RJ, Vane JR. Selectivity of nonsteroidal antiinflammatory drugs as inhibitors of constitutive and inducible cyclooxygenase. Proc Natl Acad Sci USA. 1994;90:11693–7.
23. DeWitt DL, Meade EA, Smith WL. PGH synthase isoenzyme selectivity: The potential for safer nonsteroidal antiinflammatory drugs. Am J Med. 1993;95:40s–44s.
24. Futaki N, Takahashi S, Yokoyama M, Arai I, Higuchi S, Otomo S. NS-398, a new anti-inflammatory agent, selectively inhibits prostaglandin G/H synthase (COX-2) activity in vitro. Prostaglandins. 1994;47:55–9.
25. Isakson P. Synthesis and pharmacology of selective COX-2 inhibitors. Proceedings of 208th American Chemical Society National Meeting, Division of Medicinal Chemistry; 1994 Aug 20–25; Washington, DC. Washington, DC: American Chemical Society; 1994: MEDI 270.
26. Laneuville O, Breuer DK, DeWitt DL, Hla T, Funk CD, Smith WL. Differential inhibition of human prostaglandin endoperoxide H synthasases-1 and -2 by nonsteroidal anti-inflammatory drugs. J Pharmacol Exp Ther. 1994;271:927–34.
27. Masferrer JL, Zweifel BS, Manning PT et al. Selective inhibition of inducible cyclooxygenase 2 in vivo is antiinflammatory and nonulcerogenic. Proc Natl Acad Sci USA. 1994;91:3228–332.

28. Lecomte M, Laneuville O, Ji C, DeWitt DL, Smith WL. Acetylation of human prostaglandin endoperoxide synthase-2 (cyclooxygenase-2) by aspirin. J Biol Chem. 1994;269:13207–15.
29. O'Neill GP, Mancini JA, Kargman S et al. Overexpression of human prostaglandin G/H synthase-1 and -2 by recombinant vaccinia virus: Inhibition by nonsteroidal antiinflammatory drugs and biosynthesis of 15-hydroxyeicosatetraenoic acid. Mol Pharmacol. 1994;45:245–54.
30. Garavito RM, Picot D, Loll PJ. The 3.1 Å X-ray structure of the integral membrane enzyme prostaglandin H_2 synthase. Adv Prostaglandin, Thromboxane, Leukotriene Res, 1995;23: 99–103.
31. Zeng J, Fenna RE. X-ray crystal structure of canine myeloperoxidase at 3 Å resolution. J Mol Biol. 1992;226:185–207.
32. Ruf HH, Raab-Brill U, Blau C. A model for the catalytic mechanism of prostaglandin endoperoxide synthase. Biochem Soc Trans. 1993;21:739–44.
33. Picot D, Garavito R. Prostaglandin H synthase: implications for membrane structure. FEBS Lett. 1994;346:21–5.
34. Shimokawa T, Smith WL. Prostaglandin endoperoxide synthase: The aspirin acetylation region. J. Biol Chem. 1992;267:12387–92.
35. Hsi L, Hoganson C, Babcock G, Garavito R, Smith W. An examination of the source of the tyrosyl radical in ovine prostaglandin endoperoxide-1. Biochem Biophys Res Commun. 1995; 207:652–60.
36. Wells G, Mustafi D, Makinen M. Structure at the active site of an acylenzyme of α-chymotrypsin and implications for the catalytic mechanism. J Biol Chem. 1994;269:4577–86.
37. Rotilio D, Joseph D, Hatmi M, Vargaftig BB. Structural requirements for preventing the aspirin- and the arachidonate-induced inactivation of platelet cyclooxygenase: additional evidence for distinct enzymatic sites. Eur J Pharmacol. 1984;97:197–208.
38. Humes JL, Winter CA, Sadowski SJ, Kuehl FAJ. Multiple sites on prostaglandin cyclooxygenase are determinants in the action of nonsteroidal antiinflammatory agents. Proc Natl Acad Sci USA. 1981;78:2053–6.
39. de Gaetano G, Cerletti C, Dejana E, Latini R. Pharmacology of platelet inhibition in humans: Implications of the salicylate-aspirin interaction. Circulation. 1985;72:1185–93.
40. Vargaftig B. The inhibition of cyclo-oxygenase of rabbit platelets by aspirin is prevented by salicylic acid and by phenanthrolines. Eur J Pharmacol. 1978;50:231–41.
41. Merino J, Livio M, Rajtar G, de Gaetano G. Salicylate reverses in vitro aspirin inhibition of rat platelet and vascular prostaglandin generation. Biochem Pharmacol. 1980;29:1093–6.
42. Loll P, Carrell C, Carrell H, Garavito R. 1-(4-Iodobenzoyl)-5-methoxy-2-methylindole-3-acetic acid, an iodinated indomethacin analogue. Acta Cryst C. 1996 (in press).
43. Morrison JF, Walsh CT. The behavior and significance of slow-binding enzyme inhibitors. Adv Enzymol Rel Areas Mol Biol. 1988;61:201–301.
44. Peitsch M, Jongeneel C. A 3-D model for the CD40 ligand predicts that it is a compact trimer similar to the tumor necrosis factors. Int Immunol. 1992;5:233–8.
45. Prasit P. L-745,337, a selective COX-2 inhibitor. Proceedings of 208th American Chemical Society National Meeting, Division of Medicinal Chemistry; 1994 Aug 20–25; Washington, DC. Washington, DC: American Chemical Society; 1994; MEDI 272.
46. Reitz D, Li J, Norton M et al. Novel 1,2-diarylcyclopentenes are selective, potent, and orally active cyclooxygenase inhibitors. Proceedings of 208th American Chemical Society National Meeting, Division of Medicinal Chemistry; 1994 Aug 20–25; Washington, DC. Washington, DC: American Chemical Society; 1994; MEDI 271.

3 The dilemma of two cyclooxygenases: identifying the roles of COX-1 and COX-2 in inflammation and apoptosis

D.L. SIMMONS, X. LU, W.S. BRADSHAW and W. XIE

The finding in 1991 of a second form of cyclooxygenase (COX) has opened a new era of non-steroid anti-inflammatory drug (NSAID) research[1-3]. The tremendous interest shown in comparing COX-1 and COX-2 expression has led to the generalization that COX-1, which is found in most tissues of mammals, is involved in physiological regulation of homeostasis. COX-2, on the other hand, is involved in the inflammatory response and certain physiological phenomena, such as ovulation, that respond to transitory hormonal signals[4,5]. The hallmark, therefore, of mammalian COX-1, is its widespread expression in cells and tissues. Typically, COX-1 is constitutively expressed, although increasing examples of its induction have been reported. In most cases, COX-1 is induced by agents that cause the cells in question to differentiate, reinforcing the notion that the role of COX-1 is in the maintenance of differentiated homeostasis[6,7]. In these cases, COX-1 induction is long-term or permanent.

The hallmark of COX-2 is its inducibility, which typically is large (> 10-fold), transient, and proceeds from a very low basal level to a high level of expression. In the absence of some external stimulus the level of COX-2 in mammalian tissues is generally low. High levels of COX-2 mRNA have been identified in mouse prostate, however, and levels are detectable in lung, kidney and neural tissues of mice and humans[8]. The latter finding suggests that COX-2 may play yet undefined roles in neural function, such as those that have been identified for other inducible immediate-early genes such as c-*fos*[9].

GENE STRUCTURE AND REGULATION OF COX-2

COX-2 is a prototypical immediate-early gene product which is encoded by an 8.8 kb gene in both chicken and mammals. In contrast, the gene encoding COX-1 is 24 kb in mammals and its size has not been determined in chicken[10]. The two genes encoding COX-1 and COX-2 are clearly descended from a common ancestor. Each contains near-identical intron placement, suggesting that they arose from a common gene through gene duplication[10]. Recently my laboratory cloned a cDNA for COX-1 in chicken. The finding of COX-1 in a non-mammalian species places the duplication event resulting in COX-1 and COX-2

Table 1 Evolutionary comparison of COX-1 and COX-2 amino acid sequences

	Chicken	*Mammalian*
COX-1	100%	77%
COX-2	100%	86%

Chicken COX-1 and COX-2 amino acid sequences encoded by the chicken 972 bp cDNA clone were compared with human, mouse, and for COX-1, sheep counterparts. This region is largely in the membrane binding and catalytic domains and is conserved among species. The variable regions at the carboxy- and aminoterminal ends of COX-1 and COX-2 were excluded from the comparison. Only identities were scored without attempt to assess conservative amino acid substitutions

before the arrival of the first mammals. Further evidence for a relatively ancient origin of COX-1 and COX-2 genes is that they have evolutionarily segregated onto different chromosomes: in mice, COX-1 is on chromosome 2 whereas COX-2 is on chromosome 1[10].

Comparison of the chicken COX-1 sequence with its mammalian counterparts shows that COX-1 in chicken is evolutionarily less conserved than COX-2 (Table 1). This finding is striking in that not only is the structure of COX-1 not as conserved in chicken, but neither is its pattern of expression. In chicken, COX-1 is expressed as a very rare mRNA in tissues (Figure 1). However, as in mammals, we have observed no transient induction of COX-1 by mitogens, hormones or other stimuli.

In all organisms, induction of COX-2 is largely at the mRNA level and in most cases is transcriptionally driven. Like other immediate-early genes, its transcription increases abruptly within 15 min of treatment with a mitogen or other inducer[11]. Increases in cytosolic mRNA levels lag behind transcription by hours, and protein levels reach their maximum even later. In addition to being up-regulated at the mRNA level, COX-2 is also down-regulated at this level by synthetic glucocorticoids[3], inhibitors of tyrosine phosphorylation[12], activated oxygen scavengers[13] and prostanoids[14]. Down-regulation by dexamethasone (DEX) is the most studied of these, and has been shown to be due to transcriptional[15] and post-transcriptional repression of COX-2 mRNA[11]. Both basal and induced levels of COX-2 mRNA expression are decreased by DEX, the latter typically being suppressed by 70–80%[11].

The instability of the COX-2 gene and protein make it ideal for transient expression. In all species COX-2 mRNA contains >10 copies of the Shaw/Kamen sequence, AUUUA, that is responsible for destabilizing RNA[16]. Even when placed in rabbit reticulocyte lysate, the COX-2 mRNA is extremely unstable, with a half-life of <10 min (Figure 2). However, when the 3′ untranslated region containing the multiple Shaw/Kamen sequences is removed, the mRNA half-life is dramatically increased to 60 min. The COX-2 protein is also unstable and has a half-life of 22.5 min in chicken embryo fibroblasts[11].

***Figure 1** Northern blot analysis of COX-1 RNA from chicken seminal vesicle. Chicken seminal vesicle was found to contain one of the highest levels of COX-1 mRNA even though, as shown, this was barely detectable above background. Left panel shows an ethidium bromide-stained formaldehyde denaturing gel loaded with 10 μg (right lane) of total seminal vesicle RNA. Right panel shows the autoradiogram of the Northern filter made from the gel in the left hand figure. The filter was hybridized to radiolabelled chicken COX-1 cDNA probe. Hybridization conditions were 20×10^6 cpm/ml in Church-Gilbert buffer at 65°C*[1]

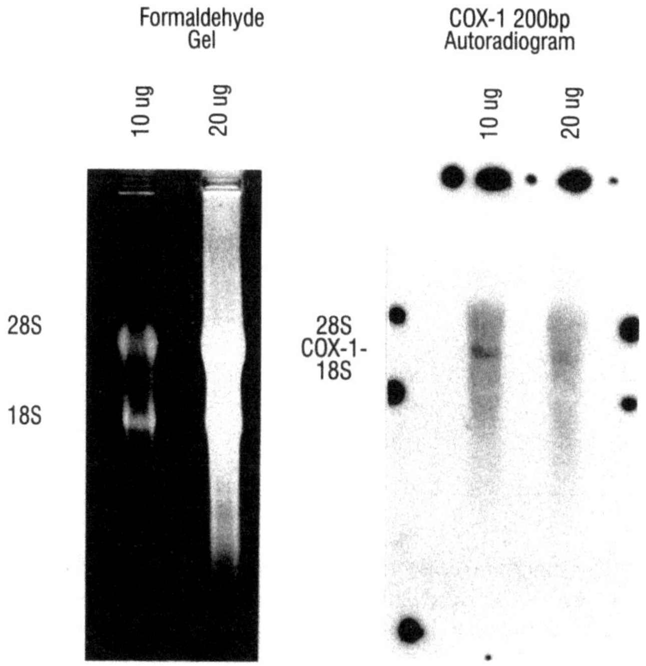

DIFFERENCES IN NSAID SENSITIVITY

The finding that aspirin treatment completely inhibited COX-1 activity, but resulted in COX-2 producing 15-R-HETE suggested that the active sites of the two isoenzymes are subtly different (reviewed by Garavito in this volume). Extensive drug screening by the pharmaceutical industry has led to the identification of multiple potential COX-2-selective inhibitors and one COX-1-selective drug[17–20]. COX-2 ultra-selective drugs show high promise of having pharmacological properties that are substantially different from current NSAIDs. Hopefully, among these properties will be low gastric and renal toxicity and high anti-inflammatory activity.

But are the dozens of currently available NSAIDs truly non-selective COX

***Figure 2** COX-2 RNA half-life determination in a cell-free system. The upper left-hand arrow designates two COX-2 transcripts (lanes 1–8 and 9–16 respectively) which differ only at their 5′ ends but contain the entire 3′ untranslated region. The lower left-hand arrow designates a COX-2 transcript lacking its 3′ untranslated region. Uniformly ^{32}P-labelled transcripts were placed in rabbit reticulocyte translation lysate for the times shown at the top of the figure. The transcripts were tested with a 5′ 7-methylguanosine cap (indicated by a +) or without a cap (indicated by a −). Transcripts with a 3′ untranslated region had a half-life of significantly less than 10 min, which was the first time point tested. Removal of the 3′ untranslated region increased the half-life to approximately 30 min*

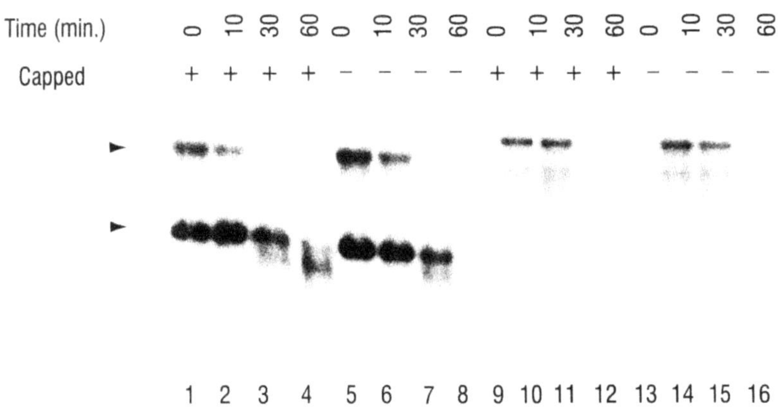

inhibitors? The enormous amount of drug testing data that has recently been presented in journals and at scientific meetings is highly contradictory. However, some consistent and prominent themes emerge from these studies. First, drug selectivity is often dependent on whether investigators used instantaneous inhibition assays or long-term (i.e. 10–30 min) exposure to drug. Second, when current NSAIDs are applied to purified COX isoenzymes, they exhibit non-selective or only moderately selective inhibitory activity. Third, current NSAIDs applied to whole cells or microsomes of cells over-expressing large amounts of isoenzymes from expression vectors show the same general pattern of activity as with purified enzymes. Fourth, when NSAIDs are applied to cells unmodified by recombinant expression of COX, enormous differences in activity, of as much as 4–5 orders of magnitude, are seen for individual drugs. Finally, some cells (e.g. macrophages, monocytes) seem to be generally more sensitive to NSAIDs, whereas others (e.g. fibroblasts) are resistant.

These properties are clearly evident for the NSAID diclofenac, which was first marketed in 1979 and is sold in the USA as Voltarin[21]. It is a bicyclic aromatic compound in the acetic acid subclass of NSAIDs. Instantaneous COX inhibition assays, in which COX activity is measured immediately after addition of the drug

Table 2 IC_{50} values of diclofenac for purified or semi-purified human COX-1 and COX-2

	IC_{50} (μM)	
Study	COX1	COX-2
Laneauville et al.[22]	2.7±1.0	20.5±6.4
Gierse et al.[24]	0.04	0.1
Barnett et al.[23]	0.9±0.04	1.5±0.13

showed IC_{50} values of 2.7 μM and 20.5 μM for COX-1 and COX-2, respectively[23], when diclofenac was applied to microsomal preparations of over-expressed COX proteins[22]. In time-dependent assays, where the drug was incubated with enzyme for 30 min prior to assay, diclofenac was found to be a time-dependent inhibitor, similar to indomethacin[22]. The latter drug showed a 700-fold higher potency toward COX-2 and a 10-fold higher potency toward COX-1 in time-dependent, as opposed to instantaneous assays respectively[22].

Diclofenac has now been measured by time-dependent and instantaneous assays in several studies using purified COX isoenzymes, or isoenzymes over-expressed in cell lines[22–24]. The results clearly show diclofenac to inhibit COX-1 and -2 at sub-micromolar concentrations, with the drug showing modest inhibitory preference toward COX-1 (Table 2).

We have tested 27 NSAIDs in time-dependent assays using two established rodent cell lines. The first, NIH3T3 cells, contains large amounts of constitutively expressed COX-1[11,25]. Treatment of these cells with serum, phorbol ester, or other mitogens produces a robust induction of COX-2. Total COX activity in the presence of exogenous arachidonate approximately doubles in these cells following mitogen treatment (Figure 3). This modest induction is due to a 10- to 20-fold increase in COX-2 from its low basal to its induced state, superimposed upon the high constitutive level of COX-1[8,11]. Levels of PGE_2 synthesized from endogenous arachidonate concomitantly rise 10- to 100-fold in these cells following treatment, the magnitude of the increase being dependent on the growth state of the cells (Figure 4).

The other cell line tested for inhibition with NSAIDs is RS-2. Like NIH3T3 cells, this is a rodent (rat) embryo fibroblast-derived line[11]. Although, unlike NIH3T3, it is neoplastically transformed by the v-*fos* oncogene, studies using a non-transformed derivative of RS-2, 208, have shown that neoplastic transformation does not alter the effectiveness of NSAIDs in the cells. RS-2 lacks detectable COX-1 mRNA but expresses inducible levels of COX-2 mRNA and protein. The level of COX-2 induction is lower in these cells, but in spite of this, total COX activity rises 5-fold after mitogen treatment[11].

NIH3T3 and RS-2 cells provide models for measuring COX-1 and COX-2, respectively, in whole cell, time-dependent assays. In the COX-1 model, NIH3T3

***Figure 3** Kinetics of serum-induced PGHS activity in serum-starved NIH3T3 cells to which 10% fetal calf serum was added for the times indicated. Culture media were then aspirated and the wells were washed once with serum-free medium. Serum-free medium (1 ml containing 30 μM arachidonate) was added to each well and the cells were incubated for an additional 10 min at 37°C. Culture media containing released prostaglandins were collected and PGE_2 levels were determined by RIA. Each test was performed in duplicate*

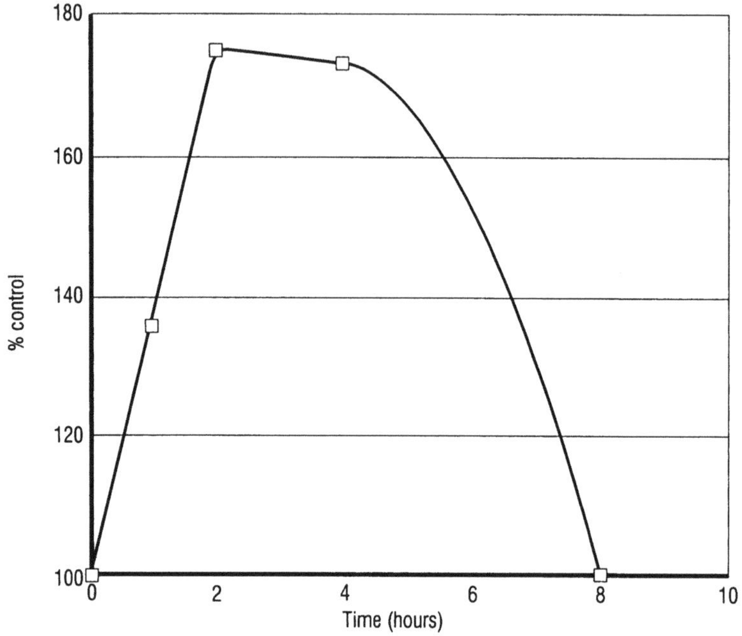

cells are grown to high density to cause contact inhibition. The cells are then deprived of growth factors and cultured in the presence of 2 μM dexamethasone (DEX) to remove any residual COX-2 expression. In the COX-2 model, RS-2 cells are stimulated with serum for 2–4 h in order to induce maximum COX-2 expression.

Measurement of COX activity in these two cell systems after treatment for 30 min with various standard NSAIDs showed that some were completely inactive at up to millimolar concentrations, whereas others showed modest to potent activity (Table 3). Here, PGE_2 synthesis was measured after the addition of exogenous arachidonic acid. Only one of the drugs, diclofenac, was highly selective for either enzyme; showing $>1\times10^4$-fold preference for inhibiting COX-2 in RS-2 cells than COX-1 in NIH3T3 cells (Figure 5). To determine whether this apparent isoenzyme-specific effect might be an artifactual result of

Figure 4 Bar graph of prostaglandin E_2 formation in serum-starved (the left bar in each bar pair) and serum-stimulated (the right bar in each bar pair) NIH3T3 cells. Prostaglandin E_2 was assayed in cellular supernatants by RIA. Cells were either cultured in 0.9% fetal calf serum (FCS) NIH3T3 or were stimulated with 10% FCS for the times indicated

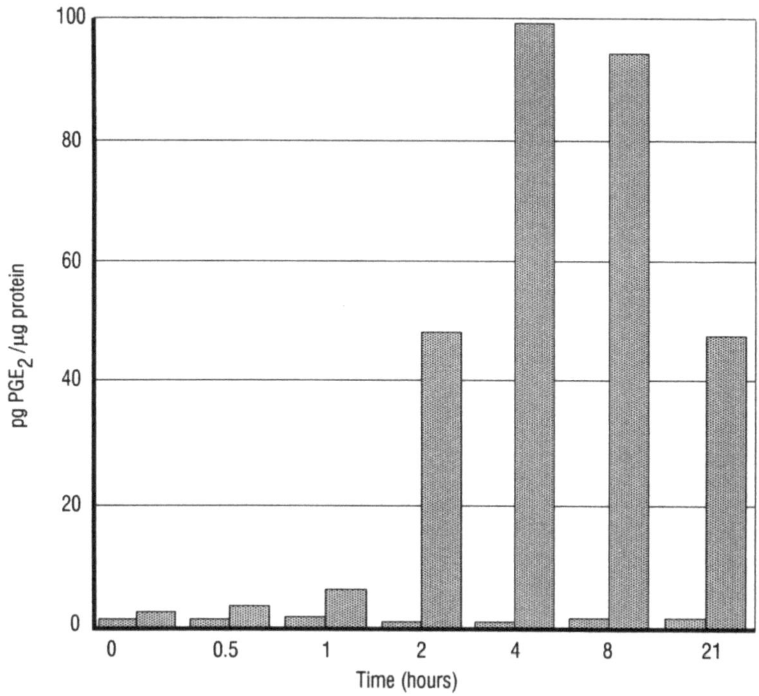

species differences between mice and rats, we measured the effect of diclofenac on serum-induced NIH3T3 cells containing both COX-1 and COX-2 (Figure 6). A clear biphasic inhibition pattern was observed. Phase one showed an IC_{50} value of 1 – 2 nM and Phase 2 an IC_{50} value near 200 μM. These are nearly identical to the IC_{50} values of 7 nM and 200 μM for COX-2 and COX-2, respectively, derived in our RS2/NIH3T3 cell assays (Figure 7).

In this assay, therefore, we have found a reversal of what would be predicted from time-dependent assays using purified protein: diclofenac is much more potent and selective toward COX-2 in fibroblasts than toward purified COX-2, and is much less potent toward fibroblast COX-1 than purified enzyme. The most compelling explanation for this is that other factors present in the cell can markedly change the response of COX enzymes to NSAIDs under normal physiological conditions. In the case of diclofenac, the effect of these yet

Table 3 Inhibitory activity of NSAIDs in NIH3T3 and RS2 cells

	IC_{50} (μM)	
NSAID	*NIH3T3*	*RS2*
Strong inhibitors		
Diclofenac	150	0.007
Indomethacin	0.05	0.28
Flurbiprofen	42	42
Aspirin	88	170
Carprofen	>500	120
Flufenamic Acid	>500	150
Niflumic Acid	>500	240
Acemetacin	N.D.	N.D.
Mefenamic Acid	N.D.	N.D.
Diflunisal	>500	N.D.
Ibuprofen	>500	330
Moderate inhibitors		
Piroxicam[a]	<500	~500
Isoxicam[a]	<500	~500
Tolemetin[a]	<500	>500
Zomepirac[a]	<500	~500
Suprofen[a]	<500	>500
Ketoprofen[a]	<500	~500
(+)Naproxen[a]	<500	~500
Sulindac[a]	<500	~500
Poor inhibitors		
Acetamidophenol	>500	>500
Acetaphenetidin	>500	>500
Fenbufen	>500	>500
(–)Naproxen	>500	>500
Phenylbutazone	>500	>500
Oxybutazone	>500	>500

NIH3T3 cells were cultured under conditions of serum deprivation and in the presence of 1 μM DEX, and therefore contained only COX-1; RS-2 cells were serum-stimulated and contained only COX-2.
N.D., not determined. Complete dose–response curves have not yet been obtained for acemetacin and mefenamic acid, and no IC_{50} is shown. However, the data available clearly show these drugs to be potent inhibitors of both COX-1 and COX-2.
[a]Determined from incomplete dose–response curves and therefore approximate values. <500 means that the IC_{50} is marginally below this value; ~500 μM indicates an IC_{50} at or near this value; >500 μM indicates an IC_{50} significantly greater than this.

unknown factors was isoenzyme specific — either conferring on COX-2 high susceptibility to inhibition or reducing the sensitivity of COX-2, or both. Because each isoenzyme in NIH3T3 or RS-2 cells has normal activity in the presence of exogenous arachidonate, and because other NSAIDs showed no similar selectivity, the diclofenac phenomenon indicates that COX-1 and COX-2 experience subtly different microenvironments within the cells.

Factors that confer the 'diclofenac effect' on COX isoenzymes in rodent

***Figure 5** Concentration-dependent inhibition of COX by diclofenac in NIH3T3 and RS-2 cells. COX inhibition curve for diclofenac in serum-starved NIH3T3 cells (top graph) containing only COX-1. Only a resistant COX pool with an IC_{50} value of approximately 150–200 μM is evident. Serum stimulated RS-2 cells (bottom graph) containing only COX-2 exhibit a monophasic inhibition curve with an IC_{50} value of 7 nM*

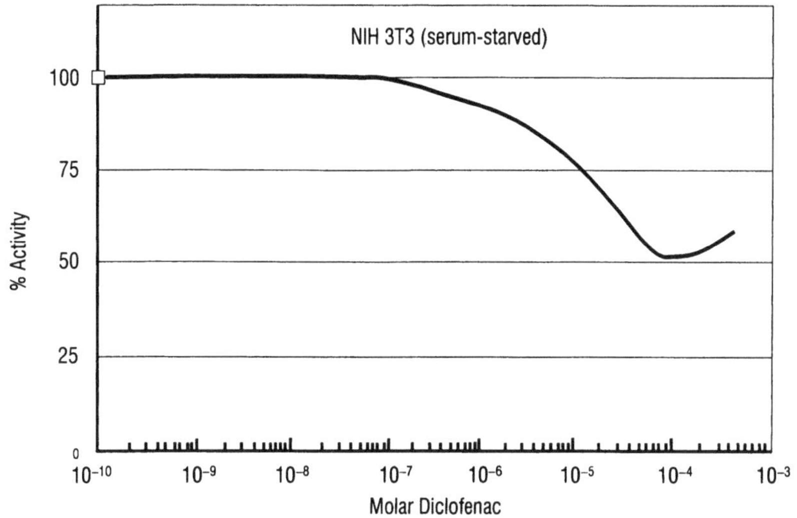

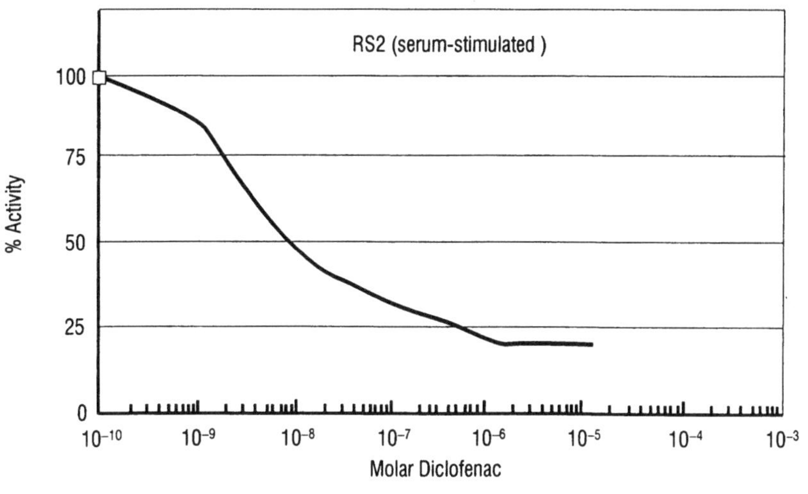

Figure 6 ***COX inhibition curve for diclofenac in serum-stimulated NIH3T3 cells containing approximately equimolar ratios of COX-1 and COX-2. The biphasic curve predicts two pools of COX, one with an IC_{50} value of 1 nM and another highly diclofenac-resistant pool with an IC_{50} value of approximately 150–200 μM***

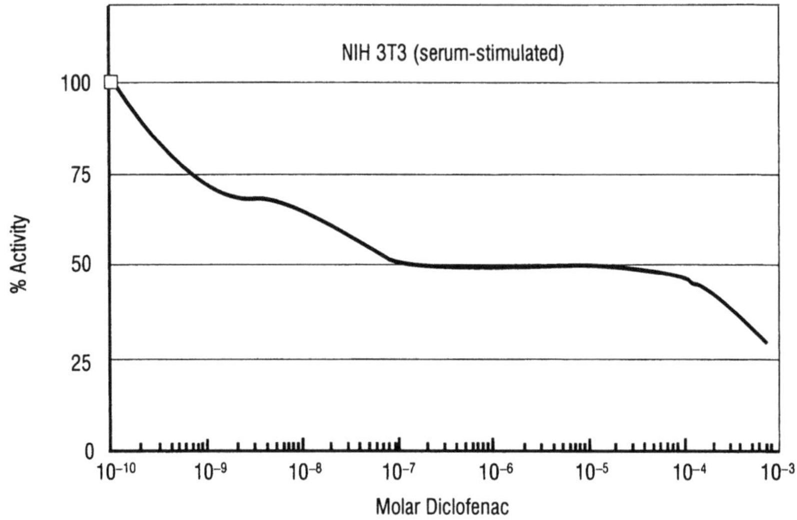

Figure 7 ***IC_{50} determination for the diclofenac-sensitive, mitogen-induced COX pool in Figure 6. The IC_{50} value of approximately 1 nM is very similar to the value of 7 nM for COX-2 inhibition determined from Figure 5***

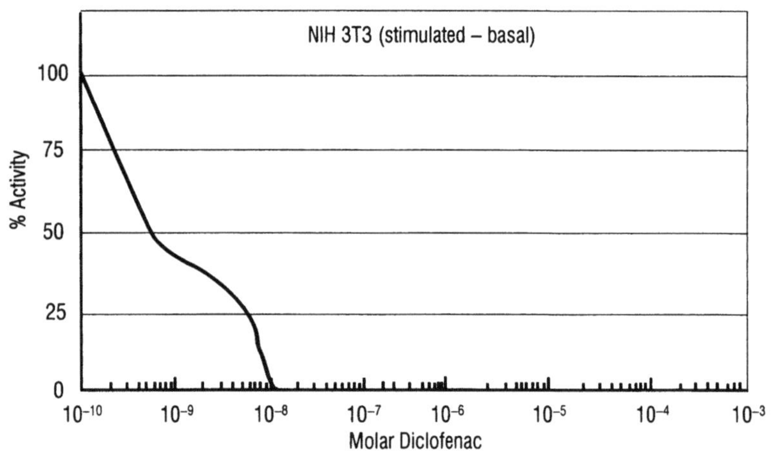

fibroblast lines are almost certainly cell specific. This is shown by the fact that measurement of COX isoenzymes in time-dependent assays shows a tremendous dependency on cell type. For example, measurements of NSAIDs in fibroblast whole-cell assays typically yield IC_{50} values in the 0.1–500 μM range, and some are inactive[25]. These same drugs, when tested in cells of macrophage lineage, inhibit at nanomolar concentrations or lower[26]! This large difference may be partially attributable to the ability of the cell to accumulate drug, as a result of membrane permeability, transport (import or export) mechanisms, or catabolism. However, these mechanisms cannot explain how COX-1 and COX-2 became differentially sensitive to diclofenac in the same NIH3T3 cell. An equally likely explanation for the differences in COX sensitivity between cell types is that cyclooxygenase is complexed with other proteins in a cell-specific fashion.

DIFFERENCES IN SUBSTRATE DELIVERY TO COX-1 AND COX-2

An additional phenomenon reinforcing the concept that COX-1 and COX-2 may differ radically in their catalytic abilities in whole cells has to do with substrate delivery. Prostaglandin release proceeds at a high rate immediately upon addition of exogenous (10–30 μM) arachidonate to cells containing substantial levels of either COX-1 or COX-2. This finding is consistent with the high catalytic activity, and low K_m of purified isoenzymes for substrate[22]. Because most cells contain significant levels of COX-1 and low levels of COX-2, basal level expression of COX products will be primarily derived from COX-1. Similarly, any arachidonic acid release mechanism that liberates substrate before COX-2 can be transcriptionally produced will result in an induction of metabolites generated from COX-1. This phenomenon was seen in studies performed by Uhlig and colleagues, which show that both PAF and LPS are potent bronchiolar constrictors in perfused rat lung[27,28]. The effects of PAF and LPS are mediated by COX-1 and COX-2, respectively, via the release of prostanoids, specifically thromboxane A_2 (Ref. 27, and personal communication). After PAF treatment, thromboxane A_2 release and accompanying bronchoconstriction is immediate, peaking within 1–2 min of treatment[27]. This effect is mediated by COX-1, since COX-2 cannot be induced this quickly. For LPS, the prostanoid release and bronchoconstriction occurs after 30 min, requires protein induction and is solely dependent on COX-2.

Following mitogen stimulation of established cell lines there is a large increase in PGE_2 release that parallels the induction of COX-2. Furthermore, this increase is inhibited by DEX. Antisense oligonucleotides to COX-2, but not those directed against COX-1, prevent this release[29], as does diclofenac at a concentration of 1 μM which is only inhibitory for COX-2. These data clearly demonstrate that PGE_2 is released solely from COX-2. The dilemma is how COX-2 'sees' substrate upon mitogen stimulation while COX-1 is blind to it. Arachidonic acid delivery proteins that selectively feed substrate to COX-2, or proteins that block the channel by which COX-1 reaches arachidonate delivered from phospholipase A_2 (PLA_2) could be involved. That 85 kDa cytosolic $cPLA_2$ is somehow coupled to COX-2 is evident from the recent finding that antisense oligonucleotides directed against the cPLA mRNA prevent the mitogen-induced PGE_2 synthesis described above[30].

A final indicator that COX-1 and COX-2 are catalytically different in intact cells may eventually come from studying prostanoid isomers arising from each isoenzyme in whole cell systems to determine whether COX-1 or COX-2 are differentially coupled to prostaglandin isomerases. However, no firm data currently exist to support this notion.

Two models for cyclooxygenase activity might therefore be hypothesized. In the first, the 'naked cyclooxygenase model', cyclooxygenases exists within the lumen of the endoplasmic reticulum/nuclear envelope (ER/NE) uncomplexed with other proteins. Differing isoenzyme concentrations, spatial location within the ER/NE, or modification (e.g. nitrosylation) cause isoenzyme-specific catalytic properties such as selective delivery of arachidonate to COX-2. Differences in sensitivity of isoenzymes to NSAID in a single cell type are due to microgradients of drug in the ER/NE. Differences between cell types are due to different drug permeabilities, drug concentration and drug metabolism. This model is illustrated in Figure 8a. The ram seminal vesicle may be a paradigm of the naked cyclooxygenase model. Here, COX-1 accounts for 1–5% of the total microsomal protein and is the predominant protein in Coomassie blue-stained microsomal protein electrophoresed on a polyacrylamide gel. Morita et al. have shown that COX-1 is located in a more perinuclear site in the cell than is COX-2[31]. This finding is consistent with the naked cyclooxygenase model. Nitric oxide (NO) has recently been implicated as a modulator of prostaglandin synthesis (reviewed by Vane in this volume). Results in this area are contradictory, since NO is found to both up-regulate and down-regulate COX activity, depending on the system[32–34]. The biochemical basis for this phenomenon has yet to be determined.

The alternative to the naked cyclooxygenase model is the 'coated cyclooxygenase model'. Here, COX enzymes exist in dynamic protein complexes, extending perhaps through the ER membrane. The composition of the complexes determines substrate delivery, product fate, and NSAID sensitivity of COX-1 and COX-2 isoenzymes. This model is illustrated in Figure 8b. The 'diclofenac effect' and selective delivery of substrate from $cPLA_2$ to COX-2 following mitogen stimulation provide the strongest evidence for this model. It is most likely that cells conforming with the coated cyclooxygenase model will contain relatively low levels of cyclooxygenase isoenzymes. Spatial localization of COX isoenzymes within the ER/NE[31] and differential NO regulation of COX-1 and COX-2[32–34] are not inconsistent with the coated cyclooxygenase model, and may require proteins to be complexed with COX.

***Figure 8** (a) The naked model of cyclooxygenase. Cyclooxygenase dimers (ellipses) are shown embedded on the luminal surface of the ER or nuclear envelope. The model conveys the idea that although the lumen of the ER contains many proteins, including those destined for export, cyclooxygenases do not associate with any of them. (b) The coated model of cyclooxygenases. Here cyclooxygenase dimers are complexed with other proteins. Theoretical associated proteins include regulatory proteins, substrate delivery or channelling proteins, and prostaglandin isomerases*

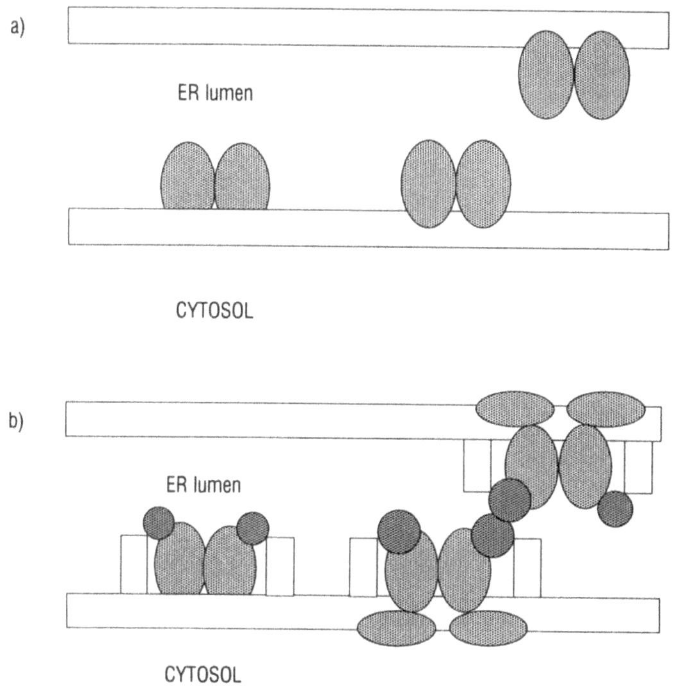

THE ROLES OF CYCLOOXYGENASES IN APOPTOSIS

NSAIDs are well known therapeutic agents for inflammation, pain, fever, clotting and premature childbirth. Epidemiological and animal studies show that NSAIDs also have an anti-neoplastic effect[35–38]. This effect of COX-2 was identified in three independent studies of cell division by ourselves and two other laboratories[1–3]. In our case, we identified COX-2 as being induced during neoplastic transformation of chicken embryo fibroblasts (CEF) by Rous sarcoma virus (RSV)[39]. Induction of COX-2 in this cell system is long-term, and COX-2 remains elevated as long as the cells are transformed by the oncogene v-*src*. The logical question is whether this long-term COX-2 induction is needed for v-*src* transformation of CEF. We

Figure 9 Apoptotic response of transformed CEFs to NSAIDs. The sequence of morphological changes occurring during transformation by v-src is shown for infected cells held at the non-permissive temperature of 42°C (A), 30 h at the permissive temperature 37°C (B), or 48 h at 37°C (C). (D) Indomethacin at 100 μM for 48 h at 37°C

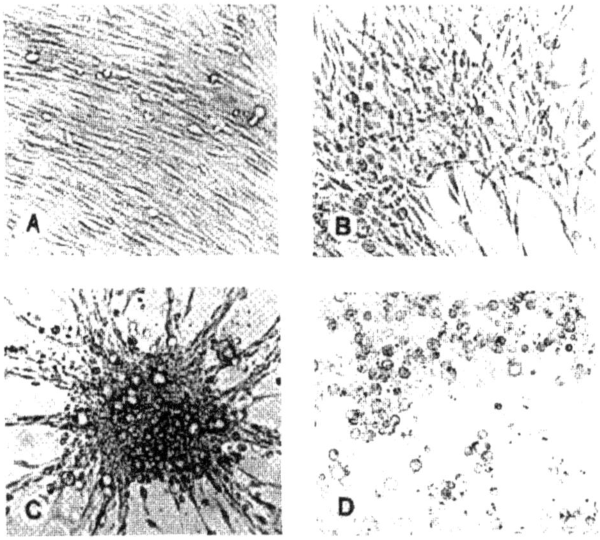

addressed this by administering NSAIDs to CEF during transformation by v-*src*. Neoplastic transformation was controlled using a temperature-sensitive mutant of RSV, tsNY72-4[39]. The 27 NSAIDs referred to in the above study of COX-1 and COX-2 in NIH3T3 and RS-2 cells were independently administered to tsNY72-4 RSV-infected CEF in doses ranging from 1 μM to 1 M. As with inhibition of COX-1 and COX-2 in rodent cell lines, some of the drugs had no effect on CEF, whereas others elicited a pronounced morphological effect (Figure 9; Table 4). The most obvious aspect of this morphological effect was that certain drugs prevented the formation of foci and, instead, rapidly induced cell rounding[40]. Close inspection revealed the presence of apoptotic bodies. Treated cells excluded Trypan blue dye, consistent with apoptosis; however, after 24–48 h the cells appeared to contain condensed chromatin and took up Trypan blue[40].

Comparison of the drugs in Table 4 with the drugs in Table 3 shows a very striking correlation between the ability of individual NSAIDs to cause apoptosis in CEF and their ability to inhibit COX-2 in rodent fibroblasts. The only drug that did not exactly fit this correlation was aspirin, which exhibited an IC_{50} toward COX-2 of 180 μM but showed no apoptotic activity at concentrations up to

Table 4 Morphological inhibition of transformation in response to NSAID treatment

	Effect	
NSAID	*100 μM*	*10 μM*
Oxicam		
Isoxicam	–	–
Piroxicam	\	–
Salicylate		
Aspirin	–	–
Diflunisal	X	–
Acetamidophenol	–	–
Acetaphenetidin	–	–
Salicylamide	–	–
Acetic acid		
Indomethacin	X	X
Acemetacin	X	\
Tolmetin	\	–
Sulindac	–	–
Diclofenac	X	\
Zomepirac	\	–
Fenamate		
Mefenamic acid	X	\
Flufenamic acid	X	\
Niflumic acid	X	\
Propionic acid		
Ketoprofen	\	–
Naproxen	\	–
Indoprofen	\	–
Ibuprofen	X	–
Flurbiprofen	\	–
Suprofen	\	–
Fenbufen	\	–
Carprofen	X	–
Pyrazole		
Phenylbutazone	–	–
Oxyphenbutazone	–	–

X, complete inhibition of focus formation by RSV; \, partial inhibition that was characterized by cell rounding and formation of small clumps of cells; –, no effect.

1 mM. This discordance could be due to the fact that induction of apoptosis, as judged by morphological criteria, takes 1–2 days to observe. Aspirin, however, decomposes within minutes to salicylate and acetic acid in warm, basic solutions such as tissue culture media. The absence of aspirin-induced apoptotic effects may therefore have been due to its inability continually to suppress COX activity in CEF growing in such media. This striking correlation between inhibition of

COX-2 and induction of apoptosis is strong evidence that NSAID-induced apoptosis (NIA) occurs through inhibition of COX, rather than through some other mechanism.

Eight NSAIDs – diflunisal, indomethacin, acemetacin, diclofenac, mefenamic acid, flufenamic acid, niflumic acid and carprofen – were chosen for intensive study. All but one, carprofen, induced endonucleolytic autodigestion of CEF DNA by 29 h, with each drug giving rise to classic nucleosomal ladders. All of the drugs induced tissue transglutaminase[40], a hallmark of apoptosis resulting in cytoskeletal crosslinking. All of the drugs were also found to decrease expression of p20, a protein secreted by CEF upon entry into cellular quiescence[40]. We speculate that this protein may play a role in protecting the cell against apoptosis during the G_0 stage of the cell cycle[40].

DEX neither caused apoptosis nor influenced NIA. From an epidemiological standpoint this finding was consonant with data in humans, where use of NSAIDs but not use of steroid anti-inflammatory drugs, was associated with a reduced incidence of tumours of the gastrointestinal tract. The inability of DEX to influence NIA would seem to suggest that inhibition of COX-2 alone would be insufficient to cause NIA. Alternatively, it is possible that DEX treatment does not fully down-regulate COX-2 below the threshold needed to induce NIA. Some other activity modulated by DEX may also counteract any apoptosis-inducing property associated with COX-2 down-regulation by this steroid.

The work of Hanafusa and co-workers has shown that transformation of CEF by v-*src* results in a large increase in PGE_2 synthesis which, as with other prostanoids, can induce apoptosis[41–45]. PGE_2 administered to v-*src*-transformed CEF caused some cell rounding and may, itself, be mildly apoptotic in this cell system[40]. However, it was incapable of preventing NIA, suggesting that NSAID inhibition of the synthesis of this prostaglandin is not responsible for NIA. Cycloheximide completely prevented NIA, indicating that protein translation is required for NIA[40].

COX-generated mediators are likely to function in signal transduction pathways leading to an ultimate regulatory pathway of apoptosis containing p53, *bcl*-2, ICE proteases, and c-*myc*. In our model CEF system, p53 was expressed at moderate to high levels, but it was not induced by NSAID-treatment. *bcl*-2, which blocks apoptosis, was almost absent from CEF and its extremely low concentration was not increased or decreased by NSAID treatment. We have not yet analysed ICE proteases, but we did find a dramatic change in c-*myc* expression. This is discussed in detail below.

In addition to these fundamental regulators of apoptosis, we also determined that v-*src* expression was absolutely required for NIA. In its absence all drugs were ineffective in causing cell death except at millimolar concentrations, where they caused necrosis. This finding is contrary to that commonly observed, where tyrosine kinase expression typically antagonizes apoptosis[46–48]. However, with regard to human disease, we believe this finding of a v-*src* requirement for NIA to be relevant, since colorectal tumours at virtually all stages of progression exhibit elevated levels of c-*src* activity[49].

Because NSAIDs and prostaglandins can transcriptionally modulate COX expression[14,50] we tested the effects of apoptotic doses of NSAIDs on COX-1 and COX-2 mRNAs. All drugs induced COX-2 mRNA and protein to some extent. Diclofenac was chosen for further study, and was found to induce COX-2 mRNA by >20-fold at a concentration of 25 μM[40]. COX-1 mRNA was induced 20-fold at a concentration of 400 μM[40]. The mechanism by which this induction occurs is unknown, but the different doses required for COX-1 and COX-2 induction is provocative. We hypothesize that a negative feed-back loop may be interrupted by drug treatment, resulting in induction of the COX-1 and COX-2 genes. The differences in diclofenac concentrations needed to cause COX-2 and COX-1 induction are qualitatively similar to the inhibitory pattern observed for this drug in NIH3T3 and RS-2 cells. Furthermore, the fact that different concentrations of drug result in COX-1 rather than COX-2 induction suggests that the COX products functioning in the feed-back loop are isoenzyme specific.

For all drugs, NIA was found to be dose dependent[40]. In our initial studies we applied NSAIDs to CEF at 12 h intervals and measured cell death by Trypan blue exclusion assays. It was clear to us at the time that our dosing regimen was more intense than the pharmacological doses of NSAIDs prescribed in humans. It was also obvious that morphometric analyses, coupled with Trypan blue staining, measured only late aspects of programmed cell death. We therefore used the sensitive DNA comet assay to measure the DNA breakage that is an irreversible step in apoptosis.

As shown in Table 5, significant cell death was detected within 6 h of treatment with a single, 32 μM dose of diclofenac. Concentrations <10 μM were ineffective at this point. Although this dose is much lower than in our previous study, it may still be higher than the concentration to which colonic and oesophageal epithelial cells are exposed during the treatment of arthritis or other pathologies in humans with NSAID. As shown above however, COX in fibroblasts requires relatively high concentrations of NSAIDs for inhibition. We suggest that cells of the gut, similar to macrophages in vitro, are more sensitive to these drugs.

HOW DO NSAIDs CAUSE APOPTOSIS?

Besides a sensitivity to inhibition of COX by NSAIDs, what else might be predicted to be needed for NIA to occur in human cells? Our studies clearly show an absolute requirement for *src* expression in order for NIA to occur. The expression of *bcl*-2 must also be low in these cells, since over-expression of *bcl*-2 in CEF completely blocks NIA. Additionally, c-*myc* was strongly up-regulated during NIA. The application of c-*myc* antisense oligonucleotides, but not scrambled mixmers of the same length, inhibited NIA by 50%. We presume, but have not yet proven, that this incomplete prevention of NIA was an artifact of

Table 5 Altered morphology, indicated as percentage rounded cells, as an indicator of diclofenac-induced apoptosis in chicken embryo fibroblasts

Diclofenac concentration (μM)	*Time* (h)				
	2.5	5	7.5	12	24
0	4.6	–	4.3	3.5	9.3
3.2	5.2	–	5.6	5.7	9.3
10.0	5.3	–	5.0	5.6	9.5
32.0	7.0	10.9	8.5	7.9	42.2
100.0	21.8	31.4	46.9	90.0	99.0
320.0	35.1	39.6	68.3	96.8	99.8

the antisense oligonucleotide technique, caused by an inability to fully down-regulate c-*myc* in all cells of the culture. NIA therefore proceeds in a *src*-mediated pathway resulting in the eventual superinduction of c-*myc*. Induction of c-*myc* has been shown to cause apoptosis in CEF and other cells[51]. In these cases, however, it was necessary to remove trophic factors such as serum in order to induce apoptosis. In NIA resulting in induction of c-*myc*, apoptosis occurs whether or not trophic factors are present, suggesting that NSAID treatment of CEF results in biochemical changes in addition to the induction of c-*myc*, that allow NIA to proceed independently of the presence or absence of trophic factors.

The effects of NSAIDs in preventing the occurrence of human gastrointestinal adenomas and adenocarcinomas are probably manifest through the induction of cell death in the neoplastic tissue. This is indicated by the disappearance of visible tumour masses following NSAID treatment, which must result from a reduction in cell number[52]. Our studies show that NSAIDs can directly induce apoptosis in neoplastic cells. We found that most NSAIDs are capable of inducing apoptosis in our model system, which parallels in many ways colonic neoplastic tissue. For example, *src* expression and COX-2 expression were induced relative to normal CEF, and colon tumours similarly show increased *src* and COX-2 compared with colonic epithelial cells[49,53,54]. COX-1 expression is very low in CEF, and neoplastic colon cells show a significant reduction compared with normal epithelial cells.

Our current data suggest that the inhibition of COX is the mechanism by which NSAIDs induce apoptosis. We suggest that the induction of apoptosis in neoplastic cells is the mechanism by which NSAIDs inhibit tumours of the gastrointestinal tract in humans. The important COX-generated metabolites, the production or inhibition of which results in NIA, remain to be determined.

References

1. Xie W, Chipman J, Robertson DL, Erikson RL, Simmons DL. Expression of a mitogen-responsive gene encoding prostaglandin synthase is regulated by mRNA splicing. Proc Natl Acad Sci USA. 1991;88:2692–6.

2. Kujubu DA, Fletcher BS, Varnum BC, Lim RW, Herschman HR. TIS10, a phorbol ester tumor promoter-inducible mRNA from Swiss 3T3 cells, encodes a novel prostaglandin synthase/cyclooxygenase homologue. J Biol Chem. 1991;266:12866–72.
3. O'Banion MK, Sadowski HB, Winn V, Young DA. A serum- and glucocorticoid-regulated 4-kilobase mRNA encodes a cyclooxygenase-related protein. J Biol Chem. 1991;266:23261–7.
4. Vane J. Towards a better aspirin. Nature. 1994;367:215–6.
5. Sirois J, Simmons DL, Richards JS. Hormonal regulation of messenger ribonucleic acid encoding a novel isoform of prostaglandin endoperoxide H synthase in rat preovulatory follicles: induction in vivo and in vitro. J Biol Chem. 1992;267:11586–92.
6. Nusing RW, Mohr S, Ullrich V. Activin A and retinoic acid synergize in cyclooxygenase-1 and thromboxane synthase induction during differentiation of J774.1 macrophages. Eur J Biochem. 1995;227:130–6.
7. Smith CJ, Morrow JD, Roberts LJ, Marnett LJ. Differentiation of monocytoid THP-1 cells with phorbol ester induces expression of prostaglandin endoperoxide synthase-1 (COX-1). Biochem Biophys Res Commun. 1993;192:787–93.
8. Simmons DL, Xie W, Chipman JG, Evett JG. Multiple cyclooxygenases: Cloning of a mitogen-inducible form. In J.M. Bailey, editor. Prostaglandins, Leukotrienes, Lipoxins, and PAF. New York: Plenum Press; 1991:67–77.
9. Yamagata K, Andreasson KL, Kaufmann WE, Barnes CA, Worley PF. Expression of a mitogen-inducible cyclooxygenase in brain neurons: regulation by synaptic activity and glucocorticoids. Neuron. 1993;11:371–86.
10. Xie W, Merrill JR, Bradshaw WS, Simmons DL. Structural determination and promoter analysis of the chicken mitogen-inducible prostaglandin G/H synthase gene and genetic mapping of the murine homolog. Arch Biochem Biophys. 193;300:247–52.
11. Evett GE, Xie W, Chipman JG, Robertson DL, Simmons DL. Prostaglandin G/H synthase isoenzyme 2 expression in fibroblasts: regulation by dexamethasone, mitogens and oncogenes. Arch Biochem Biophys. 1993;306:169–77.
12. Chanmugam P, Geng L, Liou S et al. Radicicol, a protein tyrosine kinase inhibitor, suppresses the expression of mitogen-inducible cyclooxygenase in macrophages stimulated with lipopolysaccharide and in experimental glomerulonephritis. J Biol Chem. 1995;270:5418–26.
13. Feng L, Xia Y, Garcia GE, Hwang D, Wilson CB. Involvement of reactive oxygen intermediates in cyclooxygenase-2 expression induced by interleukin-1, tumor necrosis factor-α, and lipopolysaccharide. J Clin Invest. 1995;95:1669–75.
14. Akarasereenont P, Hide E, Ney P, Thiemermann C, Vane JR. The induction of cyclooxygenase-2 elicited by endotoxin in endothelial cells and macrophages is inhibited by prostaglandin E1 and 13,14-dihydroprostaglandin E1. Agents Actions. 1995;45:59–64.
15. Kujubu DA, Herschman HR. Dexamethasone inhibits mitogen-induction of the TIS10 prostaglandin synthase cyclooxygenase gene. J Biol Chem. 1992;267:7991–4.
16. Shaw G, Kamen R. A conserved AU sequence from the 3′ untranslated region of GM-CSF mRNA mediates selective mRNA degradation. Cell. 1986;46:659–67.
17. Bhattacharyya DK, Lecomte M, Dunn J, Morgans DJ, Smith WL. Selective inhibition of prostaglandin endoperoxide synthase-1 (cyclooxygenase-1) by valerylsalicylic acid. Arch Biochem Biophys. 1995;317:19–24.
18. Copeland RA, Williams JM, Giannaras J et al. Mechanism of selective inhibition of the inducible isoform of prostaglandin G/H synthase. Proc Natl Acad Sci USA. 1994;91:11202–6.
19. Oullet M, Percival MD. Effect of inhibitor time-dependency on selectivity towards cyclooxygenase isoforms. Biochem J. 1995;306:247–51.
20. Reitz DB, Li JJ, Norton MB et al. Selective cyclooxygenase inhibitors: novel 1,2-diarylcyclopentenes are potent and orally active COX-2 inhibitors. J Med Chem. 1994;37:3878–81.
21. Robinson DR. Prostaglandins and the mechanism of action of anti-inflammatory drugs. Am J Med. 1983;75:26–31.
22. Laneuveille O, Breuer DK, DeWitt DL, Hla T, Funk CD, Smith DL. Differential inhibition of human prostaglandin endoperoxide synthases-1 and -2 by nonsteroidal antiinflammatory drugs. J Pharmacol Exp Ther. 1994;271:927–34.
23. Barnett J, Chow J, Ives D et al. Purification, characterization and selective inhibition of human prostaglandin G/H synthase 1 and 2 expressed in the baculovirus system. Biochim Biophys Acta. 1994:1209:130–9.

24. Gierse JK, Hauser SD, Creely DP, Koboldt C, Rhangwala SH, Isakson PC. Expression and selective inhibition of the constitutive and inducible forms of human cyclooxygenases. Biochem J. 1995;305:479-84.
25. Simmons DL, Xie W, Evett G, Merrill J, Robertson DL, Bradshaw WS. Drug inhibition and cellular regulation of prostaglandin G/H synthase isoenzyme 2. J Lipid Med. 1993;6:113-7.
26. Grossman CJ, Wiseman J, Lucas FS, Trevethick MA, Birch PJ. Inhibition of constitutive and inducible cyclooxygenase activity in human platelets and mononuclear cells by NSAIDs and COX2 inhibitors. Inflamm Res. 1995;44:253-7.
27. Uhlig S, Wollin L, Wendel A. Contributions of thromboxane and leukotrienes to PAF-induced impairment of lung function in the rat. J Appl Physiol. 1994;77:262-9.
28. Uhlig S, Brasch F, Wollin L, Fehrenbach H, Richeter J, Wendel A. Functional and fine structural changes in isolated rat lungs challenged with endotoxin ex vivo and in vitro. Am J Pathol. 1995;146:1235-47.
29. Reddy ST, Herschman HR. Ligand-induced prostaglandin synthesis requires expression of the TIS10-PGS-2 prostaglandin synthase gene in murine fibroblasts and macrophages. J Biol Chem. 1994;269:15473-80.
30. Roshak A, Sathe G, Marshall LA. Suppression of monocyte 85-kDa phospholipase A_2 by antisense and effects on endotoxin-induced prostaglandin biosynthesis. J Biol Chem. 1994; 269:25999-6005.
31. Morita I, Schindler M, Regier MK, Ho JC, Hori T, De Witt DL, Smith WL. Different intracellular locations for prostaglandin endoperoxide H synthase-1 and -2. J Biol Chem. 1995;270:10902-8.
32. Salvemini D, Misko TP, Masferrer J, Seibert K, Currie MG, Needleman P. Nitric oxide activates cyclooxygenase enzymes. Proc Natl Acad Sci USA. 1993;90:7240-4.
33. Salvemini D, Seibert K, Masferrer JL, Misko TP, Currie MG, Needleman P. Endogenous nitric oxide enhances prostaglandin production in a model of renal inflammation. J Clin Invest. 1994;93:1940-7.
34. Swierkosz TA, Mitchell JA, Warner TD, Botting RM, Vane JR. Co-induction of nitric oxide synthase and cyclo-oxygenase: interactions between nitric oxide and prostanoids. Br J Pharmacol. 1995;114:1335-42.
35. Rosenberg L, Palmer J, Zanber AG, Warshauer ME, Stolley PD, Shapiro S. A hypothesis: nonsteroidal anti-inflammatory drugs reduce the incidence of large-bowel cancer. J Natl Cancer Inst. 1991;83:355-8.
36. Kune G, Kune S, Watson LF. Colorectal cancer risk, chronic illnesses, operations, and medications: case control results from the Melbourne Colorectal Cancer Study. Cancer Res. 1988;48:4399-404.
37. Thun M, Namboodiri M, Heath CW. Aspirin use and reduced risk of fatal colon cancer. N Engl J Med. 1991;325:1593-6.
38. Pollard M, Luckert P. Prevention and treatment of primary intestinal tumors in rats by piroxicam. Cancer Res. 1989;49:6471-5.
39. Simmons DL, Levy DB, Yannoni Y, Erikson RL. Identification of a phorbol ester-repressible v-src-inducible gene. Proc Natl Acad Sci USA. 1989;86:1178-82.
40. Lu X, Xie W, Reed D, Bradshaw WS, Simmons DL. Nonsteroidal antiinflammatory drugs cause apoptosis and induce cyclooxygenases in chicken embryo fibroblasts. Proc Natl Acad Sci USA. 1995;92:7961-5.
41. Ackerman RC, Murdock WJ. Prostaglandin-induced apoptosis of ovarian surface epithelial cells. Prostaglandins. 1993;45:475-85.
42. Brown DM, Warner GL, Ales-Martinez JE, Scott DW, Phipps RP. Prostaglandin E_2 induces apoptosis in immature normal and malignant B lymphocytes. Clin Immunol Immunopathol. 1992;63:221-9.
43. Goetzl EJ, An S, Zeng L. Specific suppression by prostaglandin E_2 of activation-induced apoptosis of human CD4+CD8+ T lymphocytes. J Immunol. 1995;154:1041-7.
44. Mastino A, Grelli S, Piacentini M et al. Correlation between induction of lymphocyte apoptosis and prostaglandin E_2 production by macrophages infected with HIV. Cell Immunol. 1993; 152:120-30.
45. Barker K, Adrem A, Hanafusa H. Modulation of arachidonic acid metabolism by Rous sarcoma virus. J Virol. 1989;63:2929-35.

46. McGahon AJ, Nishioka WK, Martin SJ, Mahboubi A, Cotter TG, Green DR. Regulation of the Fas apoptotic cell pathway by Abl. J Biol Chem. 1995;270:22626–31.
47. Abrahamsohn PA, Zorn TM. Implantation and decidualization in rodents. J Exp Zool. 1993; 266:603–28.
48. Chiou S-K, Rao L, White E. Bcl-2 blocks p53-dependent apoptosis. Mol Cell Biol. 1994;14: 2556–63.
49. Talamonti MS, Roh MS, Curley SA, Gallick GE. Increase in activity and level of pp60c-src in progressive stages of human colorectal cancer. J Clin Invest. 1993;91:53–60.
50. Takahashi Y, Taketani Y, Takeshi E, Yamamoto S, Kumegawa M. Studies on the induction of cyclooxygenase isozymes by various prostaglandins in mouse osteoblastic cell line with reference to signal transduction pathways. Biochim Biophys Acta. 1994;1212:217–24.
51. Evans GI, Wyllie AH, Gilbert CS et al. Induction of apoptosis in fibroblasts by c-myc protein. Cell. 1992;69:119–28.
52. Labayle D, Fischer D, Vielh P et al. Sulindac causes regression of rectal polyps in familial adenomatous polyposis. Gastroenterology. 1991;101:635–9.
53. Eberhart CE, Coffey RJ, Radhika A, Giardiello FM, Ferrenbach S, Dubois RN. Up-regulation of cyclooxygenase 2 gene expression in human colorectal adenomas and adenocarcinomas. Gastroenterology. 1994;107:1183–8.
54. Kargman SL, O'Neill GP, Vickers PJ, Evans JF, Mancini JA, Jothy S. Expression of prostaglandin G/H synthase-1 and -2 protein in human colon cancer. Cancer Res. 1995;55:2556–9.

4 Inducible enzymes with special reference to COX-2 in inflammation and apoptosis

D.A. WILLOUGHBY, A. TOMLINSON, D. GILROY and D. WILLIS

Inflammation is a dynamic process of plasma-derived and cellular events occurring in response to tissue injury or infection. The early stages of acute inflammation are characterized by the sequential release of mediators including histamine, 5-hydroxytryptamine (5-HT), kinins, prostanoids, substance P and nitric oxide (NO). Prostaglandins (PGs) and thromboxanes (TXs), collectively termed prostanoids, are biologically active molecules operative in both acute and chronic inflammation. They are formed from membrane-released arachidonic acid by a series of enzymes including cyclooxygenase (COX), alternatively named prostaglandin H synthase (PGHS), or prostaglandin endoperoxidase synthase.

COX is acknowledged to be constitutively expressed in almost all cell types, releasing prostanoids which regulate gastric cytoprotection, renal function and vascular homeostasis. However, COX is also present and inducible in inflamed tissues, where inhibition of this enzyme by non-steroidal anti-inflammatory drugs (NSAIDs) alleviates the symptoms of inflammation, including oedema, pain, erythema and pyrexia. Unfortunately, the price paid for relief of the symptoms of pathology is the disruption of the physiological role of prostanoids, increasing the possibility of gastric ulceration and renal damage.

COX exists in more than one form[1,2], constitutively expressed COX-1, which is present in most cells and produces prostanoids with a physiological role and COX-2, an isoform induced by pro-inflammatory cytokines and mitogens, which appears to be present in inflamed tissue. This discovery clarified many anomalies of prostanoid synthesis, but also promised much more than this. The realization of the full potential of this breakthrough could mean selective inhibition of prostanoid formation in inflammation with sparing of the physiological functions. From the perspective of in vivo inflammation, our priorities were to define the role of COX-2 in a wide range of inflammatory events arising from differing initiating factors, to identify the cell types which expressed COX-2 in these events, to examine the time frame over which this occurred and to identify endogenous switch-on mechanisms (mediators) and switch-off mechanisms (modulators).

COX IN CHRONIC INFLAMMATION: THE MURINE AIR POUCH MODEL OF CHRONIC GRANULOMATOUS TISSUE INFLAMMATION

The murine air pouch is a model of immune inflammation which encompasses stages of both acute and chronic inflammation, followed by a phase of resolution[3]. To initiate the model, 3 ml of air are injected into the dorsal subcutaneous tissue of a mouse, followed 24h later by 0.5 ml of 0.1% (vol/vol) croton oil in Freund's complete adjuvant. Inflammatory cells migrate into the dermis of the skin and accumulate at the edge of the air pouch. During the first 24h of acute inflammation, the polymorphonuclear neutrophil (PMN) is the dominant inflammatory cell. By day 3 a distinct granulomatous tissue lines both dorsal and ventral surfaces of the pouch and the cellular population changes, becoming dominated by macrophages. Fibroblasts and endothelial cells migrate into the newly forming tissue and proliferate. This results in a highly vascularized and ultimately fibrotic resolving tissue. The air pouch forms a surrogate synovium and the granulomatous tissue formed has many similarities with the pannus tissue which invades a rheumatoid arthritic joint; indeed it was at one time described as facsimile synovium[4]. The first 48h after initiation of the air pouch is considered to constitute the acute phase; the granulomatous tissue is maximal at 7 days during the chronic phase; this is quickly followed by the resolving phase and the model is terminated at 28 days. The granulomatous tissue of the air pouch is therefore constantly changing in terms of the dominant cell type.

COX activity and expression

COX activity, measured as the capacity of homogenates of air pouch tissues to produce prostanoids from exogenous arachidonic acid, progressively rose during the first 24h of acute inflammation (Figure 1), accompanied by an increase in COX-2, protein as indicated by Western blot[5]. COX activity does not discriminate between the contributions from either of the COX isoforms to prostanoid formation; however a Western blot, using antibodies specific to COX-1 and COX-2, indicates the levels of each isoform of the protein over time. In the chronic phase of the inflammatory response COX activity was 2–3 times greater than in the acute phase, with prostaglandin E_2 (PGE_2) and prostacyclin (PGI_2) the predominant metabolites. The increase in COX activity was mirrored by an increase in COX-2 protein levels. Levels of COX-1 protein appeared unchanged throughout the time course.

Macrophages were identified as the cells which most obviously immunolabelled for COX-2 protein, with fibroblasts also strongly immunopositive by day 7[6]. Endothelial cells lining the capillaries in the granulomatous tissue were positive by day 14. Therefore, from this study we determined that COX-2 was present in acute and chronic inflammation, that COX-2 protein levels more closely followed the rise in COX activity than did COX-1 and that the inflammatory cell expressing COX-2 was the macrophage.

***Figure 1** COX and NOS activity and distribution of cytokines in the murine chronic granulomatous tissue air pouch. Neutrophils (PMNs) predominate in the acute phase, macrophages in the chronic phase and fibroblasts during resolution*

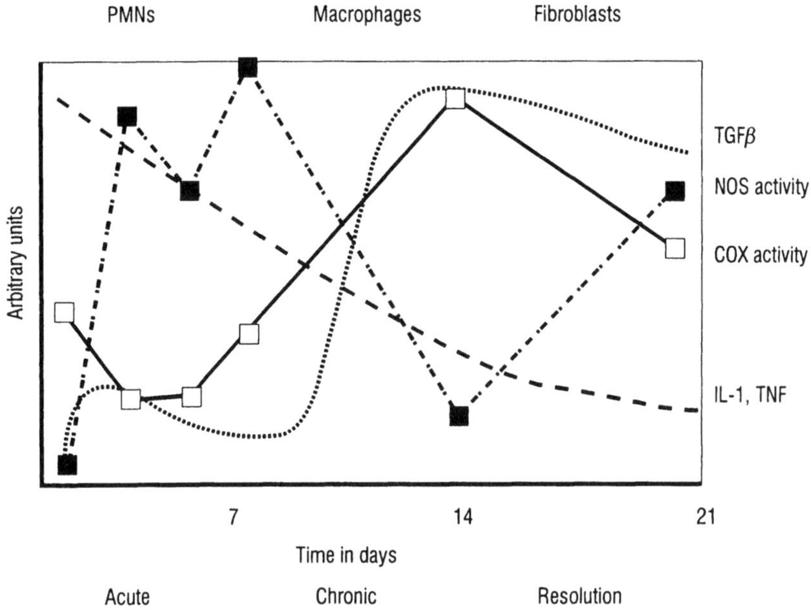

Mediators and modulators of COX

Cytokines

Cytokines are mediators and modulators of inflammation and are therefore obvious candidates for endogenous regulation of COX-2. Studies in vitro and in vivo have shown that COX-2 is highly inducible by cytokines, growth factors, hormones and oncogenes. Interleukin-1 (IL-1) induces COX-2 expression in human monocytes[7], endothelial cells[8] and rat mesangial cells[9], tumour necrosis factor α (TNFα) and basic fibroblast growth factor in mouse glial astrocytes[10], platelet-derived growth factor (PDGF) and epithelial growth factor (EGF) in 3T3 fibroblasts[11] and endothelin-1 in rat mesangial cells[12]. The expression of numerous cytokines has been investigated in the murine air pouch model of inflammation[3] (Figure 1). In the acute phase, IL-1α and β, EGF, TNFα and PDGF are at their highest levels. Any of these, alone or in synergy, may be responsible for the early rise in PGs. Expression of these COX-2-inducing cytokines falls in the chronic phase of this model, but increasing levels of transforming growth factor β (TGFβ), a cytokine which is known to induce COX-2[11], is a possible endogenous mediator in the chronic phase.

Nitric oxide

Nitric oxide (NO) is formed from L-arginine by constitutive and inducible isoforms of the enzyme nitric oxide synthase (cNOS, iNOS respectively)[13]. The inducible NOS is produced by inflammatory cells, in both acute and chronic inflammation, and is implicated in a number of inflammatory diseases and disease models including rheumatoid arthritis[14], renal inflammation[15], inflammatory bowel disease[16] and experimental allergic encephalomyelitis[17]. NO is recognized as a potent effector molecule of macrophage cytotoxicity[18] and is involved in host defence, participating in the elimination of pathogens, viruses and tumour cells. However, inappropriate or excessive production of NO may result in trauma to normal tissues. In addition, NO can combine with oxygen free radicals produced by inflammatory cells to form peroxynitrite, which decomposes to form hydroxyl radical and other reactive oxygen intermediates implicated in the destructive processes of inflammation[19].

Nitric oxide has paradoxical effects on COX activity. It has been reported to both stimulate and inhibit enzyme activity, though the isoform affected is not often specified. COX activity is stimulated by NO in rat lipopolysaccharide (LPS)-treated lungs[20] and in the hydronephrotic kidney[21]. In contrast, NO inhibits PG production in LPS-stimulated rat peritoneal cells by downregulation of the COX-2 isoform[22]. An explanation of these phenomena may lie in the levels of NO attained, with low levels increasing and high levels inhibiting PG production. High levels of sodium nitroprusside, an NO donor, inhibited COX expression and activity in LPS-stimulated J774 macrophages[23]. However, in the absence of endogenous NO, smaller amounts of exogenous NO donor increased COX activity. In an analogous manner PGs can activate or suppress NOS activity. Endogenous PGE_2 is reported to inhibit IL-1-stimulated NO production in rat mesangial cells[24] and exogenously applied to LPS-treated J774 cells has the same effect[25], but endogenous PGE_2 in LPS-treated rat Kupffer cells stimulated NO production[26].

We measured NOS activity in the murine air pouch by the conversion of [^{3}H]L-arginine to [^{3}H]L-citrulline[5]. NOS activity was induced in the acute phase, continued to rise into the chronic phase, peaking at day 7 with an 8-fold increase over levels recorded at 24h (Figure 1). Thereafter, activity was reduced dramatically by day 14. The majority of the NOS activity was attributable to iNOS and coincided with maximal immunolabelling of macrophages for iNOS protein. Both COX and NOS were co-induced up to 24h, but their profiles of activity dissociated in the chronic and resolving phases of this model. Such profiles may indicate differential regulation of the two enzyme systems. There may be reciprocal control of the enzymes by their products, or regulation may be related to a changing pattern of cytokine expression. Certainly, immunoreactive levels of TGFβ rise in the chronic and resolving stages and this cytokine inhibits NOS while stimulating COX (Figure 1). Therefore TGFβ may be a decisive cytokine of chronic inflammation. A single dose of neutralizing antibody to TGFβ will block inflammatory cell accumulation and suppress tissue pathology in an experimental model of chronic erosive polyarthritis[27].

COX ACTIVITY IN ACUTE INFLAMMATION: CARRAGEENIN-INDUCED PLEURISY IN THE RAT

Having demonstrated that the predominant isoforms of COX and NOS in the murine chronic granulomatous tissue air pouch were inducible, we extended our studies to a complement-dependent model of acute inflammation, carrageenin-induced pleurisy in the rat. This model of acute inflammation is characterized by vasodilatation, plasma extravasation and PMN influx into the pleural cavity. Damage to tissues is followed by a sequential release of mediators of the acute phase (histamine, 5-HT, kinins, prostanoids) and activation of complement. Depletion of complement has been shown to suppress this model of inflammation. Platelets aggregate and PMNs infiltrate the tissues, followed subsequently by macrophages. Vasodilatation is induced by the COX metabolites PGE_2 and PGI_2, which act directly to relax vascular smooth muscle, whilst the inflammatory mediators bradykinin, substance P, 5-HT and histamine were thought to act via the release of NO from the endothelium, resulting in increased vascular permeability. Recent studies however suggest that vascular permeability elicited by platelet activating factor or histamine appears to be independent of NO, whereas bradykinin, 5-HT and substance P have an NO-mediated component contributing to oedema formation[28].

Pleurisy was induced in rats by injecting a solution of carrageenin in saline into the pleural cavity and exudates were collected by pleural lavage at set times up to 48 h after injection of the irritant. Pleural injection of carrageenin results in an acute inflammatory episode, maximal at 24h as assessed by inflammatory cell number and exudate volume, but the lesion is significantly resolved at 48 h[29].

COX activity as measured by the production of PGE_2, peaked at 2h in the pleural cell exudates[30] (Figure 2). Western blotting confirmed that COX-2 was the predominant isoform, with maximal protein recorded at 2 h. This protein peak coincided with PMNs being the major source of COX-2 immunoreactivity, with smaller numbers of macrophages immunopositive at later times. COX activity returned to baseline levels by 24h. There was an increase in NOS activity over the period of 2–6 h, producing a mirror image of COX activity. The peak at 6 h was solely attributable to the iNOS isoform (Figure 2). At 24h activity returned to baseline and there was no further change by 48 h, at the end of the inflammatory event.

Low levels of COX-2 immunoreactivity were detected in PMNs from smears

Figure 2 ***Graph showing COX activity (□), NOS activity (■) and haem oxygenase (HO) activity (columns) in the rat carrageenin-induced pleurisy model of acute inflammation***

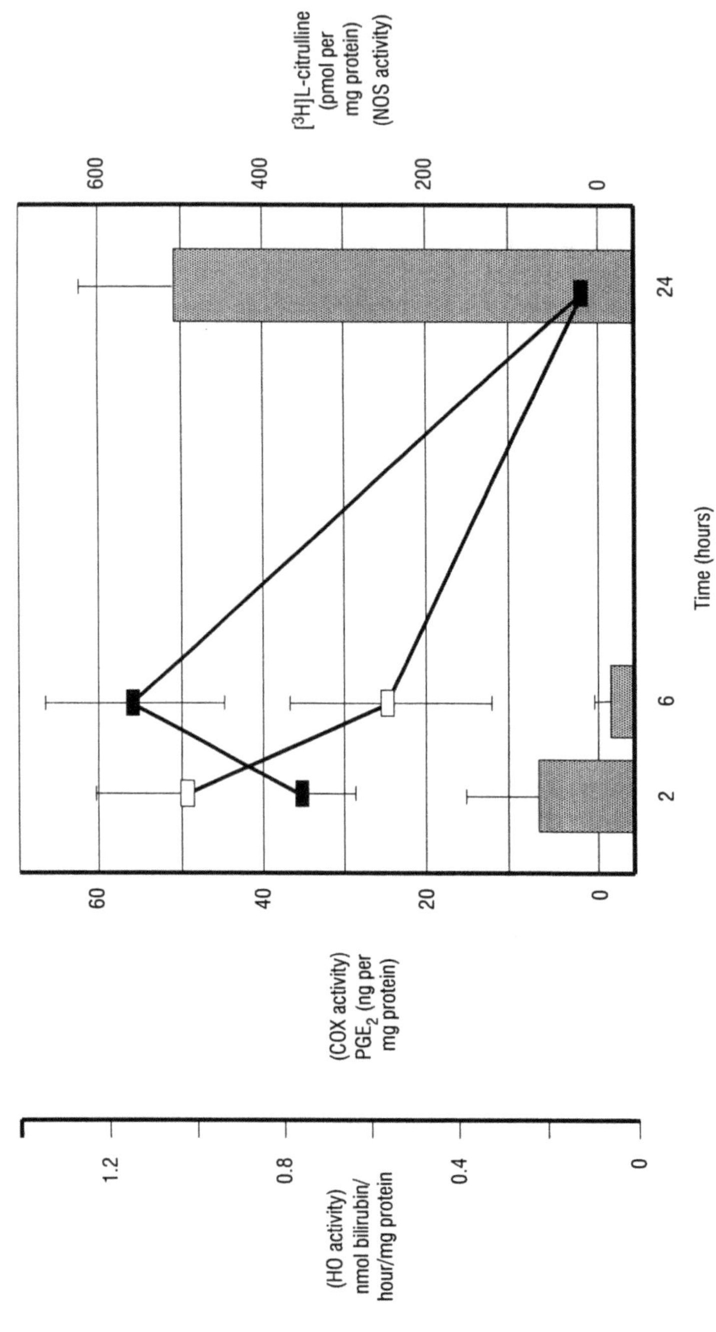

of peripheral blood leukocytes from animals without inflammation and low levels of NOS activity were recorded in cell pellets from the same source. The significance of these findings is unknown at present but we can speculate that circulating PMNs may have a basal expression of COX-2, which upon exposure to an inflammatory stimulus is rapidly recruited for prostanoid formation. Alternatively, they may represent a newly formed population of cells which require some systemic activation to migrate from the bone marrow into the circulation.

The principal findings of this study of acute inflammation were that the predominant isoforms of COX and NOS are inducible, as found in the air pouch, but that the PMN is the major source of COX-2 immunoreactivity.

COX AND NOS ACTIVITY IN THE ARTHUS REACTION: AN IMMUNE MODEL OF IMMEDIATE HYPERSENSITIVITY

The Arthus reaction is initiated by the deposition in tissues of a complex of antigen and antibody; which activates the complement system and causes a very acute inflammatory response peaking at 6h, dominated by PMN accumulation and subsequent oedema formation[31]. This reaction is suppressed by NSAIDs, and prostanoids are therefore implicated in the pathogenesis.

Rats sensitized by an injection of bovine serum albumin (BSA) into the base of the tail were challenged 12 days later with an injection of BSA into the pleural cavity. COX activity was increased, but not significantly, up to 24h and to date this model has been taken no further (Figure 3a). Analysis at later time points will determine whether there is a peak of COX activity or a subsequent return to base levels. COX-2 protein was identified in the Western blot at 2, 6 and 24h but there was little difference in protein density with time. Immunocytochemistry identified the PMN as a source of COX-2 protein[32]. NOS activity was elevated at 2h and significantly declined by 24h; again the profile of activity was the opposite of that seen for COX (Figure 3a). Cellular exudates recovered from the pleural cavity peaked at 6h and were greatly reduced by 24h (Figure 4a).

COX AND NOS ACTIVITY IN METHYL BOVINE SERUM ALBUMIN (met BSA) PLEURISY: A MODEL OF CELL-MEDIATED IMMUNITY

Rat pertussis pleurisy has been extensively used as a model of delayed type hypersensitivity reactions, but the use of a whole cell vaccine of *Bordatella pertussis* has meant that the antigens involved in the reaction are poorly understood. Adrian Moore and Dean Willis, working in our group, have recently developed a new immunological model of delayed hypersensitivity using met BSA. In contrast to the Arthus reaction this inflammatory response has a delayed reaction, peaking at 24h and is dominated by mononuclear cells. Rats were sensitized by intradermal injection of met BSA in Freund's adjuvant at the base

***Figure 3** COX activity (♦) and NOS activity (□) in (a) the Arthus reaction and (b) met BSA delayed hypersensitivity. *p < 0.05, **p < 0.01*

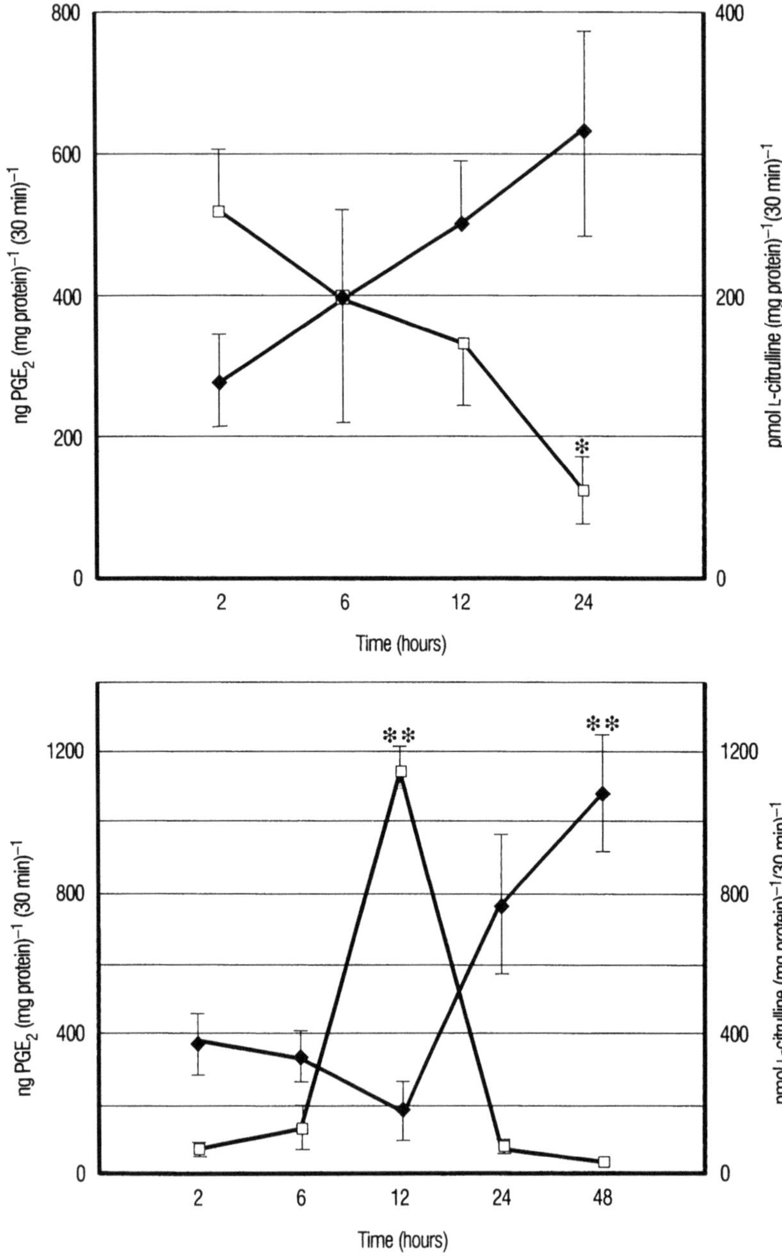

of the tail. Twelve days later they were challenged by injection of met BSA into the pleural cavity. This model produced an acute reaction over 12h and then a delayed reaction at 24h, which was suppressed by 48h, as measured by pleural exudate volumes (Figure 4b). COX activity measured as ng PGE_2/mg protein/30min, rose briefly at 2h, declined up to 12h and then reached a significantly higher level at 48h – approximately double the peak levels recorded in the Arthus reaction and over 20 times higher than activity at 2h in carrageenin pleurisy (Figure 3b). Western blotting showed COX-2 protein to be present at 2, 6, 12, 24 and 48h, with highest levels at 2 and 6h.

Measurement of NOS activity in the met BSA model showed that the majority was again derived from the inducible isoform of NOS. Between 6 and 12h activity increased 12-fold, to levels four times greater than in the Arthus reaction and twice that in carrageenin pleurisy, again forming a mirror image of the COX activity profile, before returning to base level at 24h (Figure 3b). Interestingly, the burst of NOS activity in all the acute models discussed here, whilst differing in profile, was finished by 24h.

The presence of inducible isoforms of COX and NOS in all stages of the inflammatory response and their localization in inflammatory cells is incontrovertible and they would appear to be excellent therapeutic targets for inhibition in the treatment of inflammatory disease. Nevertheless, PGs, particularly those of the E series, have important immunoregulatory properties, including the inhibition of proliferation of T and B cells and class switching of immunoglobulins[33]. Nitric oxide also has a role in host defence and the inhibitory or stimulatory interactions of COX and NOS will have to be carefully considered when selectively inhibiting these enzymes.

HEME OXYGENASE IN INFLAMMATION

In the search for endogenous mediators and modulators of the inflammatory process which may be accessible to beneficial pharmacological intervention, Willis has explored the activity of heme oxygenase (HO). This enzyme is rate limiting in the catabolism of haem derived from proteins such as haemoglobin and cytochrome p-450 to the bile pigments biliverdin and bilirubin with the production of carbon monoxide[34]. Biliverdin is rapidly converted to bilirubin by biliverdin reductase. Increased HO activity has been implicated in protecting tissues against oxidative stress[35], probably arising from the strong antioxidant properties of the bile pigments. In addition, biliverdin and conjugated bilirubin are reported to have anti-complement effects in vitro and in vivo[36].

To date, two isoforms of HO have been characterized. HO-2 is a 36kDa constitutively expressed isoform, present in high levels in the testis and brain and, under normal physiological conditions, is the predominant enzyme. HO-1, a 32kDa protein also known as heat shock protein or stress protein 32, is highly inducible and normally found in the spleen[34,37]. Levels of HO-1 are increased in

***Figure 4** Heme oxygenase activity (columns) and inflammatory response, total number of cells (■) in (a) the Arthus reaction and (b) met BSA delayed hypersensitivity. **p < 0.01*

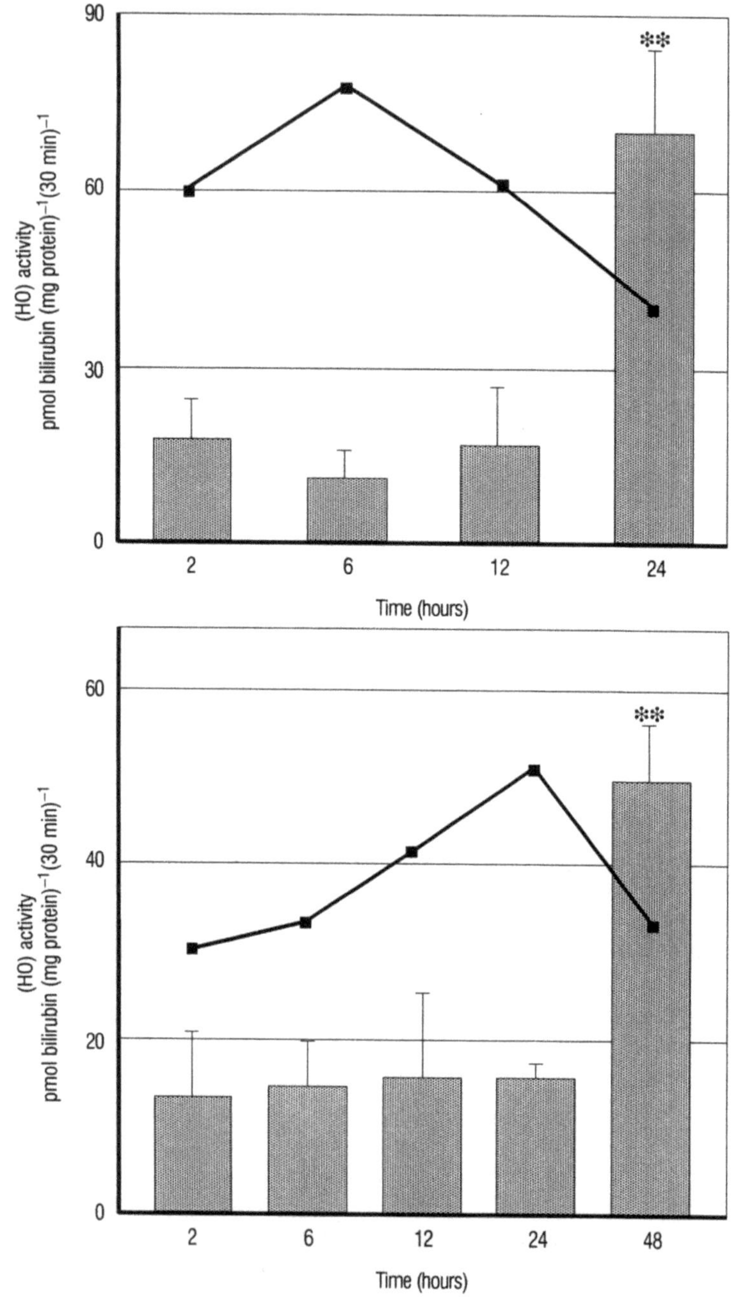

response to stressful stimuli such as heat, ultraviolet light, hypoxia, reactive oxygen species and the pro-inflammatory cytokines IL-1 and TNF. In the light of its highly inducible nature, Willis investigated HO-1 in inflammatory conditions.

HO activity in acute inflammation: the carrageenin pleural model of acute inflammation

As inflammation progressed in this model of acute inflammation, HO activity in pleural exudates increased. Unlike COX and NOS activity, however, which were maximal in the first 6h, the rise in HO activity was delayed, significantly increasing by 24h, but peaking at 48h with a 12-fold increase in specific activity of the enzyme in comparison to that at 2h[38]. HO-1 protein levels were also maximal at 48h as assessed by Western blotting. Thus the peak of HO-1 activity was coincident with the conclusion of the inflammatory response. HO-1 immunoreactivity in this model was found almost exclusively in the macrophages. HO activity is measured by its production of bilirubin. Bilirubin levels fell at 6h but increased at 24h, possibly indicating that endogenous bile pigments are sequestered or cleared from the inflammatory exudate initially, but are induced and rise in the resolving phase of the inflammation.

HO activity in the Arthus and met BSA pleurisy models of immediate and delayed type hypersensitivity

Preliminary results in these models of inflammation show a similar pattern of HO activity to that described in carrageenin pleurisy. In the Arthus reaction, HO activity was low up to 12h but significantly increased at 24h, coinciding with a reduction in the inflammatory response (Figure 4a) and a return of NOS activity towards baseline levels. An extension of the model to 48h is required to clarify interactions between HO and COX. In this inflammatory model, HO-1 protein was localized in the PMNs, in contrast to the macrophage expression in the carrageenin pleurisy. In the met BSA model of delayed hypersensitivity, HO activity was low up to 24h, but significantly elevated at 48h to coincide with the suppression of the inflammation (Figure 4b).

In all three examples of acute inflammation, increasing HO activity occurred after the peak of the inflammatory response, leading to the hypothesis that the sequential induction of enzymes with pro-inflammatory effects, including COX-2 and iNOS, is followed by an increase in the expression of one or more enzymes, with anti-inflammatory effects, including HO. It is likely that the bile pigments act both as antioxidant tissue protectors and in concert with other as yet unknown mechanisms operating as a consequence of increasing HO activity, to advance the resolution of inflammation. Thus the induction of HO-1 can potentially activate the radical scavenging and anti-complement activity of bilirubin, inactivating NO and other free radicals. In addition both Fe and CO formed in the reaction have the ability to down-regulate NOS[39,40]. In conclusion, HO may represent an endogenous mechanism for the control of acute inflammation. If this thesis holds true then pharmacological manipulation of HO to boost its activity may be a way forward in combating acute inflammation.

Modulation of heme oxygenase

Inducers and inhibitors of HO in inflammation

On the premise that the inflammatory response could be affected by the modulation of HO-1 expression, inhibitors and inducers were employed in a rat carrageenin pleurisy model[38]. An inhibitor of HO, tin protoporphyrin (SnPP), and an inducer of HO, ferriprotoporphyrin IX chloride (FePP), were administered before and at the time of induction of the inflammation. Twenty-four hours after injection the animals receiving SnPP showed a dose-dependent increase, up to 100%, in inflammatory exudate. In contrast, those receiving FePP showed a dose-dependent suppression of the inflammatory exudate. The degree of suppression achieved was greater than that seen with optimal doses of NSAIDs and steroids previously used in this model. These data suggest that modulation of HO by SnPP and FePP profoundly affects the inflammatory process, but alternative actions of these drugs cannot be discounted. However, it was confirmed that treatment with SnPP and FePP, respectively, inhibited and increased HO-1 activity in the cell pellets and this activity correlated with an exacerbation and suppression of the inflammatory response. Modulation of HO-1 activity may therefore represent an important therapeutic target for modifying the inflammatory response.

Heme oxygenase and apoptosis

Apoptosis, or programmed cell death, results in the orderly shut down and packaging of cellular contents prior to cell death. As a mechanism of cellular destruction it is distinct from necrosis. Inflammatory mediators, in particular reactive oxygen species and NO, are potential causative agents[41]. Recently NSAIDs have been implicated in the promotion of apoptosis[42], potentially involving the inhibition of a COX isoform, which may be modulating NO production. The occurrence of apoptotic profiles was examined in cell smears from the exudate produced in carrageenin-induced pleurisy and the Arthus reaction, using in situ end-labelling techniques (Figure 5). Substantial numbers of apoptotic figures were associated with the PMNs in carrageenin pleurisy, but not with macrophages. Macrophages expressed HO-1 but PMNs did not. In contrast, in the Arthus reaction, which is characterized by a persistently high level of PMNs, this cell type did express HO-1 and apoptotic profiles were sparse. These findings may suggest that the expression of the stress-related protein HO-1 may afford protection from programmed cell death. The rise in

***Figure 5** Diagram to illustrate HO activity, NOS activity and apoptosis in the rat carrageenin-induced pleurisy model. (PMN, polymorphoneutrophil, MN, mononuclear cell)*

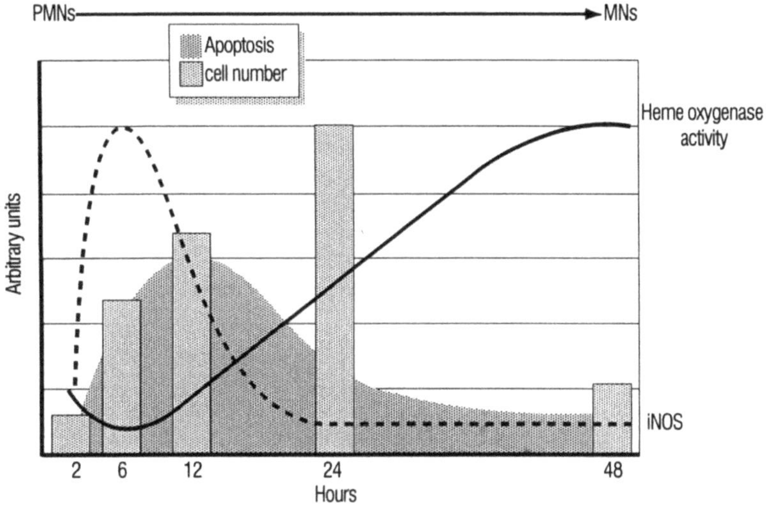

HO-1 activity following the peak of NOS activity in carrageenin-induced pleurisy (Figure 5) lends support to this hypothesis. The phenomenon of PMN apoptosis may explain in part the switch from the dominance of PMNs to the dominance of macrophages seen during the development of most inflammatory responses. However it is interesting that the Arthus reaction, which is characterized by a persistence of PMNs, is the one model in which we have not observed apoptosis of PMNs.

Modulation of heme oxygenase by nitric oxide

As NO has the capacity to activate or inhibit metalloprotein-containing enzymes, we investigated the possible modulation of HO activity by NO. Although HO is not a haem-containing protein, when the substrate haem binds to the enzyme in a 1:1 ratio, a transitory haemoprotein is formed[43]. In this respect HO may be activated or inhibited by NO. Alternatively, NO may in some other way interfere with substrate availability.

We measured HO and NOS activity in homogenates of rat brain and spleen. Brain homogenates contained both HO and NOS activity and homogenates of spleen contained twice the HO activity of brain but lacked NOS activity as determined by our assay system[44]. In homogenates of rat brain, the arginine analogue L-NAME, dose-dependently increased HO activity. L-Arginine, the

Figure 6 Known and potential reactions between COX, NOS and HO

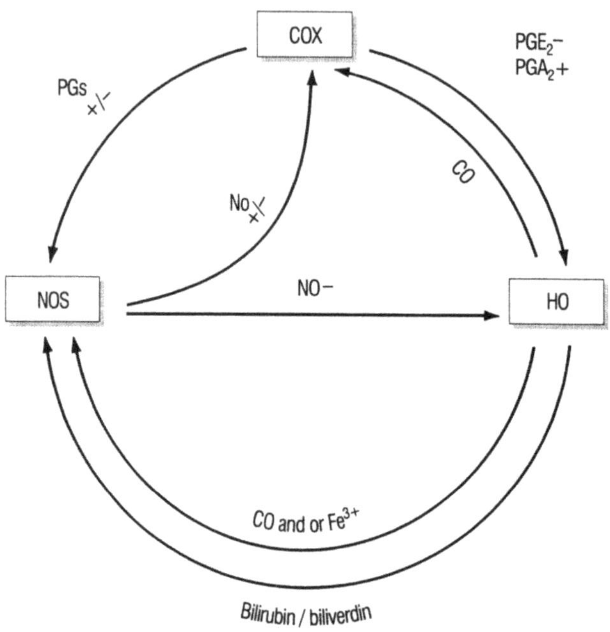

substrate for NOS, but not D-arginine suppressed HO activity. In spleen homogenates, where endogenous levels of NOS activity are low, L-NAME and L-arginine were without effect. The nitric oxide donor sodium nitroprusside, however, reduced HO activity in both spleen and brain homogenates. These results suggest that biological effects attributed to NOS may be acting through HO.

CONCLUSION

We present in Figure 6 an overview of known and potential interactions between COX, NOS and HO. COX activity can be stimulated or inhibited by NO[20–23] and NOS is a similar target for PGs[24–26]. Carbon monoxide produced by HO has the ability to inhibit cytochrome P450 enzymes including COX, whilst PGE_2 suppresses[45] and PGA_2 stimulates the activity of HO[46]. The bile salts are potent free radical scavengers with consequences for NO inactivation[35] and Fe^{3+} and CO[39,40] modulate NOS which is reciprocated by NO inhibition of HO activity[44].

From the evidence presented here we suggest that the three inducible enzymes described may represent distinct targets for the modulation of inflammation. COX-2 may well represent a safer target than COX-1, with benefits of elimination of side effects. Certainly there are reports on the efficacy of selective COX-2 inhibition in both acute and chronic models of inflammation. Time and further investigations will resolve the question of desirability or otherwise of suppressing prostanoid formation in chronic inflammation.

The case for NOS, an agent of host defence or tissue destruction, being a viable target for drug intervention has been widely discussed. The conclusion from the 1994 Inflammation Research Association meeting was that the case was not proven with the exception of endotoxic shock. However in our view, considering its possible interactions with heme oxygenase, iNOS would seem to be a potential target.

Heme oxygenase, the third enzyme, is fascinating in that induction of its activity produces a profound anti-inflammatory effect associated with the PMN in the Arthus reaction, but associated with the macrophage, a classical cell marker of chronic inflammation in other models. Suppression of HO activity increases the inflammatory response, which may be desirable in immunosuppressed individuals. It is intriguing that the rise in HO-1 appears to be associated with the switching off of apoptosis. This may have significance beyond inflammation, for example in tumours, where elevated levels of HO-1 have been observed. In conclusion, these three inducible enzymes do not exist in vacuo and a clearer understanding of the inflammatory process may be profitably gained from further investigation of their mutual interactions. Therefore we offer a cartoon of known and potential interactions of these three inducible enzymes (Figure 6), that we hope to build upon with our future research.

Acknowledgements

The work presented here constitutes the combined efforts of research from the staff of Experimental Pathology on COX, NOS and HO, including Ian Appleton, Adrian Moore, Mark Paul-Clarke, Rodney Frederick, Joanne Brown and the authors of this manuscript.

References

1. Xie W, Chipman JG, Robertson DL, Erickson RL, Simmons DL. Expression of a mitogen-responsive gene encoding prostaglandin synthase is regulated by mRNA splicing. Proc Natl Acad Sci USA. 1991;88:2692–6.
2. Kujubu DA, Fletcher S, Varnum BC, Lim RW, Herschman HR. TIS10, a phorbol ester tumor promoter-inducible mRNA from Swiss 3T3 cells, encodes a novel prostaglandin synthase/cyclooxygenase homologue. J Biol Chem. 1991;266:12866–72.
3. Appleton I, Tomlinson A, Colville-Nash PR, Willoughby DA. Temporal and spatial immunolocalization of cytokines in murine chronic granulomatous tissue. Lab Invest. 1993;69:405–14.
4. Edward JC, Sedgwick AD, Willoughby DA. The formation of a structure with the features of a synovial lining by subcutaneous injection of air: an in vivo tissue culture system. J Pathol. 1981;134:147–56.
5. Vane JR, Mitchell JA, Appleton I et al. Inducible isoforms of cyclooxygenase and nitric oxide synthase in inflammation. Proc Natl Acad Sci USA. 1994;91:2046–50.

6. Appleton I, Tomlinson A, Mitchell JA, Willoughby DA. Distributions of cyclooxygenase isoforms in murine chronic granulomatous inflammation. Implications for future anti-inflammatory therapy. J Pathol. 1995;176:413–20.
7. O'Banion MK, Winn VD, Young DA. cDNA cloning and functional activity of a glucocorticoid regulated inflammatory cyclooxygenase. Proc Natl Acad Sci USA. 1992;89:4888–92.
8. Hla T, Nielson K. Human cyclooxygenase 2 cDNA. Proc Natl Acad Sci USA. 1992;89:7384–8.
9. Rzymkiewicz D, Leinang K, Baird N, Morrison AR. Regulation of prostaglandin endoperoxide synthase gene expression in rat mesangial cells by interleukin-1β. Am J Physiol. 1994;266:F39–45.
10. O'Banion MK, Dusel JC, Chang JW, Coleman PD. Cytokine induction of prostaglandin G/H synthase 2 (PGHS 2) and inducible nitric oxide synthase (iNOS) in primary murine glial cell cultures. 9th Int Conf Prostaglandins, Italy, 1994.
11. Herschmann HR, Gilbert RS, Xie W, Luner S, Reddy S. Regulation and role of TIS10/PGS2. Adv Prost Thromb Leuk Res. 1995;23:23–8.
12. Kester M, Coroneos E, Thomas PJ, Dunn MJ. Endothelin stimulates prostaglandin endoperoxide synthase 2 mRNA expression and protein synthesis through a tyrosine signalling pathway in rat mesangial cells. J Biol Chem. 1994;269:22574–80.
13. Moncada S, Palmer RMJ, Higgs EA. Nitric oxide: physiology, pathophysiology and pharmacology. Pharmacol Rev. 1991;43:109–42.
14. Stefanovic-Racic M, Stadler J, Evans CH. Nitric oxide and arthritis. Arthritis Rheum. 1993;36: 1036–44.
15. Jansen A, Cook T, Taylor GM et al. Induction of nitric oxide synthase in rat immune complex glomerulonephritis. Kidney Int. 1994;45:1215–9.
16. Boughton-Smith NK, Evans SM, Hawkey CJ et al. Nitric oxide synthase activity in ulcerative colitis and Crohn's disease. Lancet. 1993;342:338–40.
17. Lin RF, Lin TS, Tilton RG, Cross AH. Nitric oxide localised to the spinal cords of mice with an experimental allergic encephalomyelitis: an electron paramagnetic resonance study. J Exp Med. 1993;178:643–8.
18. Nathan C, Hibbs JB Jr. Role of nitric oxide synthesis in macrophage antimicrobial activity. Curr Opin Immunol. 1991;3:65–70.
19. Radi R, Beckman JS, Bush KM, Freeman BA. Peroxynitrite oxidation of sulfhydryls: The cytotoxic potential of superoxide and nitric oxide. J Biol Chem. 1991;266:4244–50.
20. Sautebin L, Di Rosa M. Nitric oxide modulates prostacyclin biosynthesis in the lung of endotoxin-treated rats. Eur J Pharmacol. 1994;262:193–6.
21. Salvemini D, Seibert K, Masferrer JL, Misko TP, Currie MG, Needleman P. Endogenous nitric oxide enhances prostaglandin production in a model of renal inflammation. J Clin Invest. 1994;93:1940–7.
22. Habib A, Bernard C, Tedgui A, Maclouf J. Evidence of cross talk between inducible nitric oxide synthase and cyclooxygenase 2 in rat peritoneal macrophages. 9th Int Conf Prostaglandins, Italy. 1994.
23. Swierkosz TA, Mitchell JA, Warner TD, Botting RM, Vane JR. Co-induction of nitric oxide synthase and cyclooxygenase: interactions between nitric oxide and prostanoids. Br J Pharmacol. 1995;114:1335–42.
24. Tetsuka T, Daphna-Iken D, Srivastava SK, Baier LD, DuMaine J, Morrison AR. Cross talk between cyclooxygenase and nitric oxide pathways: Prostaglandin E_2 negatively modulates induction of nitric oxide synthase by interleukin-1. Proc Natl Acad Sci USA. 1994;91:12168–72.
25. Marotta P, Sautebin L, DiRosa M. Modulation of the induction of nitric oxide synthase by eicosanoids in the murine macrophage cell line J774. Br J Pharmacol. 1992;107:640–1.
26. Gaillard T, Mulsch A, Klein H, Decker K. Regulation of prostaglandin E_2 of cytokine elicited nitric oxide synthesis in rat liver macrophages. J Biol Chem. 1992;373:897–902.
27. Wahl SM, Allen JB, Costa GL, Wong HL, Dasch JR. Reversal of acute and chronic synovial inflammation by anti-transforming growth factor β. J Exp Med. 1993;177:225–30.
28. Fujii E, Irie K, Muraki T. Nitric oxide (NO) plays a role of increase in vascular permeability induced by bradykinin, substance P and 5-HT, but not by PAF and histamine in mouse skin. Can J Physiol Pharmacol. 1994;72(S1):470.
29. Velo GP, Dunn CJ, Giroud JP, Timsit J, Willoughby DA. Distribution of prostaglandins in inflammatory exudate. J Pathol. 1973;111:149–58.
30. Tomlinson A, Appleton I, Moore AR et al. Cyclooxygenase and nitric oxide synthase isoforms

in rat carrageenin-induced pleurisy. Br J Pharmacol. 1994;113:693-8.
31. Yamamoto S, Dunn CJ, Deporter DA, Capasso F, Willoughby DA, Huskisson EC. A model for the quantitative study of Arthus (immunologic) hypersensitivity in rats. Agents Actions. 1975; 5:374-7.
32. Moore AR, Willis D, Gilroy D, Tomlinson A, Appleton I, Willoughby DA. Cyclooxygenase in rat pleural hypersensitivity reactions. Adv Prost Thromb Leuk Res. 1995;23:349-51.
33. Roper RL, Phipps RP. Prostaglandin E_2 regulation of the immune response. Adv Prost Thromb Leuk Res. 1994;22:101-11.
34. Maines MD. Heme oxygenase: function, multiplicity, regulatory mechanisms and clinical application. FASEB J. 1988;2:2557-68.
35. Nath KA, Balla G, Vercellotti GM et al. Induction of heme oxygenase is a rapid protective response in rhabdomyolysis in the rat. J Clin Invest. 1992;90:267-70.
36. Nakagami T, Toyomura K, Kinoshita T, Morisawa S. A beneficial role of bile pigments as an endogenous tissue protector: anticomplement effects of biliverdin and conjugated bilirubin. Biochim Biophys Acta. 1993;1158:189-93.
37. Maines MD, Trakshel GM, Kutty RK. Characterization of two constitutive forms of rat liver microsomal heme oxygenase: only one molecular species of the enzyme is inducible. J Biol Chem. 1986;251:411-9.
38. Willis D. Expression and modulatory effects of heme oxygenase in acute inflammation in the rat. Inflam Res. 1995;44:S218-20.
39. Weiss G, Werner-Felmayer G, Werner ER, Grunewald K, Wachter H, Hemtze MW. Iron regulates nitric oxide synthase activity by controlling nuclear transcription. J Exp Med. 1994;180:969-76.
40. White KA, Marletta MA. Nitric oxide synthase is a cytochrome P450 type hemoprotein. Biochemistry. 1992;31:6627-31.
41. Albina JE, Cui S, Mateo RB, Reichner JS. Nitric oxide-mediated apoptosis in murine peritoneal macrophages. J Immunol. 1993;150:5080-5.
42. Lu X, Xie W, Reed D, Bradshaw WS, Simmons DL. Non steroidal anti-inflammatory drugs cause apoptosis and induce cyclooxygenases in chick embryo fibroblasts. Proc Natl Acad Sci USA. 1995;92:7961-5.
43. Henry Y, Lepoivre M, Drapier JC, Ducrocq C, Boucher JL, Guissani A. EPR characterization of molecular targets for NO in mammalian cells and organelles. FASEB J. 1993;7:1124-34.
44. Willis D, Tomlinson A, Frederick R, Paul-Clark MJ, Willoughby DA. Modulation of heme oxygenase activity in rat brain and spleen by inhibitors and donors of nitric oxide. Biochem Biophys Res Commun. 1995;214:1152-6.
45. Tetsuka T, Daphna-Iken D, Srivastava SK, Morrison AB. Regulation of heme oxygenase mRNA in mesangial cells: prostaglandin E_2 negatively modulates IL-1 induced heme oxygenase-1 mRNA. Biochem Biophys Res Commun. 1995;212:617-23.
46. Santoro MG, Garaci E, Amici C. Induction of heat shock protein synthesis by prostaglandins with antineoplastic and antiviral activity. Adv Prost Thromb Leuk Res. 1990;21:867-74.

5 NSAID mechanism of action: the role of intracellular pharmacokinetics

L.G. HERBETTE, M. VECCHIARELLI and G. TRUMMLITZ

Nonsteroid anti-inflammatory drugs (NSAIDs) are a structurally diverse group of agents with similar therapeutic effects. They reduce pain, fever and inflammation, and are also associated with lowered risks of cardiovascular disease[1] and colon cancer[2,3]. The biological basis for the therapeutic effects of NSAIDs is their ability to inhibit prostaglandin biosynthesis. The NSAIDs specifically target the bifunctional cyclooxygenase enzyme (COX) which is responsible for the initial rate-limiting conversion of arachidonic acid to prostaglandin G (PGG) and its subsequent conversion to PGH_2. This is then converted to other prostanoids[4,5].

The COX enzyme exists in two forms encoded by separate genes, and have 60% homology in their amino acid sequences[6]. COX-1, first isolated from ram seminal vesicles, is constitutively expressed and responsible for the production of homeostatic prostanoids in tissues such as the stomach mucosa and kidney[7]. COX-2 is the inducible isoform of the enzyme, the expression of which is glucocorticoid sensitive[8] and can be stimulated by mitogens[9], cytokines[10,11], inflammation and tissue injury. The unwanted side effects of the NSAIDs, including gastrointestinal distress, are thought to be due to the inhibition of COX-1, while their primary anti-inflammatory effects are due to inhibition of COX-2[12].

COX is an integral membrane protein located primarily in the endoplasmic reticulum/nuclear membrane network of the cell. The X-ray crystal structure of COX-1 has been determined and indicates that the enzyme is a monotopic dimer, that is, the binding surface of the protein extends through only one leaflet of the membrane with the bulk of the protein facing the lumen[13]. The active site of the enzyme at which NSAIDs are thought to bind exists as a long narrow hydrophobic channel (8×25 Å) extending from the outer surface to the centre of the protein. Interestingly, this active site structure of COX is believed to be located in the hydrocarbon domain of the lipid bilayer: endogenous arachidonic acid may gain access to the active site of the COX enzyme via the lipid bilayer structure of the membrane, as with other ligand/membrane receptor systems[14].

Recently it has been found that some NSAIDs appear to show significant selectivity towards the inhibition of COX-2 rather than COX-1[15–17]. In vivo, these compounds demonstrate good anti-inflammatory effects with little unwanted ulcerogenicity[18]. Copeland et al.[19] suggested that this selective inhibition is due to a slow structural transition induced in the COX-2 enzyme upon binding of the drug. Although these compounds initially inhibit both isozymes with equal potency, the COX-1 enzyme fails to undergo such a time-dependent transition and is only moderately inhibited.

When Reddy and Herschman[20] inhibited COX-2 with an antisense oligonucleotide in macrophages, COX-1 was unable to convert the released arachidonic acid to prostaglandins. This suggested that there may be two distinct endogenous pools of arachidonic acid, one constantly available to COX-1 and its housekeeping production of prostaglandins, and a second pool which may be released upon induction and available only to COX-2. This may be related to the recent findings of two different intracellular locations for COX-1 and COX-2[21]: COX-2 is much more concentrated in the nuclear envelope rather than in the endoplasmic reticulum where COX-1 predominantly resides.

Regardless of the preferential binding to COX-1 or COX-2, an NSAID must move from within the plasma compartment of the circulatory system, through tissue membrane structures, and eventually across the plasma membrane of the target cell, which usually contains relatively high amounts of cholesterol, on average 0.3–0.4 mol cholesterol per mol lipid[22]. It then must traverse many intracellular barriers before being incorporated into the endoplasmic reticulum membrane network, which contains low amounts of cholesterol, or further, within the nuclear envelope. There is a stringent requirement, therefore, for NSAIDs to have good amphiphillic properties so that they are able to be transported easily across several membrane barriers to their site of action. NSAIDs must also possess a high lipophilic character in order to reside in the target membranes at sufficient concentrations to inhibit the COX enzyme system. This means that in order to gain access to the intrabilayer active site of the COX enzyme, the NSAID must partition well into the membrane. The ideal NSAID must therefore be both amphiphilic for rapid membrane transport and lipophilic or membrane soluble (Figure 1)[23].

PREPARATION OF MODEL PHOSPHOLIPID MEMBRANE VESICLES

For partitioning experiments, large unilamellar vesicles (LUV) and multilamellar vesicles (MLV) formed from egg phosphatidylcholine (Egg PC) in the presence and absence of cholesterol were utilized. Egg PC and cholesterol were obtained from Avanti Polar Lipids, Inc. (Alabaster, AL) in powder form and stored dessicated in chloroform (Egg PC at 20 mg/ml and cholesterol at 25 mg/ml) at −20°C. TLC was used to ascertain purity and the presence of degradative products in the lipid and cholesterol suspensions.

Large unilamellar vesicles (LUV)

LUVs were prepared using a detergent dialysis method[24]. Cholesterol: phospholipid (molar ratio 0: 1) was dried to a thin film on the walls of a glass test tube (13×100 mm) by evaporation under nitrogen gas and the residual solvent

***Figure 1** The membrane bilayer hypothesis. Drug–receptor binding models illustrating a single step aqueous pathway to receptor binding (A) and a two-step bilayer pathway (M). The components of the two-step model are ligand partitioning into the membrane followed by lateral diffusion and subsequent interaction with a binding domain within the membrane bilayer. An additional kinetic component could be associated with diffusion (flip-flop) across the bilayer leaflet*

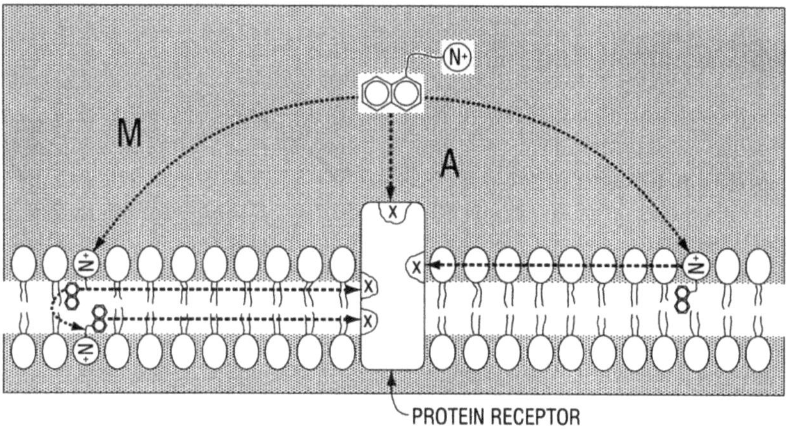

was removed by lyophilization overnight. HEPES buffer (10 mM HEPES, 150 mM NaCl, pH 7.0) was then added (979 μl) to the dried lipid and vortexed for 3 min at high speed to produce multilamellar vesicles. The MLV suspension was sonicated in a cold room (4°C) for 1.5–2 h until the suspension became clear, indicating the formation of small unilamellar vesicles (SUV). After sonication, 21 μl of a 10% solution of deoxycholate was added to bring the volume to 1.0 ml. The sample was vortexed gently for 5–10 s and left to incubate at room temperature for 30 min. The LUV sample was then added to a Sepharose 4B (Sigma Chemical Co, St. Louis, MO) column (12 mm diameter). The sample was collected on a fraction collector set for 40 drops per tube.

The LUV fractions were recognized by their slight turbidity. As a result of the detergent being retained longer on the column, the LUV are relatively detergent free. To determine the final ratio of cholesterol:phospholipid (C:PL) in the membrane vesicles, the 4–5 visible fractions were assayed for phosphate[25] and cholesterol[26]. The fractions were combined and diluted with HEPES buffer for a final LUV stock of 0.2 mg/ml.

Multilamellar vesicles (MLV)

To prepare the MLV, 3.95 μmol (150 μl of a 20 mg/ml stock in chloroform) of Egg PC and the appropriate molar ratio of cholesterol were dried to a thin film by evaporation under nitrogen on the sides of a test tube and lyophilized overnight. The lipid was then reconstituted with 1.0 ml of HEPES buffer and vortexed on high for 3 min. The MLV were then diluted with 14 ml of HEPES buffer to make a 0.2 mg/ml stock solution.

EQUILIBRIUM AND KINETIC MEMBRANE PARAMETERS – RADIOLABEL METHODS

Membrane partition coefficient

The membrane partition coefficient *K*p[mem] is an equilibrium value expressing the relative amount, by mass, of a drug in the membrane vs that in the aqueous buffer. This distribution of the drug between the aqueous buffer and membrane lipid is an expression of the drug's true lipophilicity or affinity for the membrane bilayer.

*K*p[mem] was experimentally measured using vacuum filtration as previously described in detail[27]. This technique is able rapidly and efficiently to separate membrane-bound radioligand from free radioligand. All solutions were filtered through Whatman GF/C glass fibre filters on a Brandel Cell Harvester model M-48 (Brandel, Gaithersburg, MD). All filters were counted for radioactivity using a Tracor Analytic Delta 300/6891 Liquid Scintillation system.

The incubation reaction consisted of a fixed phospholipid concentration of 2.63 μM Egg PC and known amounts of cholesterol. The pH of the reaction was maintained at pH 7.0, unless otherwise specified, using HEPES buffer. Radiolabelled drug was added for a final drug concentration of 2.5×10^{-8} M.

Meloxicam (*N*-methyl-^{3}H] (specific activity 81 Ci/mmol) and diclofenac [phenyl ring-^{3}H(N)] (specific activity 50.2 Ci/mmol) were provided by Boehringer Ingelheim (Germany). Each compound had a radiochemical purity >98.5% in high performance liquid chromatography and proved stable over the testing period.

Reaction mixtures containing drug, but no membrane were used to correct for the total non-specific binding of drug directly to the filters. The amount of free drug in the filtrate is determined by subtracting the amount of drug bound to the membrane (CPM of lipid + drug + filter – CPM of filter + drug) from the total amount of drug added to the reaction mixtures (CPM in reaction mixture with drug not run through the filtration). The amount of lipid bound to the filters was corrected for by the recovery of membrane on the filters determined by lipid retention experiments using vesicles labelled with [^{3}H]cholesterol (Dupont NEN Research Products, Boston, MA). The membrane partition coefficient is calculated using the following equation:

$$K\text{p[mem]} = \frac{\text{(g drug bound to membrane/g lipid)}}{\text{(g free drug/g buffer)}}$$

'Wash-in' assay

The 'wash-in' assay measures the rate of drug partitioning into model membranes by filtering the partitioning reaction mixture at time points prior to equilibrium. The earliest time point presented here was 5 min and the longest 3 h.

Drug release ('wash-out') from membranes

The time dependence of drug release from membranes was measured by incubating the tritiated drug (2.5×10^{-8} M) with MLV cholesterol: Egg PC (0: 1) in HEPES buffer (pH 4.0) for 1 h and filtering the solutions through Whatman GF/C glass fibre filters on a Brandel cell harvester. Control reactions contained drug but no membranes. Three filters with membranes and three control filters were immediately counted for radioactivity, the difference representing maximal binding of drug to membranes. The remaining filters are impaled in groups of three on 25 gauge needles mounted on a flat plexiglass 'donut'. The filters on each needle were spaced with pieces of tubing (length 1 cm, OD 1 mm) to prevent them from touching. The plexiglass structure was then placed near the base inside a 3 l round plastic container situated on a magnetic stirrer at medium speed, and the container filled with HEPES buffer (pH 4.0). At 2.5, 5, 10, 15, 30, 60 and 120 min, filters with and without membranes were removed from the buffer and counted for radioactivity.

The percentage of drug remaining bound to membranes was calculated for each time point. Separate washout experiments using control filters containing [^{3}H]cholesterol-labelled lipid were performed to determine lipid loss over the duration of the washout. This was determined to be 10% in these experiments and accounted for in the final calculations.

POTENTIOMETRIC METHODS

*K*p[mem] was also determined by potentiometry using the PCA101 pK_a log P Analyzer designed and manufactured by Sirius Analytical Instruments Ltd. (Forest Row, East Sussex, UK). This non-radiolabel method is a derivation of the log P function in octanol which is a specialized application of the determination of the pK_a using this apparatus.

The PCA101 uses volumetric analyses where precisely known volumes of standardized strong acid (0.25 M HCl) or base (0.25 M KOH) are added to a solution of protogenic substance, during which the pH is continuously measured with a combination glass electrode within the interval of pH 1 to 13 at a constant temperature of 25°C. The PCA101 then derives the pK_a from the resulting titration curve (pH versus volume of titrant). A second titration is then done with the substance in model membranes (Egg PC). When a weak acid or a weak base partitions into the lipid phase, the titration curve will shift, producing a p[mem]K_a. The larger the difference between the pK_a and the p[mem]K_a, the larger the Kp[mem]. The PCA101 refines the pK_a and Kp[mem] (actually the log Kp[mem]) values taking into consideration such parameters as purity, titrant strength, acidity and CO_2 errors[28]. A significant correlation (r^2=0.98) has been shown between the log Kp[mem] determined by the above radiotracer method and the potentiometric method under a variety of cholesterol: lipid ratios (data not shown for meloxicam and diclofenac).

The Pka

All NSAIDs were provided by Boehringer Ingelheim (Germany). To ensure solubility in the entire pH range of 2.5–8.5, the pK_a of piroxicam, tenoxicam, naproxen, indomethacin Na, ibuprofen (purchased at RBI, Natick, MA), 6-methoxy-naphthylacetic acid (the active metabolite of nabumetone, 6-MNA), and diclofenac were measured in a mixed solvent system of methanol and water. The pK_a of meloxicam was measured in ethanol. Three assays of 2–4 mg of drug in various mixed solvent ratios were performed and pK_a values determined. The PCA101 extrapolated these values to the aqueous pK_a using the Yasuda–Shedlovsky method[29,30].

Log *K*p[mem]

The PCA101 determines the log P[mem] in a MLV system. The MLV preparation is made by drying Egg PC (100 mg/ml in chloroform) with or without cholesterol to a thin film on the side of a round bottom PCA101 sample vial with nitrogen gas. For drugs insoluble in the 150 mM ionic strength KCl water used in this method a stock solution in chloroform or methanol (8 mg/ml) was made and the appropriate amount dried with the lipid. This was required for naproxen, 6-MNA, ibuprofen, piroxicam, tenoxicam and meloxicam. The sample was left under vacuum overnight and then reconstituted with 1 ml of KCl water and vortexed on high for 3 min. Diclofenac stocks were made in KCl water (2 mg/ml) and added to the lipid when reconstituted. The sample was put into a temperature controlled vessel at 25°C. To start, the titration was run in both directions, from 3.5 to 10.5 and then in the reverse. The data were taken from the direction which resulted in the most reproducible curve. This seemed to be dictated by the solubility of the drug at a low or high pH. Meloxicam, piroxicam and tenoxicam titrations were performed from pH 10.5 to 3.5. Diclofenac, ibuprofen, naproxen, 6-MNA titrations were performed from pH 3.5 to 10.5. Each sample was run with 0.5–2 mg drug in 10–50 mg Egg PC (Egg PC: drug molar ratio ranged from 4.4 to 46.2). Data not shown for diclofenac showed that the log Kp[mem] is independent of the amount of Egg PC (10–50 mg) with a constant drug amount (2 mg) and independent of drug amount (0.25–2 mg) with a constant amount of Egg PC (30 mg).

Table 1 IC_{50} *(mol/l) for inhibition of different cyclooxygenases in vitro*

Test substance	*COX-1: BSV cell free*[a]	*COX-1: GPMPH*[b]	*COX-2: GPMPH*[c]
Meloxicam	4.0×10^{-6}	5.8×10^{-9}	1.9×10^{-9}
Piroxicam	2.0×10^{-5}	5.3×10^{-9}	1.8×10^{-7}
Diclofenac	1.4×10^{-7}	8.6×10^{-10}	1.9×10^{-9}

[a]Inhibition of PGE_2 production in a cell free system: enzyme, isolated from bull seminal vesicle.
[b]Inhibition of PGE_2 production of non stimulated peritoneal macrophages isolated from guinea pigs, incubated for 6 h together with the test substance.
[c]Inhibition of PGE_2-production of peritoneal macrophages, isolated from guinea pigs, stimulated by LPS for 6 h together with the test substance
Table taken from Engelhardt G. Meloxicam: a potent inhibitor of COX-2. 9th International Conference on Prostaglandins and related compounds, Florence, Italy, 6–10 June 1994.

Statistical evaluation

Means and SD are reported for radiotracer and potentiometric *K*p[mem]. SEM are used in wash-in data. MANOVA and Tukey's HSD test for equal *n* or Spijotvoil/Stoline's test for unequal *n* were performed to determine significant differences between *K*p[mem] in varying pH and cholesterol. Linear correlations were determined by a simple linear regression analysis.

ACTIVITY OF NSAIDs

Table 1 shows the IC_{50} (mol/l) for NSAID inhibition of PGE_2 production to be much greater in a cell-free system than in guinea pig peritoneal macrophages. This indicates that the NSAIDs experience different components of the overall mechanism when in the cell compared with the cell-free system. Unlike in the cell-free system, the NSAID must cross both intracellular membranes, as well as the plasma membrane in order to reach its target site of action. Furthermore, NSAIDs may be stored in cellular membranes to eventually inhibit COX. Therefore, how the NSAIDs interact with the membrane lipid bilayer may play an important role in their molecular mechanism of action.

NSAID equilibrium membrane parameters

The pK_a determinations for the NSAIDs are given in Table 2. All compounds except for meloxicam were extrapolated (Yasuda-Shedlovsky) from the pK_a in methanol. The pK_a for meloxicam was extrapolated from ethanol. The r^2 relates to correlation coefficients of these extrapolations, determined by the PCA101 itself. The NSAIDs show broad differences in pK_a which may relate to terminal plasma half-life, potency, and possibly selectivity for COX-2.

Table 3 is the summary of all log *K*p[mem] ± SD in MLV with cholesterol : Egg PC molar ratio (0 : 1) as determined by the potentiometric method (Egg PC : drug molar ratio 4.4–46.2). The log *K*p[mem] as determined by both this method and

Table 2 pK_a determinations

Drug	*pK_a*	*r^2*
Tenoxicam	5.32 ± 0.03	0.9892
Piroxicam	5.39 ± 0.04	0.9813
Naproxen	4.57 ± 0.01	0.9922
6-MNA	4.42 ± 0.01	0.9958
Ibuprofen	4.35[a]	
Diclofenac	4.14 ± 0.01	0.9902
Meloxicam[b]	4.03 ± 0.02	0.9188
	4.04 ± 0.03	0.6739

r^2 relates to the Yasuda–Shedlovsky extrapolation fit from the pK_a in methanol to the aqueous pK_a
[a]Data from Sirius Analytical Instruments Ltd.
[b]The pK_a for meloxicam used in the Log *K*p[mem] determination (4.08 ± 0.07) is an average pK_a of the UV spectrophotometric results of Tsai et al.[31] and Boehringer Ingelheim (Germany) and the two potentiometric results extrapolated from ethanol above.

Table 3 Summary of log Kp[mem] in MLV cholesterol : Egg PC (0 : 1)

Drug	*n*	*Log Kp[mem]*	*Radiotracer log Kp[mem]*
Tenoxicam	3	1.72 ± 0.07	
Piroxicam	6	2.24 ± 0.27	
6-MNA	5	3.11 ± 0.14	
Naproxen	5	3.29 ± 0.10	
Meloxicam	8	3.43 ± 0.27	3.57 ± 0.05[a]
Ibuprofen	6	3.97 ± 0.10	
Diclofenac	9	4.59 ± 0.11	4.61 ± 0.02[b]

[a]Radiotracer data for meloxicam is a mean of the *K*p[mem] at all time points 5–180 min.
[b]Radiotracer data for diclofenac is a mean of the *K*p[mem] from 15–180 min.

the radiotracer method for meloxicam and diclofenac in MLV at pH 4.0 are in good agreement. There is a broad difference in the membrane properties of these various NSAIDs.

Figure 2 shows a correlation ($r^2 = 0.800$) between the pK_a of the NSAIDs and their log *K*p[mem] where the membrane system was 0:1 cholesterol : Egg PC.

Figure 3 shows the *K*p[mem] at 60 min in MLV cholesterol : Egg PC molar ratio (0:1) for meloxicam as a function of pH over the range 3.0–7.0 ($n \geq 2$). There is a statistical difference between the *K*p[mem] at pH ≤ 4.0 and the *K*p[mem] determined at pH ≥ 5.0 (ANOVA and Spijotvoil/Stoline test, $p < 0.05$). Meloxicam prefers to partition into membranes in its acidic form, which includes three tautomeric forms: the enol, the zwitterion and the tautomer. Figure 4 shows data for diclofenac under the same conditions. Diclofenac also prefers to partition into membranes as an acidic species.

Figure 5 shows the log *K*p[mem] as a function of the amount of cholesterol in the membrane for three NSAIDs. Interestingly, there is no statistical significance in the differences in drug partitioning for meloxicam and piroxicam over the

***Figure 2** pK_a versus log Kp[mem]. The linear regression of the pK_a vs log Kp[mem] for all NSAIDs in Table 2 (excluding indomethacin Na) results in an $r^2 = 0.800$*

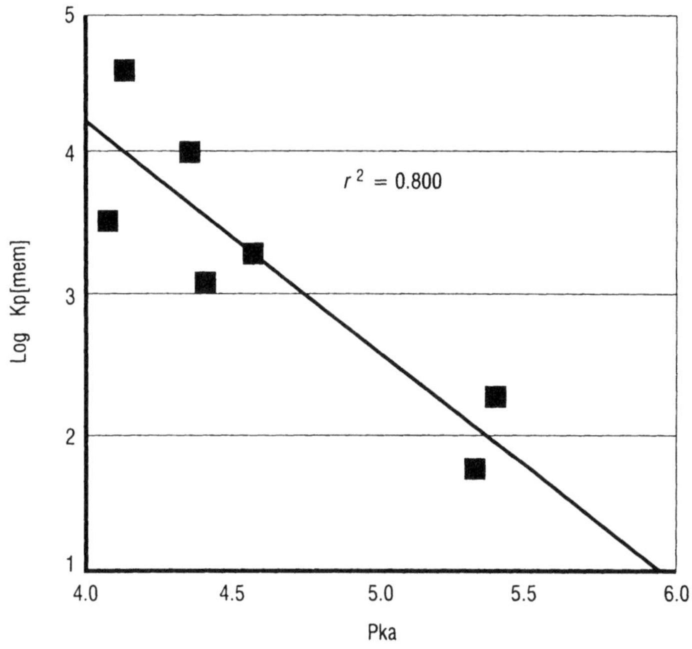

entire cholesterol range, indicating that these drugs may be located more in the upper phospholipid headgroup/glycerol backbone region of the lipid bilayer. In the case of diclofenac, a significant difference exists between 0 cholesterol and 0.6:1 cholesterol: Egg PC ($p<0.05$). Diclofenac may be penetrating more deeply into the hydrocarbon core, consistent with an overall higher *K*p[mem].

NSAID kinetic membrane parameters

Figure 6 shows the 'wash-in' curve for meloxicam in cholesterol: Egg PC (0:1) LUV at pH 4.0 and 7.0. Figure 7 shows the wash-in for meloxicam in cholesterol: Egg PC (0:1) MLV at pH 4.0 and 7.0. The time points are 5, 15, 30, 60, 120, and 180 min ($n \geq 4$ at each time point). These curves indicate a lack of a kinetic wash-in for both the LUV and MLV systems. Thus meloxicam equilibrates rapidly within membranes in <5 min, indicative of a rapid penetration into the lipid bilayer structure. Since no kinetics are observed in MLV, meloxicam must rapidly and passively transport across membranes. These data also show meloxicam to have a greater effect in MLV than in LUV, as well as at pH 4.0

Figure 3 Meloxicam Kp[mem] with varying pH. The Kp[mem] of meloxicam as determined by the radiotracer method at cholesterol : Egg PC (0 : 1) and pH 3.0–7.0. The mean Kp[mem] ($n \geq 2$) determined at pH $\leq$ 4.0 is significantly greater than that at pH > 4.0 (*$p < 0.05$)

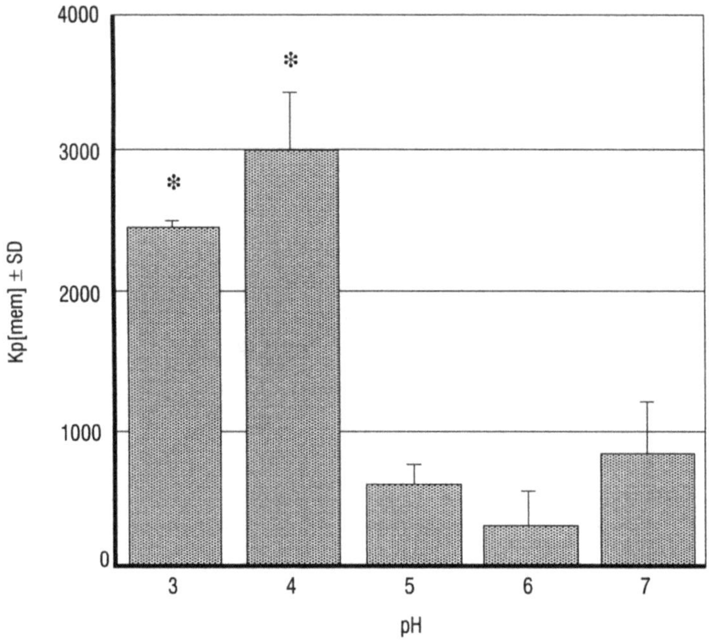

rather than pH 7.0. The most stable and consistent results for the partition coefficient of meloxicam were achieved in MLV at pH 4.0. It is important to note that the measured pK_a of meloxicam is 4.08, again indicating that the Zwitterionic species of meloxicam prefers to partition into the membrane. Figure 8 is the wash-in curve for diclofenac in cholesterol : Egg PC (0 : 1) MLV at pH 4.0. Diclofenac, like meloxicam, equilibrates rapidly into membranes with a lack of kinetics. It has a much greater *K*p[mem] than meloxicam at 30 min, by a factor of 10.

Figure 9 shows the wash-out curves for both meloxicam and diclofenac ($n = 3$ wash-out experiments per time point for each) in MLV cholesterol : Egg PC (0 : 1) at pH 4.0. The $t_{1/2}$ (time for 50% of the drug to leave the membrane) for meloxicam is 108 s (1.8 min). The $t_{1/2}$ for diclofenac is approximately twice as long at 225 s (3.75 min). Therefore, meloxicam transports more rapidly across membranes than diclofenac, even though it has a lower *K*p[mem].

*Figure 4 Diclofenac Kp[mem] with varying pH. The Kp[mem] of diclofenac as determined by the radiotracer method at cholesterol:Egg PC (0:1) and pH 3.0–7.0. The mean Kp[mem] ($n \geq 2$) determined at pH 3.0 and 4.0 (*) are significantly greater than at pH > 4.0 ($p < 0.05$), with the Kp[mem] the greatest at pH 3.0 (**$p < 0.01$)*

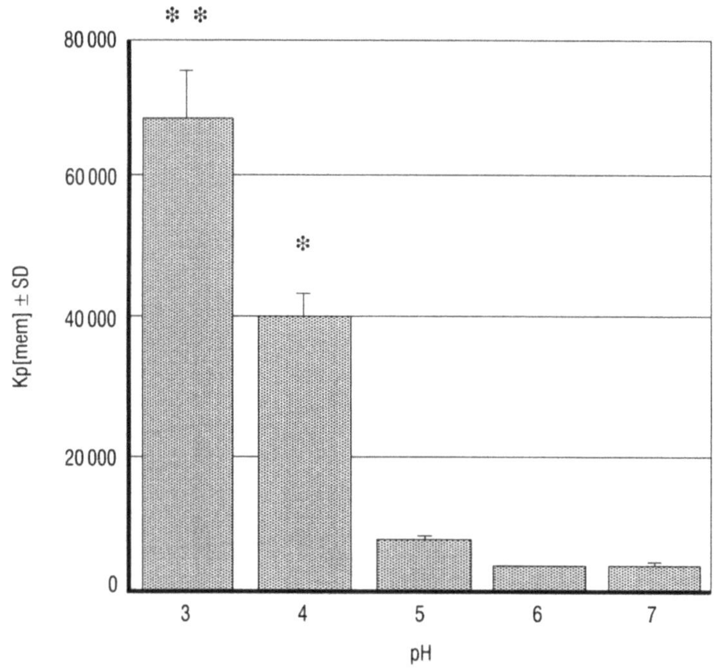

INTRACELLULAR TARGET SITE

NSAIDs are believed to target the COX enzyme system with different affinities for COX-1 and COX-2. These enzyme targets are localized in the endoplasmic reticulum/nuclear membrane network, clearly defining their localization within the cell. Interestingly, this intracellular membrane network is characterized as containing low amounts of cholesterol. NSAIDs must therefore have amphiphilic properties so that they can easily cross several membrane barriers to reach their site of action. Once administered, the concentration of NSAIDs within the plasma compartment increases rapidly and is then sustained for different periods of time, depending on their chemical structure. The NSAID must then transfer through tissue membrane structures, interacting with the plasma membrane of different cells. NSAIDs must be able to cross the plasma membrane, which usually contains relatively high amounts of cholesterol (average 0.3–0.4 mol cholesterol per mol lipid) and then traverse many intracellular barriers before

***Figure 5** The effect of cholesterol on NSAID log Kp[mem]. The molar ratio of cholesterol:Egg PC versus the log Kp[mem] of diclofenac, meloxicam and piroxicam determined potentiometrically in MLV at pH 4.0. There is no statistical significance over the entire cholesterol range for meloxicam and piroxicam. Diclofenac shows a significant difference between no cholesterol and 0.6:1 cholesterol:Egg PC*

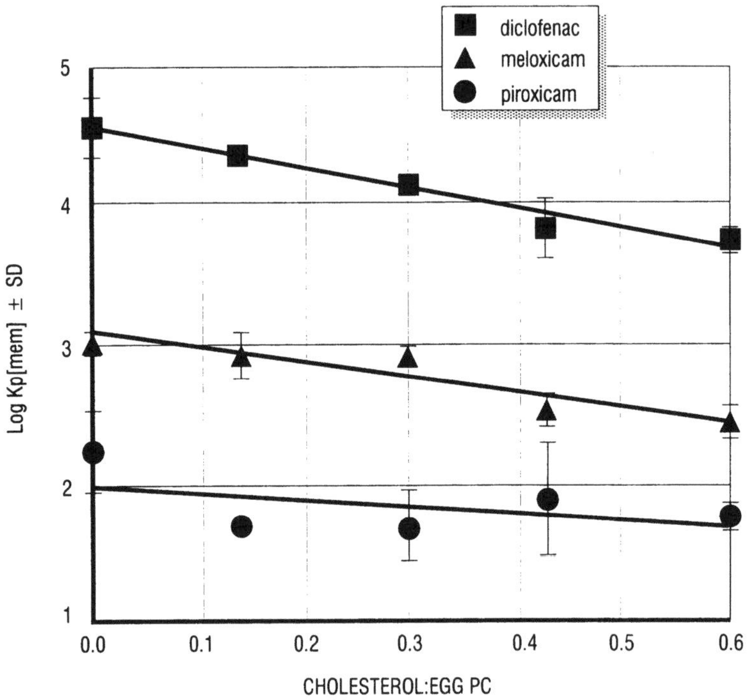

being incorporated into the endoplasmic reticulum/nuclear membrane network (Figure 10*).

In addition to this intracellular pathway, the enzyme site inhibited by NSAIDs are believed to be on the opposite side of the membrane from which the drug enters. Thus, the NSAID must exhibit other properties that clearly define its membrane interactiveness, that is, it must have good partitioning properties into the membrane environment. This allows the molecule to reach active sites on the protein from within the membrane bilayer compartment, as is believed to be the case for both COX-1 and COX-2, according to the membrane bilayer hypothesis (see Figure 1).

In summary, NSAIDs require effective intracellular transport in order to reach intracellular target membranes as part of their mechanism of action. There is also a stringent structural requirement for NSAIDs to interact strongly with cell

*See frontispiece

Figure 6 Meloxicam wash-in in LUV. The wash-in curve for meloxicam in LUV with no cholesterol at pH 4.0 and 7.0 shows meloxicam to equilibrate rapidly into membranes with a lack of kinetics

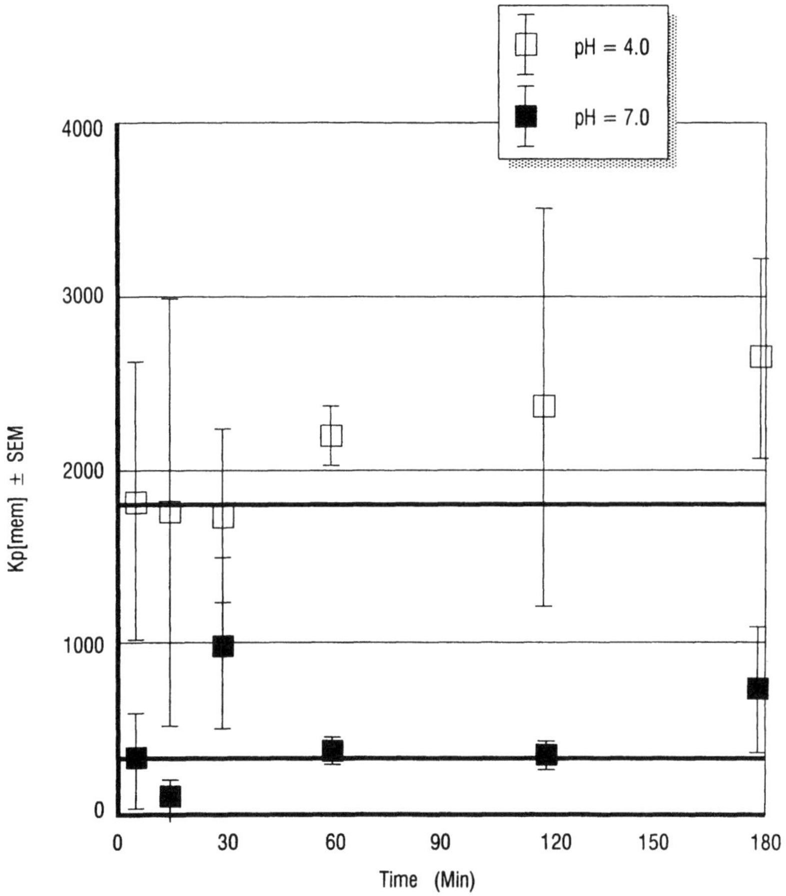

membranes in order to gain access to the COX binding site within the membrane bilayer. The ideal NSAID must both be amphiphilic (rapid membrane transport; see Figure 10) and lipophilic or membrane soluble (intrabilayer concentration of NSAID; see Figure 1).

MEMBRANE KINETICS/SOLUBILITY

The NSAIDs under study clearly show a variety of membrane interactions. It appears that the membrane partition coefficient correlates with the more acidic

Figure 7 Meloxicam wash-in in MLV. The wash-in curve for meloxicam in MLV with no cholesterol at pH 4.0 and 7.0 shows meloxicam to equilibrate rapidly into membranes with a lack of kinetics

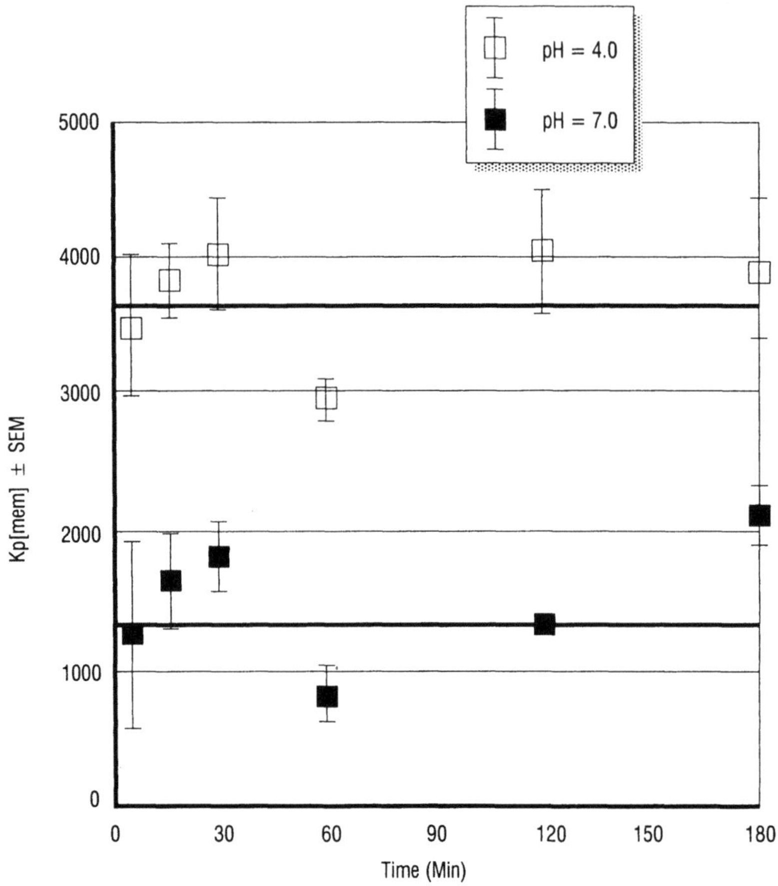

pK_a of these drugs (Figures 3 and 4). This would mean that an NSAID with a more acidic pK_a may partition more into a membrane and thus 'load' the intracellular compartment of cellular membranes more effectively.

Meloxicam has interesting membrane properties having a combination of kinetic and equilibrium parameters that result in good transport across, and solubility within, membranes. By comparison, meloxicam can enter and leave a biological membrane rapidly, indicating that it has a very high membrane transport capability. In comparative studies with diclofenac, meloxicam exhibited

***Figure 8** Diclofenac wash-in in MLV. The wash-in curve for diclofenac in MLV with no cholesterol at pH 4.0 shows diclofenac to equilibrate rapidly into membranes with a lack of kinetics. The Kp[mem] of diclofenac is approximately 10 times greater than that of meloxicam under the same conditions (see Figure 7)*

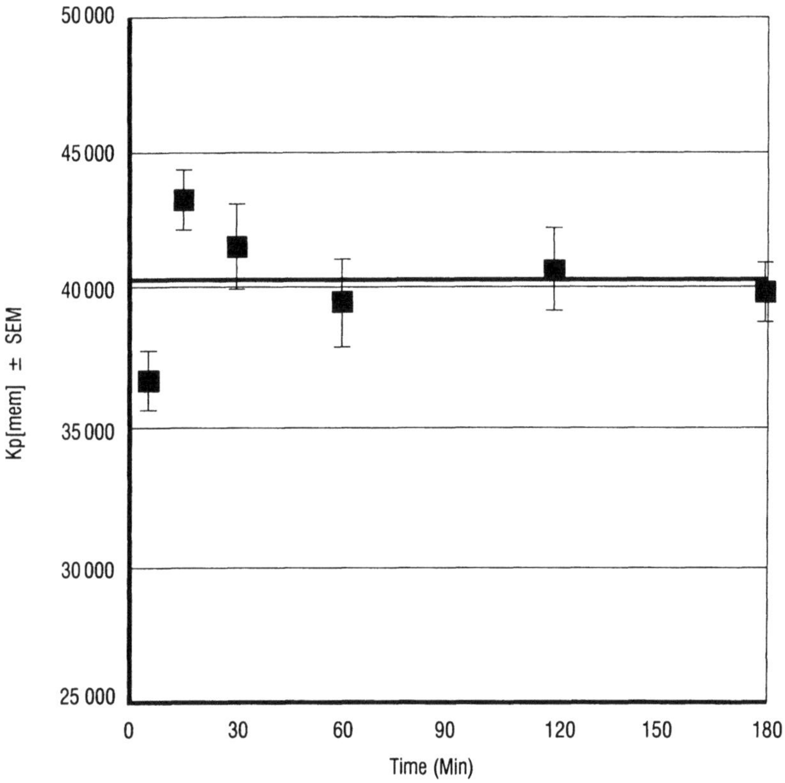

a similar transport rate into membranes, but left membranes twice as fast as diclofenac. Meloxicam also exhibits very high membrane solubility characteristics. The membrane partition coefficient of meloxicam is in the middle range: not so low that it is prevented from traversing and interacting with membranes, and not so high (as is the case with diclofenac) that it may be retained for too long in the biological membrane.

These properties fulfil the necessary criteria for the mechanism of action of NSAIDs as stated above. In addition, meloxicam exhibits the ability to be retained in multiple membrane complexes, which probably helps to prolong its duration of action in target tissues over a reasonable but not excessively long period. At the same time, meloxicam has a shorter plasma half-life than certain

Figure 9 Meloxicam and diclofenac wash-out. The wash-out curves for meloxicam and diclofenac in MLV with no cholesterol at pH 4.0 shows the $t_{1/2}$ of diclofenac (225 s) to be twice as long as that of meloxicam (108 s)

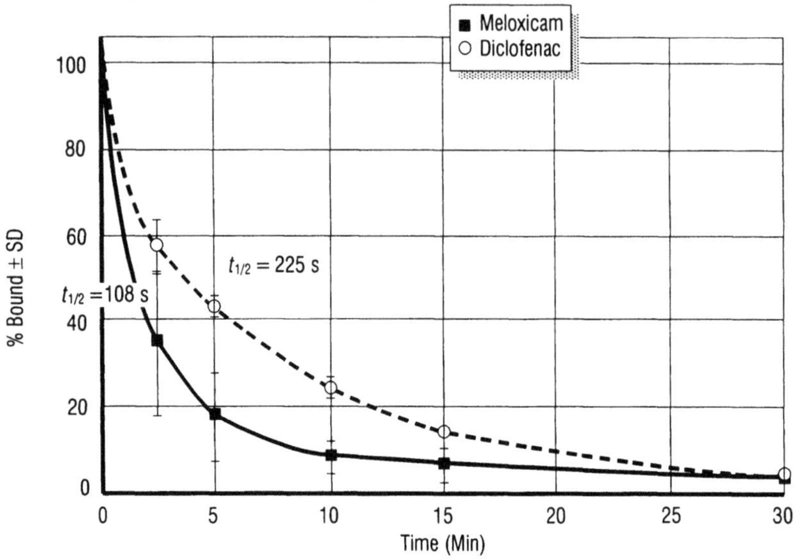

other NSAIDs. Thus, meloxicam is not retained in the plasma compartment for too long. This ensures it does not enter non-specific pathways that may lead to enhanced side effects.

NSAIDs show differential partitioning into membranes containing different amounts of cholesterol. The partitioning of diclofenac, which is highly membrane soluble, shows an inverse dependency on increasing cholesterol in membranes that is significantly different at low and high cholesterol levels. This may indicate a deeper location of diclofenac in the membrane bilayer structure. The partitioning of piroxicam and meloxicam shows no significant dependence on increasing membrane cholesterol, which may indicate a more shallow location within the membrane bilayer structure.

Partitioning of NSAIDs shows a dependence on the pH of the environment. In the case of meloxicam, there is a preference for partitioning into low pH environments which may exist intracellularly, at the target site of action. In addition, there is a large difference in the measured pK_a for piroxicam and meloxicam. The membrane partitioning coefficient of meloxicam is more than 10-fold greater than that of piroxicam which correlates with both their pK_a and their COX-2 inhibition activities as measured in vitro.

Thus, overall it appears that NSAIDs exhibit a broad range of membrane interactions which provide for differences in their intracellular pharmacokinetics.

There may be a combination of membrane properties that are optimal for NSAIDs. For example, the NSAID should exhibit efficient membrane transport in order to access target active sites, reasonable membrane solubility so that it can act on the target site, and limited retention in membranes so that high levels that lead to side effects will not be attained. It may therefore be more desirable for NSAIDs to have their pharmacokinetic control not in the plasma compartment but in the tissue/membrane compartment at the site of action, which could potentially provide a better side effect profile.

Acknowledgements

We would like to thank Boehringer Ingelheim (D-88397 Biberach, Germany) for providing the NSAID compounds and [^{3}H]meloxicam and [^{3}H]diclofenac. Also we would like to thank the staff of Sirius Analytical Ltd. (Forest Row, East Sussex, UK) and Cindy Berger of Water Technologies Inc. (Reading, PA) for their assistance and comments regarding the log *K*p[mem] titration analyses with the PCA101. Finally we would like to thank the staff of the Biomolecular Structure Analysis Center (University of Connecticut Health Center, Farmington, CT) for their dedication in keeping the facilities in optimal running condition, and especially Andrea DiMichele for her assistance with these studies.

References

1. Willard J, Lange RA and Millis LD. The use of aspirin in ischemic heart diseases. N Engl J Med. 1992;327:175–81.
2. Thun J, Namboodusi MM. Aspirin use and reduced risk of fatal colon cancer. N Engl J Med. 1991;325:1593–6.
3. Rosenberg L, Palmer JR, Zauber AG, Warshauer ME, Stolley PD, Shapiro S. A hypothesis: non-steroidal anti-inflammatory drugs reduce the incidence of large-bowel cancer. J Natl Cancer Inst. 1991;83:355–8.
4. Needleman P, Turk J, Jakschik BA, Morrison AR, Lefkowith JB. Arachidonic acid metabolism. Annu Rev Biochem. 1986;55:69–102.
5. Cashman J, McAnulty G. Nonsteroidal anti-inflammatory drugs in postsurgical pain management. Drugs. 1995;49:51–70.
6. Otto JC, DeWitt DL, Smith WL. N-glycosylation of prostaglandin endoperoxide synthases-1 and -2 and their orientations in the endoplasmic reticulum. J Biol Chem. 1993;268:18234–42.
7. Smith WL, Marnert LJ. Prostaglandin endoperoxide synthase: structure and catalysis. Biochem Biophys Acta. 1991;1083:1–17.
8. Masferrer JL, Seibert K, Zweifel B, Needleman P. Endogenous glucocorticoids regulate an inducible cyclooxygenase enzyme. Proc Natl Acad Sci USA. 1992;89:3917–21.
9. O'Banion MK, Winn VD, Young DA. cDNA cloning and functional activity of a glucocorticoid-regulated inflammatory cyclooxygenase. Proc Natl Acad Sci USA. 1992;89:4888–92.
10. Jones DA, Carlton DP, McIntyre TM, Zimmerman GA, Prescott SM. Molecular cloning of human prostaglandin endoperoxide synthase type II and demonstration of expression in response to cytokines. J Biol Chem. 1993;268:9049–54.
11. Maier JAM, Hla T, Maciag T. Cyclooxygenase is an immediate-early gene induced by interleukin-1 in human endothelial cells. J Biol Chem. 1990;265:10805–8.
12. Herschman MR. Regulation of prostaglandin synthase-1 and prostaglandin synthase-2. Cancer Metastasis Rev. 1994;13:241–56.

13. Picat S, Patrick JL, Garavito RM. The X-ray crystal structure of the membrane protein prostaglandin H_2 synthase-1. Nature. 1994;367:243–9.
14. Herbette LG. Membrane pathways for drug/ion channel interactions: molecular basis for pharmacokinetic properties. Drug Dev Res. 1994;33:214–24.
15. Meade EA, Smith WL, DeWitt DL. Differential inhibition of prostaglandin endoperoxide synthase (cyclooxygenase) isozymes by aspirin and other non-steroidal anti-inflammatory drugs. J Biol Chem. 1993;268:6610–4.
16. Mitchell J, Akarasereenont P, Thiemerman C, Flower RJ, Vane JR. Selectivity of nonsteroidal anti-inflammatory drugs as inhibitors of constitutive and inducible cyclooxygenase. Proc Natl Acad Sci USA. 1994;90:11693–7.
17. Gierse JK, Hauser SD, Creely DP et al. Expression and selective inhibition of the constitutive and inducible forms of human cyclooxygenase. Biochem J. 1995;305:479–84.
18. Masferrer JL, Zweifel BS, Manning PT et al. Selective inhibition of inducible cyclooxygenase-2 in vivo is anti-inflammatory and non-ulcerogenic. Proc Natl Acad Sci USA. 1994;91:3228–32.
19. Copeland RA, Williams JM, Giannaras J et al. Mechanism of selective inhibition of the inducible isoform of prostaglandin G/H synthase. Proc Natl Acad Sci USA. 1994;91:11202–6.
20. Reddy ST, Herschman HK. Ligand-induced prostaglandin synthase requires expression of the TIS10/PGS-2 prostaglandin synthase gene in murine fibroblasts and macrophages. J Biol Chem. 1994;269:15473–80.
21. Morita I, Schindler M, Regier MK et al. Different intracellular locations for prostaglandin endoperoxide H synthase-1 and -2. J Biol Chem. 1995;270:10902–8.
22. Colvin RA, Ashauaid TF, Herbette LG. Structure function studies of canine cardiac sarcolemmal membranes. Estimation of receptor site densities. Biochim Biophys Acta. 1985;812:601–8.
23. Rhodes DG, Sarmiento JG, Herbette LG. Kinetics of binding of 1,4-dihydropyridine to cardiac sarcolemmal receptors: diffusion limited rates for a membrane bilayer approach to the active site. Mol Pharmacol. 1985;27:612–23.
24. Enoch HG, Strittmatter P. Formation and properties of 100-Å-diameter single-bilayer phospholipid vesicles. Proc Natl Acad Sci USA. 1979;76:145–9.
25. Chester DW, Herbette LG, Mason RP, Joslyn AF, Triggle DJ, Koppel DE. Diffusion of dihydropyridine calcium channel antagonists in cardiac sarcolemmal lipid multilayers. Biophys J. 1987;52:1021–30.
26. Heider JG, Boyett RL. The picamole determination of free and total cholesterol in cells in culture. J Lipid Res. 1978;19:514–8,
27. Herbette LG, Van Erve YMH, Rhodes DG. Interaction of 1,4-dihydropyridine calcium channel antagonists with biological membranes: lipid bilayer partitioning could occur before drug binding to receptors. J Mol Cardiol. 1989;21:187–201.
28. Avdeef A. pH-Metric log P. II: Refinement of partition coefficients and ionization constants of multiprotic substances. J Pharm Sci. 1993;82:1–8.
29. Shedlovsky T. The behavior of carboxylic acids in mixed solvents. In: Pesce B, editor. Electrolytes. New York: Pergamon Press; 1962:146–51.
30. Yasuda M. Dissociation constants of some carboxylic acids in mixed aqueous solvents. Bull Chem Soc Jpn. 1959;32:429–32.
31. Tsai Ruey-Shivan, Carrupt P, Tayar NE, Giroud Y, Andrack P, Testa B. Physiochemical and structural properties of non-steroidal anti-inflammatory oxicams. Helv Chim Acta. 1993;76: 842–54.

6 Differential inhibition of COX-1 and COX-2 in vitro and pharmacological profile in vivo of NSAIDs

M. PAIRET and G. ENGELHARDT

Non-steroid antiinflammatory drugs (NSAIDs) are among the most commonly prescribed medicines. However, their therapeutic use is limited by significant adverse effects on the gastrointestinal (GI) tract[1,2] and the kidneys[3,4]. Since the demonstration by Vane[5] that inhibition of prostanoid synthesis through cyclo-oxygenase blockade is the mechanism of action of aspirin and related NSAIDs, it has been widely accepted that the mechanisms underlying both the therapeutic (i.e. anti-inflammatory) actions and the side effects of NSAIDs on the gastric mucosa, renal function and platelet aggregation are closely related.

Cyclooxygenase (COX) is part of a bifunctional enzyme, prostaglandin H synthase (PGHS), which catalyses the first step in the conversion of arachidonic acid (AA) to prostanoids, including prostaglandins (PGs), prostacyclin (PGI_2) and thromboxane A_2 (TXA_2) (Figure 1). Prostanoids (mainly prostaglandin E_2; PGE_2) are key mediators of inflammation. In addition, they have important and diverse physiological properties. PGE_2 and PGI_2 facilitate renal function and are cytoprotective for the stomach. PGI_2 released from the endothelium is also antithrombogenic, a potent vasodilator and helps maintain a non-thrombotic barrier between blood and the vessel wall. In contrast, TXA_2, which is released by platelets in response to vessel injury, is prothrombotic and acts to prevent blood loss. A new impetus has been given to the field of inflammation research by the key finding that cyclooxygenase activity can be strongly stimulated in various cell types in vitro[6–10] as well as in vivo[11]. Importantly, this increase was associated with the de novo, glucocorticoid-regulated synthesis of new COX protein[11,12]. This inducible COX protein was characterized as a distinct isoform of cyclooxygenase, named COX-2, which is encoded by a gene different from that producing the constitutive enzyme, COX-1[13–20].

The COX gene and protein structures have been reviewed by others[21–24]. COX-1 and COX-2 genes have been found on distinct chromosomes: chromosome 2 and 9 for murine and human COX-1, respectively, and chromosome 1 for both murine and human COX-2. The COX-2 gene is smaller than the COX-1 gene: 8.3 vs. 22 kb. However the size of the mRNA for COX-2 is ~4.5 whereas that for COX-1 is 2.8 kb. COX-1 and COX-2 are only 60% homologous, the residues lining the active site are almost entirely conserved and both enzymes have similar K_m and V_{max} for the metabolism of arachidonic acid. Despite the overall enzymatic similarities, there are some differences between the two isoforms. The

Figure 1 Conversion of arachidonic acid to prostaglandins, prostacyclins and thromboxanes

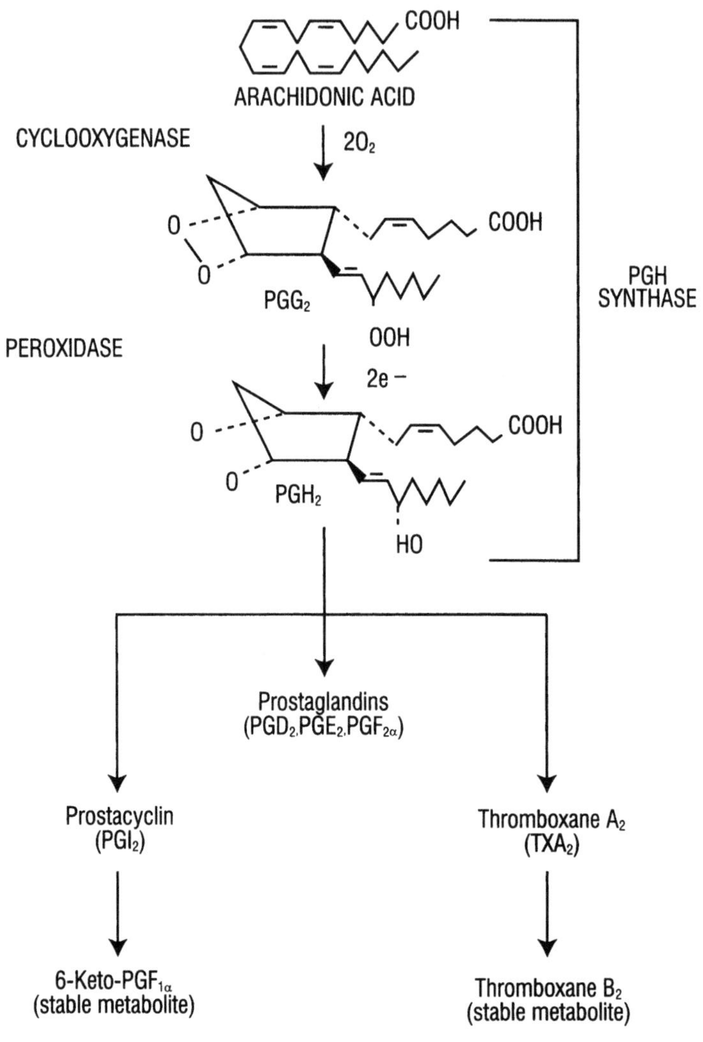

active site of COX-2, for example, seems to be larger than that of COX-1. Furthermore, the expression of COX-2 can be induced by inflammatory stimuli, hormones or mitogens, which is not the case for COX-1 (the constitutive form). Finally, glucocorticoids inhibit COX-2 but not COX-1 expression. The physicochemical properties and tissue distribution of COX-1 and COX-2 are summarized in Table 1.

Table 1 Summary of the structure, distribution and regulation of COX-1 and COX-2

	COX-1	*COX-2*
cDNA	Chromosome 2 (rodent) or 9 (human) 22 kB	Chromosome 1 8.3 kB
mRNA	2.8 kB	4.5 kB
Protein	72 kDa; 600–602 amino acids; X-ray crystal structure known	72 kDa; 603–604 amino acids
Homology	Amino acids: 90% between species for both enzymes COX-1 and COX-2: approx 60% identical, 75% similar. Similar V_{max} and K_m values for arachidonic acid	
Differences	Glucocorticoids inhibit expression of COX-2, not COX-1; the active site of COX-2 is larger than that of COX-1	
Regulation	Constitutive	Inducible
Tissue expression	Most tissues, but particularly platelet, stomach, kidney	Induced by inflammatory stimuli and mitogens in macrophages/ monocytes, synoviocytes, chondrocytes, fibroblasts, endothelial cells. Induced by hormones in the ovaries and fetal membranes. Constitutive in the CNS

Both COX-1 and COX-2 isoforms are expressed under physiological conditions in rat[25] and human[26] tissues. However, although COX-2 expression can be upregulated more than 20-fold during the inflammatory process[27–32], COX-1 activity remains unaffected or is only marginally increased (2- to 3-fold). It has therefore been proposed that COX-2 is responsible for the synthesis of inflammatory prostaglandins whereas COX-1 is a house-keeping enzyme, producing physiologically important prostanoids, for example in stomach and kidney. Consequently COX-2 is nowadays considered to be the relevant target for the therapeutic (i.e. anti-inflammatory) effects of NSAIDs, whereas inhibition of constitutive COX-1 is thought to be responsible for the gastric and renal side effects of these agents (Figure 2)[33,34]. The aim of this review is to analyse the relationship between preferential inhibition of COX-2 in vitro and improved side effect profile in vivo for NSAIDs which are commercially available or in development.

DIFFERENTIAL INHIBITION OF COX-1 AND COX-2 BY NSAIDs IN CLINICAL USE

Although standard NSAIDs are either equipotent on both COX-1 and COX-2 or preferentially inhibit COX-1, depending on the in vitro model used, some

Figure 2 Pathways of constitutive (COX-1) and inducible (COX-2) cyclooxygenases (from Ref. 33, with permission)

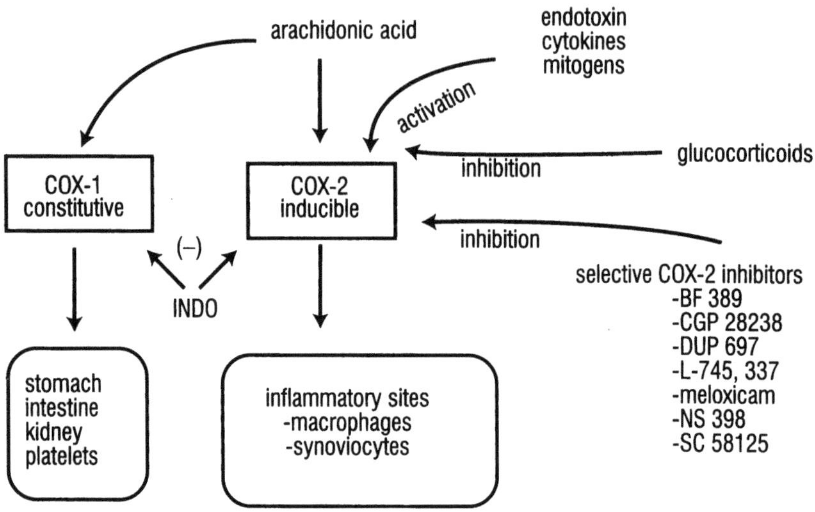

differences exist between these compounds which might explain their differing severity of gastrointestinal side effects at anti-inflammatory doses.

Various experimental models are used to test for COX-1 and COX-2 activity in vitro, including purified enzymes, cells transfected with recombinant enzymes and intact cell systems. The selectivity of the test compounds is evaluated by calculating a ratio of the IC_{50} values (concentrations which reduce prostaglandin biosynthesis by 50%) for COX-2 relative to COX-1. A ratio <1 indicates a preferential inhibition of COX-2, while a ratio >1 indicates a greater inhibitory effect on COX-1 than on COX-2. Depending on the model used, absolute IC_{50} values as well as values for the IC_{50} ratio of COX-2 vs. COX-1 vary greatly and should not be compared directly. The rank order of selectivity for COX-2 vs COX-1 within a range of compounds, however, seems to be reproducible from one model to another. This is illustrated in columns 2 and 3 of Table 2, in which IC_{50} ratios for COX-2 selectivity, obtained using two different models, are given for various NSAIDs[35,36]. Mitchell et al.[35] used bovine aortic endothelial cells as a source of COX-1 activity and endotoxin-stimulated mouse macrophages as a source of COX-2 activity. Engelhardt et al.[36] used unstimulated and lipopolysaccharide (LPS)-stimulated guinea pig macrophages to test for COX-1 and COX-2 activity, respectively. According to the figures presented, diclofenac and naproxen are approximately equipotent in inhibiting COX-1 and COX-2, ibuprofen preferentially inhibits COX-1 with a COX-2/COX-1 ratio of 15,

***Table 2** Comparison of the incidence of gastrointestinal adverse events in case control studies or spontaneous report systems and IC_{50} ratios for COX-2 relative to COX-1, for various NSAIDs in clinical use*

	Mitchell et al.[35] COX-2/COX-1 ratio	Engelhardt et al.[36] COX-2/COX-1 ratio	CSM[40] Number of ADRs per 10^6 prescriptions	Garcia Rodriguez and Jick[41] odds ratio (risk)	Langman et al.[42] odds ratio (risk)
Diclofenac	0.7	2.2	20.9	3.9	4.2
Naproxen	0.6		32.8	3.1	9.1
Ibuprofen	15		6.6		2.0
<1500 mg				2.1	
>1500 mg				6.5	
Indomethacin	60	30		6.3	11.3
Piroxicam		34	58.7	18.0	13.7

COX-2 selectivity in vitro is estimated by the ratio of the IC_{50} values of COX-2 relative to COX-1. The risk of serious clinical gastrointestinal adverse events is estimated by the number of reports per million prescriptions for spontaneous report systems[40] and by the odds ratio for case control studies[41,42]

whereas indomethacin and piroxicam, whose IC_{50} ratios vary between 30 and 60 depending on the model used, are substantially more active on COX-1 than on COX-2. Thus, it seems that some NSAIDs differentially inhibit COX-1 and COX-2. A similar conclusion can be drawn from studies using human recombinant enzymes[37,38] or human cells[39].

An important issue is the possible clinical relevance of these in vitro findings. From case control studies and spontaneous report systems published recently, it seems that the risk of GI toxicity varies markedly between the clinically available NSAIDs[2,40–42]. A comparison between COX-2 selectivity in vitro and the incidence of GI ulceration and bleeding shows that compounds which inhibit COX-1 and COX-2 with similar potency, such as diclofenac and naproxen, seem to have a lower risk of inducing serious GI adverse events than do compounds which are clearly more selective for COX-1, such as indomethacin and piroxicam. Ibuprofen is the exception since, in doses currently used in the clinic, this compound has the lowest incidence of GI toxicity in spite of preferential inhibition of COX-1 in vitro. This apparent discrepancy might be explained by the use of relatively low doses of ibuprofen (<1500 mg/day) in the clinic. When clearly anti-inflammatory doses (i.e. >1500 mg/day) were used the risk for GI toxicity was substantially higher[41]. The relationship between COX-2/COX-1 ratios in vitro and the incidence of GI side effects in the clinic is summarized in Table 2 for diclofenac, naproxen, ibuprofen, indomethacin and piroxicam.

Although high COX-2/COX-1 ratios may be related to high risks of GI side effects, the clinical efficacy and tolerability of selective COX-2 inhibition cannot yet be assessed since none of the NSAIDs in clinical use have COX-2 selectivity.

PREFERENTIAL INHIBITORS OF COX-2 IN DEVELOPMENT

A number of compounds have been described which preferentially inhibit COX-2 rather than COX-1 (Figure 3). Schematically, these compounds can be classified into two groups: substances which have been initially selected for development by drug companies because of an improved pharmacological profile in animal models, and were only later shown to preferentially inhibit COX-2 relative to COX-1; and newly designed COX-2 inhibitors, i.e. substances screened in vitro for their selectivity for COX-2, such as SC 58125 (Searle Monsanto) and L-745,337 (Merck Frosst). The former group of compounds includes meloxicam (Boehringer Ingelheim), CGP 28238 (Flosulide, Ciba Geigy Corp), NS-398 (Taisho Pharmac Co) and DuP 697 (Dupont Co). Although the development of some of these compounds has been discontinued, the pharmacological results published are useful to analyse the relationship between preferential inhibition of COX-2 in vitro and improved GI and renal tolerability in vivo. These compounds have been chosen to illustrate this review since meloxicam and flosulide are the only agents for which clinical data are available and NS-398 and DuP 697 are widely accepted pharmacological tools and have been used as lead compounds in the structure–activity relationship studies leading to the synthesis of L-745,337 and SC 58125, respectively.

Meloxicam (Boehringer Ingelheim)

Meloxicam has shown potent anti-inflammatory activity in all standard models of inflammation[43]. Comparison of the ulcerogenic dose and the effective anti-inflammatory dose in a rat model of adjuvant arthritis indicated a superior therapeutic margin in comparison with standard NSAIDs[43,44] (Table 3). This improved therapeutic margin has been correlated with preferential inhibition of COX-2 by meloxicam in various cell systems. Using unstimulated and LPS-stimulated guinea pig macrophages as sources of COX-1 and COX-2 activity, respectively, a selectivity ratio of 0.3 was found. In contrast, under the same experimental conditions, diclofenac, indomethacin and piroxicam had selectivity ratios of 2.2, 30 and 33, respectively[36] (Table 4). Using bovine aortic endothelial cells and LPS-stimulated guinea pig or mouse macrophages to test for COX-1 and COX-2 activity, respectively, a selectivity ratio of 0.2–0.8 was obtained[45]. This preferential inhibition of COX-2 has also been confirmed in studies with recombinant human enzymes[46].

Effects of meloxicam on COX-1 and COX-2 were also investigated using human intact cells, according to the model first described by Patrignani et al.[39]. Human platelets were used to test for COX-1 inhibitory activity and LPS-stimulated whole blood, i.e. mainly monocytes, were used to test for COX-2 inhibitory activity. In this model, a COX-2 to COX-1 ratio of 0.09 was found (IC_{50} values of 0.15 and 1.67 μg/ml for COX-2 and COX-1, respectively; Figure 4,

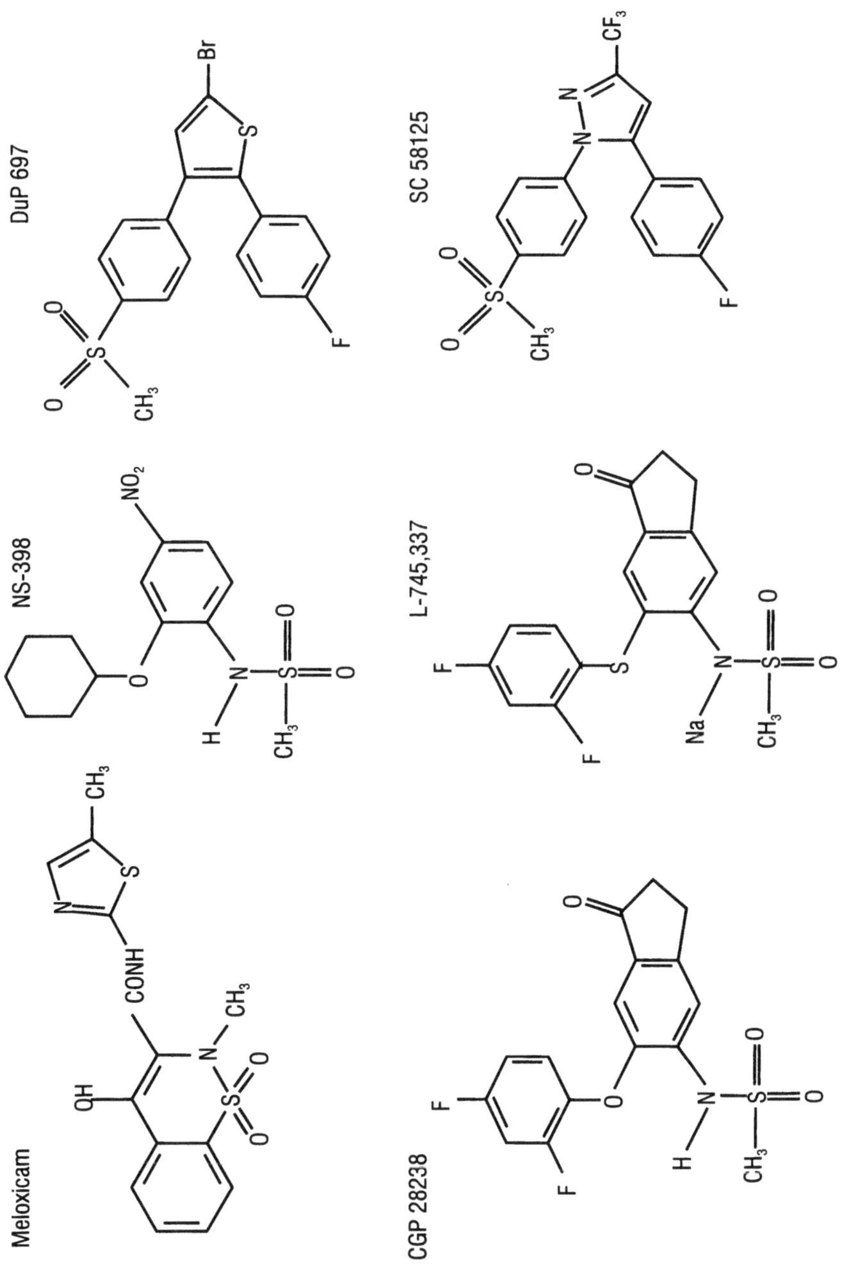

Figure 3 Some preferential inhibitors of COX-2 in development

***Table 3** Comparison of the oral therapeutic indices of test compounds with respect to their ulcerogenic effects on the stomach of the rat and their inhibitory effects on the secondary reaction (swelling) to adjuvant of rat hind paw (from Ref. 43)*

NSAID	*ED_{50} ulcer (mg/kg/day)*	*ID_{50} swelling (mg/kg/day)*	*Therapeutic index*
Meloxicam	2.47 (1.64–3.56)	0.12 (0.09–0.14)	20
Piroxicam	1.07 (0.86–1.41)	0.76 (0.49–1.52)	1.4
Indomethacin	2.35 (1.96–2.82)	0.67 (0.50–0.95)	3.5
Diclofenac	2.71 (2.38–3.09)	1.24 (0.84–2.68)	2.2
Naproxen	11.1 (7.84–15.6)	11.8 (8.12–14.9)	0.9

***Table 4** Selectivity of various NSAIDs against COX-1 and COX-2 in guinea pig macrophages (from Ref. 36)*

	Inhibition of COX-1 and COX-2: IC_{50} (nmol/l)				
	Meloxicam	*Diclofenac*	*Indomethacin*	*Piroxicam*	*Flurbiprofen*
COX-1 (no LPS)	5.77 (4.56–7.21)	0.86 (0.58–1.17)	0.21 0.13–0.31)	5.27 (3.58–7.41)	15.0 (8.6–28.2)
COX-2 (+LPS)	1.91 (1.40–2.69)	1.91 (1.47–2.39)	6.39 (4.97–8.04)	175 (149–202)	4760 (1270–12700)
Ratio COX-2/COX-1	0.33	2.2	30	33	317

Values are mean (95% confidence limit)

and unpublished data). In vivo, in the rat, meloxicam inhibited prostaglandin biosynthesis more potently at the site of inflammation than in the gastric mucosa or the kidney[47]. Data comparing the inhibitory activity of some NSAIDs on PG synthesis in the rat, in an inflammatory exudate (carrageenan-induced pleurisy) and in kidney (urine levels) are summarized in Table 5. A ratio was calculated by dividing the ID_{50} (i.e. the dose reducing PG concentration in the urine by 50%) by the ID_{50} for reducing PG concentration in the exudate. Meloxicam was shown to affect renal PG synthesis less than diclofenac, naproxen, flurbiprofen and tenidap. The preferential inhibition of COX-2 and the improved side effect profile of meloxicam were shown to be highly dependent on the specific molecular structure of the drug, since even minor chemical modifications led to a loss of COX-2 selectivity and to a less favourable side effect profile[48] (Figure 5). IC_{50} values for COX-1 and COX-2 as well as effective anti-inflammatory doses, doses inducing GI erosions and reducing urinary excretion of prostaglandins are summarized in Tables 6 and 7 for piroxicam, meloxicam and the 4′-isomer of meloxicam. An improved side effect profile over standard NSAIDs has been confirmed in man in an endoscopy study[49] and in clinical trials[50].

***Figure 4** Effects of meloxicam on the activity of platelet COX-1 and monocyte COX-2. COX-1 and COX-2 activities were investigated in a 'human whole blood assay'. Briefly, peripheral blood samples were drawn from healthy volunteers before and 48 h after the oral administration of 300 mg of aspirin. Aliquots of blood from donors who had not taken aspirin were immediately transferred into glass tubes and allowed to clot at 37°C for 60 min. TXB2 production, measured in serum, was taken as a reflection of platelet COX-1 activity. Aliquots of heparinized blood from donors who had taken aspirin (to suppress the contribution of platelet COX-1 activity) were incubated in the presence of 10 μg/ml LPS for 24 h at 37°C (to induce COX-2 in monocytes). Plasma was then separated by centrifugation and PGE_2 production was taken as a marker of COX-2 activity. Results are presented as mean percentage inhibition of cyclooxygenase activity with n = 4 for each concentration*

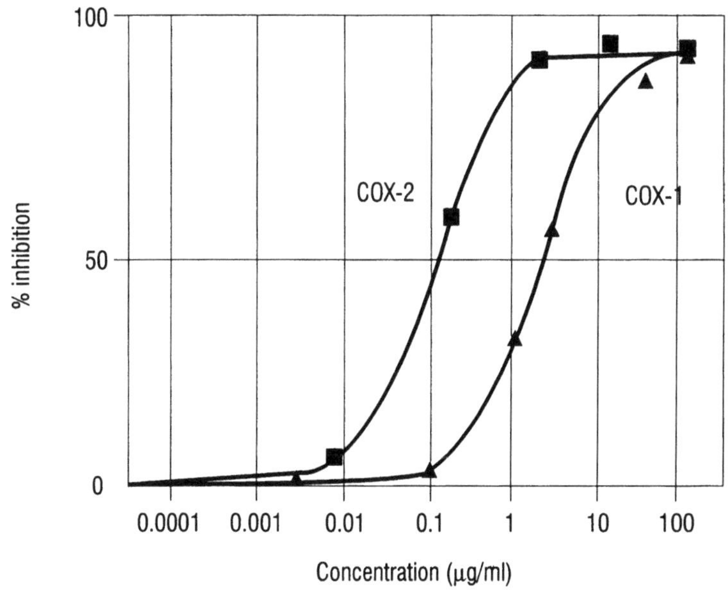

***Table 5** Comparison of PG biosynthesis inhibition by NSAIDs in pleuritic exudate and in urine (from Ref. 47)*

	Inhibition of PGE_2 synthesis in vivo: ID_{50} (mg/kg)				
	Meloxicam	*Diclofenac*	*Piroxicam*	*Flurbiprofen*	*Tenidap*
Pleuritic exudate	0.65 (0.54–0.78)	5.06 (3.72–6.63)	0.85 (0.60–1.09)	2.18 (1.78–2.75)	12.8 (9.62–18.0)
Urinary excretion	1.85 (1.05–2.78)	1.86 (1.23–2.55)	0.24 (0.10–0.41)	0.26 (0.11–0.58)	0.64 (0.23–1.50)
Safety ratio	2.9	0.4	0.3	0.1	<0.1

Values are mean (95% confidence limits)

Figure 5 Structure of meloxicam and its 4′ isomer

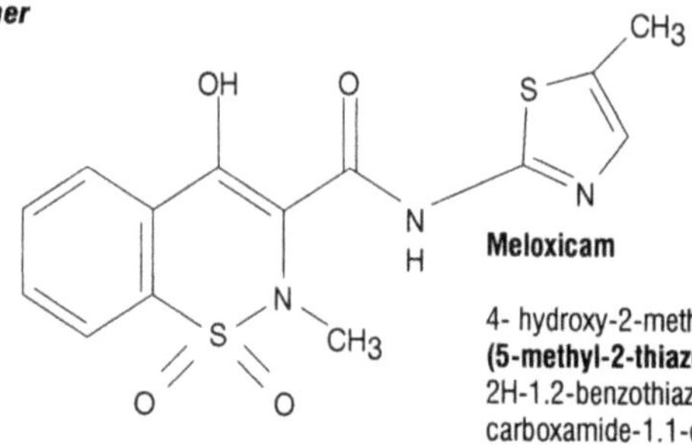

Meloxicam

4- hydroxy-2-methyl-N-
(5-methyl-2-thiazolyl)
2H-1.2-benzothiazine-3-
carboxamide-1.1-dioxide

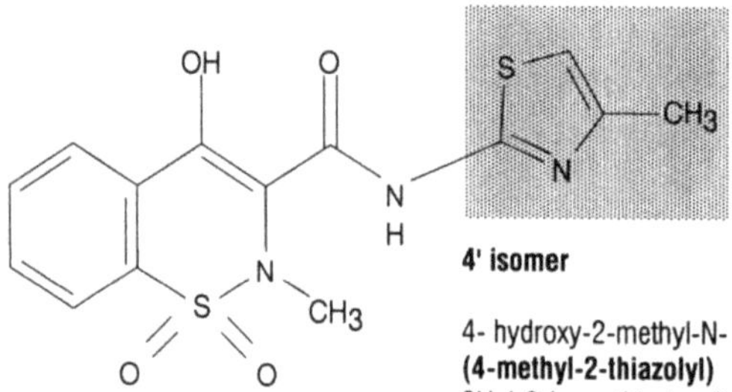

4′ isomer

4- hydroxy-2-methyl-N-
(4-methyl-2-thiazolyl)
2H-1.2-benzothiazine-3-
carboxamide-1.1-dioxide

Table 6 Summary of IC_{50} values for piroxicam, the 4′-isomer of meloxicam and meloxicam on cyclooxygenase activity in BAEC (COX-1), mouse and guinea pig macrophages (COX-2)

		Piroxicam	*4′-isomer*	*Meloxicam*
BAEC	IC_{50}	$2.4 \pm 0.2 \times 10^{-9}$ M	$4.3 \pm 1.0 \times 10^{-9}$ M	$2.1 \pm 0.4 \times 10^{-7}$ M
Mouse macrophages	IC_{50}	$6.0 \pm 0.8 \times 10^{-7}$ M	$5.7 \pm 1.5 \times 10^{-7}$ M	$1.7 \pm 0.3 \times 10^{-7}$ M
Guinea pig macrophages	IC_{50}	$1.7 \pm 0.1 \times 10^{-7}$ M	$1.3 \pm 0.2 \times 10^{-7}$ M	$0.5 \pm 0.1 \times 10^{-7}$ M

IC_{50} values, calculated from at least 4 drug concentrations, are given as mean ± SE, $n = 8-18$ for each concentration

Table 7 Effect of piroxicam, the 4′-isomer of meloxicam and meloxicam on adjuvant arthritis, induction of GI erosions and urinary excretion of PGE_2 in the rat. 95% confidence limits are given in brackets

	ED_{50} (mg/kg/day)		
	Piroxicam	*4′-isomer*	*Meloxicam*
Adjuvant arthritis			
Primary reaction	0.7 (0.5–1.1)	0.4 (0.3–0.5)	0.3 (0.1–0.6)
Secondary reaction	0.8 (0.5–1.8)	0.2 (0.1–0.3)	0.1 (0.0–0.2)
GI erosions	1.1 (0.9–1.4)	0.4 (0.2–0.6)	2.4 (1.6–3.5)
Urinary excretion	0.3 (0.1–0.5)	0.2 (0.0–0.5)	1.1 (0.5–1.7)

CGP 28238 (Flosulide: Ciba Geigy Corp)

Like meloxicam, the in vivo pharmacology of CGP 28238 was known before COX-2 was characterized and cloned. As early as 1989 the compound was described as a potent NSAID with an improved gastric tolerance which did not inhibit cyclooxygenase in a bovine seminal vesicle preparation[51]. A relative lack of activity against COX-1 was later found when using human washed platelets (IC_{50} 72 μM), whereas COX-2 activity from IL-1-stimulated mesangial cells was inhibited with an IC_{50} of 25 nM. This yields a COX-2/COX-1 ratio of 0.0002[52]. Under these experimental conditions, however, the COX-2/COX-1 ratios are consistently rather low, as illustrated by a 0.07 value for diclofenac. Nevertheless, the improved gastric tolerance of CGP 28238 has been confirmed in humans, in a comparative endoscopy study with naproxen[53].

NS-398 (Taisho Pharmac Co)

NS-398 was also first characterized in vivo where it inhibited prostanoid production in inflamed tissue (rat carrageenan air pouch) more potently (ID_{50} 0.2 mg/kg p.o.) than in the gastric mucosa (ID_{50} 62 mg/kg) or the renal papillary tissue (ID_{50} 262 mg/kg)[54]. In standard models of inflammation in the rat it was almost as potent as indomethacin, whereas no gastric ulcerations were seen at doses up to 1000 mg/kg (single oral dose)[55]. It was later shown to inhibit COX-2 activity of sheep placenta with an IC_{50} of 4 μM whereas COX-1 activity of ram seminal vesicle was unaffected at this concentration[56]. This COX-2 selectivity has been confirmed using human recombinant enzymes[57,58] as well as in human cells[59].

DuP 697 (Dupont Co)

DuP 697 was reported some years ago to be a potent inhibitor of paw swelling in adjuvant arthritis with an ID_{50} of 0.2 mg/kg/day p.o., but it did not cause gastric ulcers or alter renal blood flow in rats at doses up to 400 mg/kg[60]. A preferential inhibition of COX-2 relative to COX-1 was later demonstrated using human recombinant enzymes expressed in insect cells[57,61].

L-745,337 (Merck Frosst)

In whole cell assays, this compound inhibited COX-2 with a selectivity ratio of <0.01[59,62]. In the rat, it inhibited carrageenan-induced paw oedema with an ED_{50} of 2.0 mg/kg p.o. and prevented hyperalgesia with an ED_{50} of 0.4 mg/kg p.o. but caused no gastric ulceration at doses up to 30 mg/kg[62,63]. No gastrointestinal bleeding was detected in a ^{51}Cr excretion assay in the monkey at doses of 10 mg/kg twice daily for 5 days[62]. This compound is in preclinical development.

SC 58125 (Searle Monsanto)

SC 58125 is the prototype of a series of pyrazole derivatives which exhibited COX-2 selectivity in mouse[64] or human recombinant enzymes[65], with a COX-2/COX-1 ratio of <0.001. SC 58125 inhibited oedema in a rat model of acute inflammation (injection of carrageenan into the footpad) but had no effect on PG production in the stomach and did not cause gastric toxicity[64]. A follow-up compound, SC 58635, has been selected for clinical development.

SOME CRITICAL ISSUES

The good relationship found between preferential inhibition of COX-2 relative to COX-1 in vitro and improved pharmacological profile in vivo for various NSAIDs supports the hypothesis that preferential inhibition of COX-2 may maximize (or at least retain) the anti-inflammatory activity while minimizing the gastric and renal side effects of anti-inflammatory drugs, some critical issues still remain, however, concerning the predictive value of the in vitro models used to test for COX-2 selectivity, the role of COX-1 in inflammation and the physiological and pathophysiological relevance of COX-2 expression in conditions other than inflammatory states.

In vitro models

Various experimental models are used to test for COX-1 and COX-2 activity in vitro, including purified enzymes, cells transfected with recombinant enzymes and intact cell systems. The experimental conditions may vary greatly from one model to the other: various COX-2-inducing agents (lipopolysaccharide, IL-1, etc.) have been used, different incubation times with the test compounds (from a few seconds to 24h) or the COX-2-inducing agent (from 1 to 24h) have been reported, finally COX activity has been evaluated by measuring prostaglandin or thromboxane synthesis from arachidonic acid, whether endogenous or exogenously administered. Depending on the model used, absolute IC_{50} values, as well as values for the IC_{50} ratio of COX-2 vs COX-1, vary greatly and should not be compared directly. The rank order of selectivity for COX-2 vs COX-1 within a range of compounds, however, seems to be reproducible from one model to another. Preferential inhibition of COX-2 can only be assumed when converging comparative data are available from several models.

Role of COX-1 in inflammation?

It is currently accepted that only COX-2 expression can be upregulated >20-fold by inflammatory stimuli whereas COX-1 activity is only marginally affected. This theory is supported by several studies using various cell types, including macrophages/monocytes[9,11,12,29,66–70], synoviocytes[71,72] or endothelial cells[20,73,74]. Contradictory results also exist from rat macrophages, however. These demonstrate that COX-1 plays a major role in prostaglandin synthesis in both the basal and stimulated states[75], suggesting a possible role for COX-1 also in inflammation. Furthermore, a positive feedback mechanism between PGE_2 and COX-2 has been described, suggesting that COX-1 inhibitors may down-regulate COX-2 expression through inhibition of basal PGE_2 synthesis[76].

Physiological relevance of COX-2 expression in various tissues?

Although COX-1 functions predominantly in the stomach and the kidney, a certain amount of COX-2 has also been observed in both organs[26,77,78]. The physiological relevance of COX-2 expression in these organs has still to be more thoroughly investigated. A role for COX-2 has been suggested in the reproductive tract, in the induction of ovulation[79] and parturition[80], in the CNS, in the processing of visceral and special sensory inputs[81] and during neuronal injury and necrosis[82], in respiratory inflammatory diseases such as asthma[83] and in intestinal tumour growth[84,85].

CONCLUSIONS

The discovery of an inducible isoform (COX-2) of cyclooxygenase necessitates a reinterpretation of the theory that both the therapeutic (i.e. anti-inflammatory) activity and the gastric and renal side effects of NSAIDs are due to a common mechanism of action. The good relationship found between preferential inhibition of COX-2 relative to COX-1 in vitro and improved pharmacological profile in vivo for various NSAIDs supports the hypothesis that preferential inhibition of COX-2 may maximize (or at least retain) the anti-inflammatory activity while minimizing the gastric and renal side effects of anti-inflammatory drugs. However, a role of COX-1 in inflammation cannot be excluded, since a positive feedback mechanism has been shown to exist between PGE_2 and COX-2 and COX-1 activity has been shown during prostaglandin synthesis in both the basal and stimulated states in rat macrophages. Furthermore, the physiological relevance of COX-2 expression in the gastric mucosa and the kidney has still to be more thoroughly investigated. Therefore the optimal selectivity ratio for COX-2 over COX-1 is not yet known. The development of compounds which preferentially inhibit COX-2 relative to COX-1 will provide the opportunity to evaluate such issues.

Finally, experimental results on COX-2 expression during various pathological conditions suggest that new potential therapeutic indications might emerge in the future for selective COX-2 inhibitors, including neuronal injury, pain, asthma, management of preterm delivery as well as adjunctive therapy in the management of large bowel adenomas and/or carcinomas.

References

1. Lichtenstein DR, Syngal S, Wolfe M. Nonsteroidal antiinflammatory drugs and the gastrointestinal tract. Arthritis Rheum. 1995;1:5-18.
2. Rainsford KD, Quadir M. Gastrointestinal damage and bleeding from non-steroidal antiinflammatory drugs. I. Clinical and epidemiological aspects. Immunopharmacology. 1995;3: 169-90.
3. Carmichael J, Shankel SW. Effects of nonsteroidal anti-inflammatory drugs on prostaglandins and renal function. Am J Med. 1985;78:992-1000.
4. Murray MD, Brater DC. Renal toxicity of nonsteroidal anti-inflammatory drugs. Annu Rev Pharmacol Toxicol. 1993;32:435-65.
5. Vane JR. Inhibition of prostaglandin synthesis as a mechanism of action of aspirin-like drugs. Nature (New Biol). 1971;231:232-5.
6. Raz A, Wyche A, Siegel N, Needleman P. Regulation of fibroblast cyclooxygenase synthesis by interleukin-1. J Biol Chem. 1988;263:3022-5.
7. Raz A, Wyche A, Needleman P. Temporal and pharmacological division of fibroblast cyclooxygenase expression into transcriptional and translation phases. Proc Natl Acad Sci USA. 1989;86:1657-61.
8. Rosen GD, Birkenmeier TM, Raz A, Holtzman MJ. Identification of cyclooxygenase-related gene and its potential role in prostaglandin formation. Biochem Biophys Res Commun. 1989; 164:1358-65.
9. Fu JY, Masferrer JL, Seibert K, Raz A, Needleman P. The induction and suppression of prostaglandin H_2 synthase (cyclooxygenase) in human monocytes. J Biol Chem. 1990;265: 16737-40.
10. Wong WYL, DeWitt DL, Smith WL, Richards JS. Rapid induction of prostaglandin endoperoxide synthase induced by luteinizing hormone and cAMP is blocked by inhibitors of transcription and translation. Mol Endocrinol. 1989;3:1714-23.
11. Masferrer JL, Zweifel BS, Seibert K, Needleman P. Selective regulation of cellular cyclooxygenase by dexamethasone and endotoxin in mice. J Clin Invest. 1990;86:1375-9.
12. Masferrer JL, Seibert K, Zweifel BS, Needleman P. Endogenous glucocorticoids regulate an inducible cyclooxygenase enzyme. Proc Natl Acad Sci USA. 1992;89:3917-21.
13. Kujubu DA, Fletcher BS, Varnum BC, Lim RW, Herschman HR. TIS10, a phorbol ester tumor promoter-inducible mRNA from Swiss 3T3 cells, encodes a novel prostaglandin synthase/cyclooxygenase homologue. J Biol Chem. 1991;266:12866-72.
14. Xie W, Chipman JG, Robertson DL, Erikson RL, Simmons DL. Expression of a mitogen-responsive gene encoding prostaglandin synthase is regulated by mRNA splicing. Proc Natl Acad Sci USA. 1991;88:1692-6.
15. Hla T, Neilson K. Human cyclooxygenase-2 cDNA. Proc Natl Acad Sci USA. 1992;89:7384-8.
16. Kujubu DA, Herschman HR. Dexamethasone inhibits mitogen induction of the TIS10 prostaglandin synthase/cyclooxygenase gene. J Biol Chem. 1992;267:7991-4.
17. O'Banion MK, Winn VD, Young DA. cDNA cloning and functional activity of a glucocorticoid-regulated inflammatory cyclooxygenase. Proc Natl Acad Sci USA. 1992;89:4888-92.
18. Sirois J, Simmons DL, Richards JS. Hormonal regulation of messenger ribonucleic acid encoding a novel isoform of prostaglandin endoperoxide H synthase in rat preovulatory follicles. J Biol Chem. 1992;267:11586-92.
19. DeWitt DL, Meade EA. Serum and glucocorticoid regulation of gene transcription and expression of the prostaglandin H synthase-1 and prostaglandin H synthase-2 isozymes. Arch Biochem Biophys. 1993;306:94-102.
20. Jones DA, Carlton DP, McIntyre TM, Zimmerman GA, Prescott SM. Molecular cloning of human prostaglandin endoperoxide synthase type II and demonstration of expression in response to cytokines. J Biol Chem. 1993;268:9049-54.
21. Smith WL, Marnett LJ. Prostaglandin endoperoxide synthase: structure and catalysis. Biochim Biophys Acta. 1991;1083:1-17.
22. Xie W, Robertson DL, Simmons DL. Mitogen-inducible prostaglandin G/H synthase: a new target for nonsteroidal antiinflammatory drugs. Drug Dev Res. 1992;25:249-65.
23. Loll PL, Garavito RM. The isoforms of cyclooxygenase: structure and function. Curr Opin Invest Drugs. 1994;3:1171-80.

24. Goppelt-Struebe M. Regulation of prostaglandin endoperoxide synthase (cyclooxygenase) isozyme expression. Prostaglandins Leukotrienes Essential Fatty Acids. 1995;52:213–22.
25. Feng L, Sun W, Xia Yet al. Cloning two isoforms of rat cyclooxygenase: differential regulation of their expression. Arch Biochem Biophys. 1993;307:361–88.
26. O'Neill GP, Ford-Hutchinson AW. Expression of mRNA for cyclooxygenase-1 and cyclooxygenase-2 in human tissues. FEBS Lett. 1993;330:156–60.
27. Sano H, Hla T, Maier JAM et al. In vivo cyclooxygenase expression in synovial tissues of patients with rheumatoid arthritis and rats with adjuvant and streptococcal cell wall arthritis. J Clin Invest. 1992;89:97–108.
28. Hla T, Ristimäki A, Appleby S, Barriocanal JG. Cyclooxygenase gene expression in inflammation and angiogenesis. Ann NY Acad Sci. 1993;696:197–204.
29. Masferrer JL, Zweifel BS, Manning PT et al. Selective inhibition of inducible cyclooxygenase 2 in vivo is antiinflammatory and nonulcerogenic. Proc Natl Acad Sci USA. 1994;91:3228–32.
30. Vane JR, Mitchell JA, Appleton I et al. Inducible isoforms of cyclooxygenase and nitric-oxide synthase in inflammation. Proc Natl Acad Sci USA. 1994;91:2046–50.
31. Cavanaugh PF Jr, McDonald JS, Pavelic L, Limardi RJ, Gluckman JL, Pavelic ZP. Immunohistochemical localization of prostaglandin H synthase isoenzyme proteins in the gingival tissue of patients with periodontitis. Immunopharmacology. 1995;3:109–19.
32. Harada Y, Hatanaka K, Saito M et al. Cyclooxygenase-2 in the rat carrageenin-induced pleurisy [abstract]. Jpn J Pharmacol. 1995;67(Suppl 1):S43–4.
33. Battistini B, Botting R, Bakhle YS. COX-1 and COX-2: toward the development of more selective NSAIDs. Drug News Perspect. 1994;7:501–12.
34. Vane JR. Towards a better aspirin. Nature. 1994;367:215–6.
35. Mitchell JA, Akarasereenont P, Thiemermann C, Flower RJ, Vane J. Selectivity of nonsteroidal antiinflammatory drugs as inhibitors of constitutive and inducible cyclooxygenase. Proc Natl Acad Sci USA. 1994;90:11693–7.
36. Engelhardt G, Bögel R, Schnitzler C, Utzmann R. Meloxicam: Influence on arachidonic acid metabolism. Part I. In vitro findings. Biochem Pharmacol. 1995 (in press).
37. Laneuville O, Breuer DK, Dewitt DL, Hla T, Funk CD, Smith WD. Differential inhibition of human prostaglandin endoperoxide H synthases-1 and -2 by nonsteroidal anti-inflammatory drugs. J Pharmacol Exp Ther. 1994;271:927–34.
38. O'Neill GP, Mancini JA, Kargman S et al. Overexpression of human prostaglandin G/H synthase-1 and -2 by recombinant vaccinia virus: inhibition by nonsteroidal anti-inflammatory drugs and biosynthesis of 15-hydroxyeicosatetraenoic acid. Mol Pharmacol. 1994;45:245–54.
39. Patrignani P, Panara MR, Greco A et al. Biochemical and pharmacological characterization of the cyclooxygenase activity of human blood prostaglandin endoperoxide synthases. J Pharmacol Exp Ther. 1994;271:1705–10
40. CSM update. Non-steroidal anti-inflammatory drugs and serious gastrointestinal adverse reactions-2. Br Med J. 1986;292:1190–91.
41. Garcia Rodriguez LA, Jick H. Risks of upper gastrointestinal bleeding and perforation associated with individual non-steroidal anti-inflammatory drugs. Lancet. 1994;343:769–72.
42. Langman WJ, Weil J, Wainwright P et al. Risks of bleeding peptic ulcer associated with individual non-steroidal anti-inflammatory drugs. Lancet. 1994;343:1075–8.
43. Engelhardt G, Homma D, Schlegel K, Utzmann R, Schnitzler C. Anti-inflammatory, analgesic antipyretic and related properties of meloxicam, a new non-steroidal anti-inflammatory agent with favourable gastrointestinal tolerance. Inflammation Res. 1995;44:423–33.
44. Engelhardt G, Homma D, Schnitzler C. Meloxicam: a potent inhibitor of adjuvant arthritis in the Lewis rat. Inflammation Res. 1995. (in press).
45. Pairet M, Engelhardt G, Lidbury P, Vane JR. Meloxicam: cyclooxygenase selectivity, anti-inflammatory activity and gastric and renal safety. Inflamm Res. 1995;44(Suppl. 3):S274.
46. Churchill L, Graham A, Garina P, Grob P. Inhibition of human cyclooxygenase-2 (COX-2) by meloxicam. Rheumatol Eur. 1995;24(Suppl. 3):D205.
47. Engelhardt S, Bögel R, Schnitzler C, Utzmann R. Meloxicam: Influence on arachidonic acid metabolism. Part II. In vivo findings. Biochem Pharmacol. 1995 (in press).
48. Pairet M, Engelhardt G. The preferential inhibition of COX-2 by meloxicam is highly dependent of the structure of the drug. Rheumatol Eur. 1995;24(Suppl. 3):D204.
49. Patoia L, Santucci L, Furno P et al. Comparison of gastrointestinal tolerability of meloxicam,

piroxicam and placebo by fecal blood loss, endoscopy and symptom evaluation. Rheumatol Eur. 1995;24(Suppl. 3):E258.
50. Distel M, Mueller C, Blumkhi E. Global analysis of safety of a new NSAID, meloxicam. Rheumatol Eur. 1995;24(Suppl. 3):E259.
51. Wiesenberg-Boettcher I, Schweizer A, Green JR, Mueller K, Maerki F, Pfeilschifter J. The pharmacological profile of CGP 28238, a novel highly potent anti-inflammatory compound. Drugs Exp Clin Res. 1989;15:501-9.
52. Klein T, Nüsing RM, Pfeilschifter J, Ullrich V. Selective inhibition of cyclooxygenase 2. Biochem Pharmacol. 1994;48:1605-10.
53. Bjarnason I, Hayllar J, Parker J, Schupp J, Macpherson A. A randomised, double blind, crossover comparative endoscopy study on gastroduodenal tolerability of flosulide and naproxen. Gastroenterology. 1994;106(Suppl. 4):A53.
54. Futaki N, Arai I, Hamasaka Y, Takahashi S, Higuchi S, Otomo S. Selective inhibition of NS-398 on prostanoid production in inflamed tissue in rat carrageenan-air-pouch inflammation. J Pharm Pharmacol. 1992;45:735-55.
55. Futaki N, Yoshikawa K, Hamasaka Y et al. NS-398, a novel non-steroidal anti-inflammatory drug with potent analgesic and antipyretic effects, which causes minimal stomach lesions. Gen Pharmacol. 1993;24:105-10.
56. Futaki N, Takahashi S, Yokoyama M, Arai I, Higuchi S, Otomo S. NS-398, a new anti-inflammatory agent, selectively inhibits prostaglandin G/H synthase/cyclooxygenase (COX-2) activity in vitro. Prostaglandins. 1994;47:55-9.
57. Gierse JK, Hauser SD, Creely DP et al. Expression and selective inhibition of the constitutive and inducible forms of human cyclo-oxygenase. Biochem J. 1995;305:479-84.
58. Ouellet M, Percival MD. Effector of inhibitor time-dependency and selectivity towards cyclo-oxygenase isoforms. Biochem J. 1995;306:247-51.
59. Patrignani P, Panara M, Greco A et al. The antiinflammatory compounds L-745,337 and NS-398 are selective inhibitors of prostaglandin endoperoxide synthase-2 in human blood monocytes. Pharmacol Res. 1995;31(Suppl):311.
60. Gans KR, Gabraight W, Roman RJ et al. Anti-inflammatory and safety profile of DuP 6976, a novel orally effective prostaglandin synthesis inhibitor. J Pharmacol Exp Ther. 1990;254:180-7.
61. Copeland RA, Williams JM, Giannaras J et al. Mechanism of selective inhibition of the inducible form of prostaglandin G/H synthase. Proc Natl Acad Sci USA. 1994;91:11202-6.
62. Chan CC, Boyce S, Brideau C et al. Pharmacology of a selective cyclooxygenase-2 inhibitor, L-745,337: a novel nonsteroidal anti-inflammatory agent with an ulcerogenic sparing effect in rat and nonhuman primate stomach. J Exp Pharmacol Ther. 1995;274:1531-7.
63. Boyce S, Chan CC, Gordon R et al. L-745,337: a selective inhibitor of cyclooxygenase-2 elicits antinociception but not gastric ulceration in rats. Neuropharmacology. 1994;33:1609-11.
64. Seibert K, Zhang Y, Leahy K et al. Pharmacological and biochemical demonstration of the role of cyclooxygenase 2 in inflammation and pain. Proc Natl Acad Sci USA. 1994;91:12013-7.
65. Seibert K, Gierse J, Zhang Y et al. Expression and selective inhibition of constitutive and inducible forms of cyclooxygenase. Proceedings of the 9th International Conference on Prostaglandins and Related Compounds: 1994 June 6-10; Florence, Milan: Giovanni Lorenzini Medical Foundation, 1994.
66. Riese J, Hoff T, Nordhoff A, DeWitt DL, Resch K, Kaever V. Transient expression of prostaglandin endoperoxide synthase-2 during mouse macrophage activation. J Leuk Biol. 1994; 55:476-82.
67. Akarasereenont P, Mitchell JA, Bakhle YS, Thiemermann C, Vane JR. Comparison of the induction of cyclooxygenase and nitric oxide synthase by endotoxin in endothelial cells and macrophages. Eur J Pharmacol. 1995;273:121-8.
68. Lee SH, Soyoola E, Chanmugam P et al. Selective expression of mitogen-inducible cyclo-oxygenase in macrophages stimulated with lipopolysaccharide. J Biol Chem. 1992;267:24934-8.
69. O'Sullivan MG, Chilton FH, Huggins EM Jr, McCall CP. Lipopolysaccharide priming of alveolar macrophages for enhanced synthesis of prostanoids involves induction of a novel prostaglandin H synthase. J Biol Chem. 1992;267:14547-550.
70. Hempel SL, Monick MM, Hunninghake GW. Lipopolysaccharide induces prostaglandin H synthase-2 protein and mRNA in human alveolar macrophages and blood monocytes. J Clin Invest. 1994;93:391-6.

71. Angel J, Berenbaum F, Le Denmat C, Nevalainen T, Masliah J, Fournier C. Interleukin-1-induced prostaglandin E_2 biosynthesis in human synovial cells involves the activation of cytosolic phospholipase A_2 and cyclooxygenase-2. Eur J Biochem. 1994;226:125–31.
72. Knott I, Dieu M, Burton M, Houbion A, Remacle J, Raes M. Induction of cyclooxygenase by interleukin 1: comparative study between human synovial cells and chondrocytes. J Rheumatol. 1994;21:462–6.
73. Habib A, Créminon C, Frobert Y, Grassi J, Pradelles P, Maclouf J. Demonstration of an inducible cyclooxygenase in human endothelial cells using antibodies raised against the carboxyl-terminal region of the cyclooxygenase-2. J Biol Chem. 1993;268:23448–54.
74. Szczepanski A, Moatter T, Carley WW, Gerritsen ME. Induction of cyclooxygenase II in human synovial microvessel endothelial cells by interleukin-1. Arthritis Rheum. 1994;37:495–503.
75. Wilborn J, DeWitt DL, Peters-Golden M. Expression and role of cyclooxygenase isoforms in alveolar and peritoneal macrophages. Am J Physiol. 1995;268:L294–301.
76. Mertz PM, DeWitt DL, Stetlet-Stevenson WG, Wahl LM. Interleukin 10 suppression of monocyte prostaglandin H synthase-2. J Biol Chem. 1994;269:21322–9.
77. Harris RC, McKanna JA, Akai Y, Jacobson HR, Dubois RN, Breyer MD. Cyclooxygenase-2 is associated with the macula densa of rat kidney and increases with salt restriction. J Clin Invest. 1994;94:2504–10.
78. Iseki S. Immunocytochemical localization of cyclooxygenase-1 and cyclooxygenase-2 in the rat stomach. Histochem J. 1995;27:323–8.
79. Sirois J, Levy LO, Simmons DL, Richards JS. Characterization and hormonal regulation of the promoter of the rat prostaglandin endoperoxide synthase 2 gene in granulosa cells. J Biol Chem. 1993;268:7384–5.
80. Slater D, Berger L, Newton R, Moore G, Bennett P. The relative abundance of type 1 to type 2 cyclo-oxygenase mRNA in human amnion at term. Biochem Biophys Res Commun. 1994; 198:304–8.
81. Breder CD, DeWitt D, Kraig RP. Characterization of inducible cyclooxygenase in rat brain. J Comp Neurol. 1995;355:196–315.
82. Bazan NG, Fletcher BS, Herschman HR, Mukherjee PK. Platelet-activating factor and retinoic acid synergistically activate the inducible prostaglandin synthase gene. Proc Natl Acad Sci USA. 1994;91:5252–6.
83. Mitchell JA, Belvisi MG, Akarasereenont PA et al. Induction of cyclo-oxygenase-2 by cytokines in human pulmonary epithelial cells: regulation by dexamethasone. Br J Pharmacol. 1994;113: 1008–14.
84. Eberhardt CE, Coffey RJ, Radhika A, Giardiello FM, Ferrenbach S, Dubois R. Up-regulation of cyclooxygenase 2 gene expression in human colorectal adenomas and carcinomas. Gastroenterology. 1994;107:1183–8.
85. Kargman SL, O'Neill GP, Vickers PJ, Evans JF, Mancini JA, Jothy S. Expression of prostaglandin G/H synthase-1 and -2 protein in human colon cancer. Cancer Res. 1995;55:2556–9.

7 COX-2 expression and inhibition in human monocytes

C. PATRONO, P. PATRIGNANI, M.R. PANARA, F. CIPOLLONE, G. SANTINI, M.G. SCIULLI, M.T. ROTONDO, R. PADOVANO and M. DI GIAMBERARDINO

The conversion of arachidonic acid to prostaglandin (PG) H_2 is catalysed by PG-endoperoxide synthase (PGHS) which exhibits both cyclooxygenase (COX) and peroxidase activities[1]. PGH_2 is further metabolized by other enzymes to various prostanoids (PGs, prostacyclin and thromboxane A_2). Two isozymes of PGHS exist, referred to as PGHS-1 and PGHS-2 or COX-1 and COX-2[2]. COX-1 is a constitutive enzyme present in almost all cell types[3], and is the major isoform found in gastrointestinal tissue[4]. Prostanoid production by COX-1 is involved in physiological functions such as vascular homeostasis, control of kidney function and gastric cytoprotection[2]. COX-2 is induced in a more restricted, cell-specific fashion by mitogenic and inflammatory stimuli[5–12].

Cyclooxygenase activity is inhibited by aspirin and related non-steroid anti-inflammatory drugs (NSAIDs)[13]. Inhibition of prostanoid formation by NSAIDs is the basis for their therapeutic actions as well as their side effects. In fact, it has been suggested that the anti-inflammatory action of NSAIDs is due to inhibition of COX-2, whereas the toxic effects on the stomach and kidney are due to inhibition of the constitutive isozyme, COX-1[14]. Since COX-1 and COX-2 are structurally distinct proteins with only 60% homology[15], the development of drugs that selectively inhibit the cyclooxygenase activity of COX-2 might lead to a new generation of anti-inflammatory drugs with improved tolerability[14].

In this chapter, we will review the development of analytical tools for assessing the expression and pharmacological inhibition of COX-2 in human blood monocytes and their application to studies in vitro, ex vivo and in vivo.

IN VITRO STUDIES

Expression of COX-2 in human blood monocytes

Different methods have been developed to study the effects of NSAIDs on the cyclooxygenase activity of COX isozymes in vitro. Thus, inhibition of the cyclooxygenase activity of COX-1 and COX-2 has been evaluated in purified enzyme systems, in microsomal membranes from cos-1 cells transfected with the murine[16] or human isozymes[17], cultured cells selectively expressing COX-1 and COX-2 and in cultured intact cells, such as bovine aortic endothelial cells and endotoxin-activated J774.2 macrophages[18]. In many such systems arachidonate concentrations are used that are artificially high compared with those occurring in intact cells. Moreover, measurement of instantaneous inhibition of COX activity may underestimate the potency of some NSAIDs, which are time-dependent inhibitors[17]. Measuring prostaglandin production in intact cells that selectively express COX-2 using arachidonate released from endogenous lipid stores would therefore be a more suitable screening method for selective inhibitors than is measuring instantaneous inhibition of COX-2 in a recombinant system[17].

We have recently described a relatively simple model of human COX-2 expression in lipopolysaccharide (LPS)-stimulated whole blood[12]. This method is suitable for evaluating the extent of COX-2 inhibition both in vitro and after oral administration of NSAIDs in humans. LPS-stimulated blood cells produced large amounts of PGE_2 in a time-dependent fashion that correlated with the accumulation of a protein doublet of approximately 72kDa in monocytes, as detected by Western blot using antibodies directed against a synthetic COX-2 specific amino acid sequence. Conversely, COX-1 expressed in unstimulated monocytes was not affected by incubation with LPS for up to 24h. Dexamethasone, a selective inhibitor of COX-2 expression in monocytes/macrophages[7,8,19] profoundly suppressed PGE_2 production in LPS-stimulated whole blood both at 4 and 24h[12]. The contribution of platelet COX-1 to total COX activity measured in whole blood was suppressed selectively by treating the subjects with 300mg aspirin[20]. Aspirin was administered 48h before sampling because of previous evidence that the return of intact platelet protein and enzyme activity after a single dose of aspirin only begins after a 2-day lag, probably reflecting the acetylation by aspirin of COX-1 in megakaryocytes[21,22].

Inhibition of monocyte COX-2

To test the biochemical selectivity of various NSAIDs towards COX-2 and COX-1, we compared their inhibitory effects on PGE_2 production by LPS-stimulated whole blood at 4 and 24h and on TXB_2 production by platelets during 1 h clotting of whole blood. The production of TXB_2 in this setting has been previously demonstrated to represent an index of platelet COX-1 activity in response to endogenously formed thrombin[20,22,23]. The IC_{50} values for inhibition of the cyclooxygenase activity of platelet COX-1 and monocyte COX-2 by non-selective and selective inhibitors are given in Table 1. NS-398 and L-745,337 are novel anti-inflammatory and analgesic agents that do not produce gastrointestinal lesions following oral administration to experimental animals[24–27]. NS-398, at doses that completely inhibited PGE_2 synthesis in the fluid exudate that is formed following carrageenan injection into a subcutaneous air pouch (ED_{50} 0.3mg/kg), did not inhibit PGE_2 synthesis in the stomach, nor were gastric lesions observed when NS-398 was administered to rats at a dose of 30mg/kg[25]. NS-398 was reported selectively to inhibit the activity of recombinant and purified COX-2

Table 1 Inhibition of platelet COX-1 and LPS-induced monocyte COX-2 by cyclooxygenase inhibitors

Inhibitor	*IC_{50} for COX-1 (μM)*	*IC_{50} for COX-2 (μM)*	*IC_{50} (COX-1) / IC_{50} (COX-2)*
S-Indobufen	0.68±0.22	14.9±8	0.05
R-Indobufen	38±18	230±68	0.16
R-Ketoprofen	7.5±0.73	16±4.7	0.47
S-Ketoprofen	0.11±0.04	0.18±0.06	0.6
6-MNA	278±96	187±96	1.49
Flurbiprofen	1.1±0.13	0.69±0.08	1.59
Indomethacin	0.70±0.20	0.36±0.10	1.94
NS-398	16.8±11.8	0.10±0.03	163
L-745,337	367.7±60.5	1.5±0.34	245

COX, cyclooxygenase; LPS, lipopolysaccharide; IC_{50}, concentration required to inhibit enzyme activity by 50%.

without affecting COX-1. Baculovirus-expressed recombinant murine COX-2 was inhibited with an IC_{50} of 30nM while COX-1 activity was not affected at concentrations as high as 100 μM[25]. Using purified enzymes (COX-1 and COX-2 from ram seminal vesicles and sheep placenta, respectively), NS-398 selectively inhibited COX-2 (IC_{50} 3.8 μM)[24] but was approximately 100-fold less potent than with the recombinant enzyme. In our study, NS-398 inhibited platelet COX-1 activity and monocyte COX-2 in human whole blood in vitro with an IC_{50} of 17 and 0.1 μM, respectively[28]. Variable IC_{50} values for inhibition of COX-2 activity by NS-398 in vitro probably reflect the different experimental conditions used in the various assay systems. In our system, the effects of inhibitors were evaluated in intact cells expressing the human isozyme in the presence of plasma proteins which, by binding the compounds, may influence their concentration at the active site of the enzyme. Thus, NS-398 was approximately 70-fold more potent in inhibiting COX-2 activity when assessed in isolated monocytes than when studied in whole blood[28].

Similarly to NS-398, L-745,337 was approximately 200-fold better as an inhibitor of monocyte COX-2 than in inhibiting COX-1 (Figure 1). In human osteosarcoma cells selectively expressing COX-2[27], L-745,337 inhibited PGE_2 production in response to exogenous arachidonic acid with an IC_{50} (23nM) quite similar to that measured by us in human monocytes (45nM). In contrast, the compound did not affect the production of PGE_2 by arachidonic acid-challenged U-937 cells expressing COX-1 at concentrations up to 10 μM[27].

As distinct from dexamethasone, which inhibits the biosynthesis of prostanoids by suppressing the induction of COX-2, L-745,337 and NS-398 selectively block its cyclooxygenase activity. Copeland et al.[29] have recently demonstrated that NS-398 and DuP 697, compounds of the general form of aryl methyl sulphonamides and aryl methyl sulphonyls, irreversibly inactivate COX-2 in a time-dependent fashion while showing minimal reversible inhibition

***Figure 1** Dose–response curves for inhibition of human whole blood COX-1 and COX-2 by L-745,337. Increasing concentrations of L-745,337 were incubated with 1 ml heparinized whole blood samples (drawn from healthy volunteers pretreated with 300 mg of aspirin 48 h before sampling) in the presence of LPS (10 μg/ml) for 24 h, and plasma PGE_2 levels were assayed as a reflection of monocyte COX-2 activity (■). L-745,337 was also incubated with 1 ml whole blood samples (drawn from the same donors when they had not taken any NSAIDs during the 2 weeks preceding the study) allowed to clot for 1 h, and serum TXB_2 levels were measured as a reflection of platelet COX-1 activity (●). Results are depicted as percentage inhibition (mean ± SD) from six separate experiments. (Data from Ref. 28)*

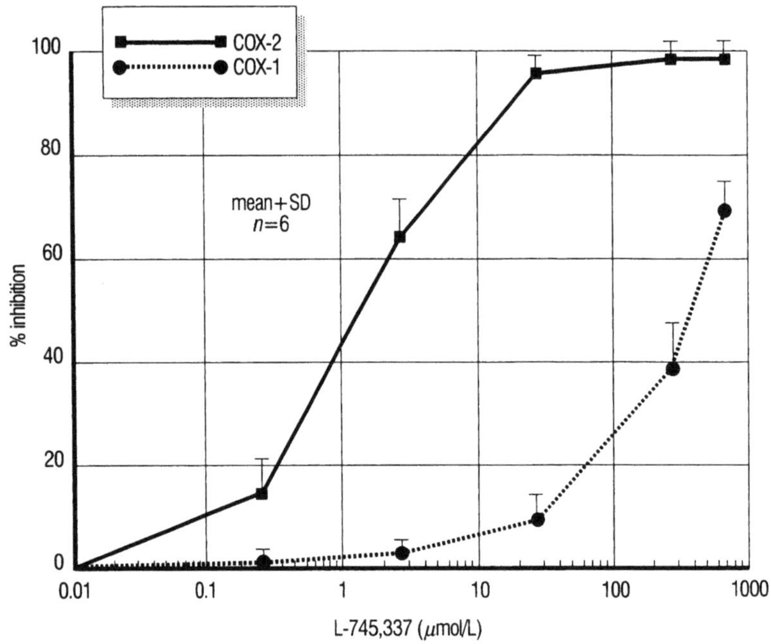

of COX-1. They suggested that binding of these inhibitors to COX-2 induces a slow structural transition of the enzyme that results in its selective inactivation[29].

COX-2-dependent formation of F_2-isoprostanes in human monocytes

Isoprostanes represent a newly characterized family of vasoactive eicosanoids that are formed by a non-cyclooxygenase, free radical-catalysed mechanism involving peroxidation of arachidonic acid[30]. One of these compounds is 8-epi-$PGF_{2\alpha}$ which has attracted considerable attention because of its biological activity: it is a potent vasoconstrictor in the rat and its action is mediated, at least in part, through the vascular PGH_2/TXA_2 receptor[31]. Moreover, 8-epi-$PGF_{2\alpha}$ induces platelet shape change but not aggregation[32].

In contrast to lipid hydroperoxides, which decompose rapidly in human body fluids, F_2-isoprostanes are chemically stable end-products of lipid peroxidation that are easily detectable in human plasma and urine[30]. Recent evidence suggests that 8-epi-$PGF_{2\alpha}$ may also be formed as a minor product of platelet COX-1 activity[33]. We have investigated 8-epi-$PGF_{2\alpha}$ production associated with induction of COX-2 in human blood monocytes and its pharmacological modulation. Heparinized whole blood samples were drawn from healthy volunteers, 48 h following oral dosing with aspirin 300 mg to suppress platelet cyclooxygenase activity. Aliquots of 1 ml were incubated with LPS (0.5–10 μg/ml) for 0–24 h at 37°C. PGE_2 and 8-epi-$PGF_{2\alpha}$ were measured in separated plasma by previously validated radioimmunoassay techniques[12,34]. Levels of both eicosanoids were undetectable (i.e. <60 pg/ml) at time 0. LPS induced the formation of PGE_2 and 8-epi-$PGF_{2\alpha}$ in a time- and concentration-dependent fashion, coincident with the induction of COX-2, as detected by Western blot analysis of monocyte lysates. After 24 h at 10 μg/ml LPS, PGE_2 and 8-epi-$PGF_{2\alpha}$ levels averaged $10\,480 \pm 4643$ and 295 ± 140 pg/ml respectively (mean ± SD, $n=6$). Dexamethasone and L-745,337 reduced PGE_2 and 8-epi-$PGF_{2\alpha}$ production in response to LPS. These novel findings suggest that inhibition of the biosynthesis of the vasoconstrictor and mitogenic 8-epi-$PGF_{2\alpha}$ may enlarge the spectrum of pharmacological effects of selective COX-2 inhibitors (Figure 2).

Three distinct mechanisms of F_2-isoprostane biosynthesis have thus been characterized in man: free radical-catalysed lipid peroxidation[30], platelet COX-1[33] and monocyte COX-2[35]. Although indirect pharmacological evidence suggests that free radical-catalysed lipid peroxidation is the prevailing mechanism of 8-epi-$PGF_{2\alpha}$ biosynthesis in healthy subjects[34], the relative contribution of the other mechanisms in various pathophysiological settings remains to be investigated.

EX VIVO STUDIES

The same method of COX isozyme inhibition assessment described above allows evaluation of the clinical pharmacology of selective COX inhibitors during phase I/II studies. We have used this approach to examine the alleged selectivity of nabumetone in inhibiting COX-2 rather than COX-1 in healthy subjects[36]. Nabumetone is a non-acidic NSAID with an unusual pharmacological profile[37]. After absorption, it is converted in the liver to the active metabolite 6-methoxy-2-naphthyl acetic acid (6-MNA)[38], which reaches maximum plasma concentrations within 2–4 h. Its elimination half-life is approximately 24 h. 6-MNA is hepatically, not renally, cleared from the circulation and it does not undergo enterohepatic recirculation. It is further metabolized in the liver to an inactive form (6-hydroxy-2-naphthyl acetic acid) which is excreted in the urine[39].

***Figure 2** Enzymatic and non-enzymatic pathways of arachidonic acid metabolism. PG, prostaglandin; TX, thromboxane; LT, leukotriene; COX, cyclooxygenase; TXR, thromboxane receptor*

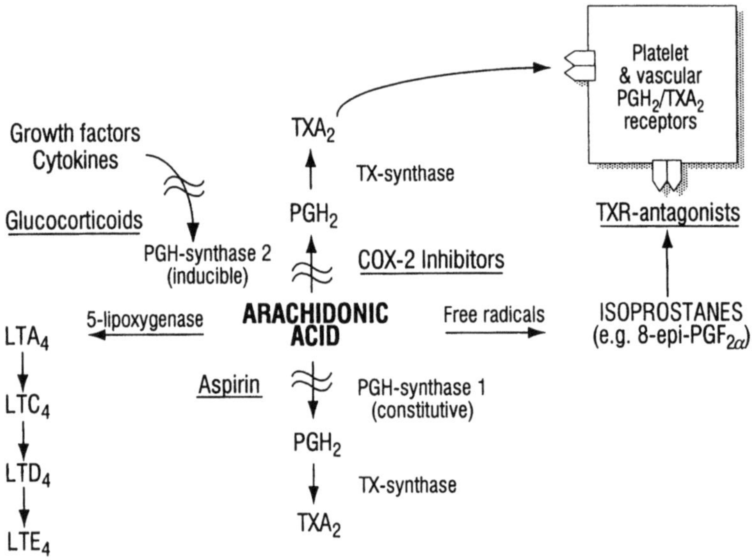

Studies in laboratory animals demonstrated that nabumetone is as effective an anti-inflammatory agent as traditional NSAIDs[40]. In clinical trials, nabumetone was effective in the treatment of patients with osteoarthritis and rheumatoid arthritis[41]. The administration of nabumetone was associated with less gastric and renal adverse events than other NSAIDs[42].

In cos-1 cells transfected with the plasmid expression constructs for murine COX-1 and COX-2, 6-MNA was about 7-fold better as an inhibitor of the inducible enzyme[16], and it was suggested that this biochemical selectivity might contribute to the safety profile of nabumetone[43]. However, when tested in a human whole blood model of COX-2 expression, 6-MNA was equally potent in inhibiting activity of platelet COX-1 and monocyte COX-2[12].

When given to healthy volunteers, nabumetone (500 and 1000 mg/day for 7 days) caused comparable suppression of COX-1 and COX-2 activities in whole blood ex vivo[12,36]. These results are consistent with previously reported circulating plasma levels of 6-MNA (i.e. 20–70 μg/ml) after oral dosing with 500 and 1000 mg of nabumetone[39,44] and with the dose–response relationship established in vitro for inhibition of human COX-1 and COX-2 (IC_{50} 52 and 35 μg/ml, respectively). It is likely that different inhibitor sensitivities of the mouse and human COX isozymes might account for the apparent discrepancy between our results[12] and those of Meade et al.[16]. The consistency between the results obtained with 6-MNA added in vitro and nabumetone administered in vivo suggests that this method of assessing the pattern of relative inhibition for human blood COX-1 and COX-2 may reliably predict the in vivo selectivity of novel NSAIDs.

IN VIVO STUDIES

For studies of pharmacological modulation of cyclooxygenase activity in vivo, we have monitored the urinary excretion of major enzymatic metabolites of TXB_2 (e.g. 11-dehydro-TXB_2). It should be emphasized that, although platelet COX-1 contributes the vast majority (70–80%) of TXA_2 biosynthesis under physiological circumstances, the contribution of extra-platelet sources, including inflammatory cells expressing COX-2, may vary in pathophysiological settings.

The comparative assessment of the relationship between inhibition of platelet cyclooxygenase activity and reduction in thromboxane metabolite excretion, carried out with two consecutive doses of nabumetone and a low-dose aspirin regimen in the same subjects, strongly suggests that the effect of therapeutic doses of nabumetone on the basal rate of in vivo TXA_2 biosynthesis in healthy subjects can be largely accounted for by reversible inhibition of platelet COX-1 activity by 6-MNA[36]. In order to explore such a relationship over varying degrees of enzyme inhibition we measured serum TXB_2 levels and urinary 11-dehydro-TXB_2 excretion six times during increasing and three times during decreasing plasma levels of 6-MNA. The same indices were measured five times during cumulative inhibition and four times during recovery of platelet cyclooxygenase activity following low-dose aspirin. The cumulative suppression of the platelet biosynthetic capacity and total body TXA_2 biosynthesis during daily dosing with 40 mg aspirin, as well as their slow pattern of time-dependent return towards control levels after aspirin withdrawal (Figure 3) confirm earlier findings suggesting that urinary 11-dehydro-TXB_2 excretion is largely a reflection of platelet TXA_2 production[45]. Similar results were obtained during and after dosing with nabumetone, although we could not explore such a relationship beyond the 70% level of inhibition of platelet cyclooxygenase activity since 6-MNA is a relatively weak inhibitor of platelet COX-1[12].

Overall, the results of our study[36] demonstrated a measurable impact of therapeutic doses of nabumetone on constitutive eicosanoid biosynthesis of healthy subjects, making it unlikely that its safety profile in patients is related to a selective inhibition of the inducible COX-2, as suggested by Meade et al.[16]. Alternative explanations related to its metabolism and tissue distribution and clearance of its active metabolite are perhaps more likely and should be further investigated.

The evidence supporting the platelet origin of urinary 11-dehydro-TXB_2 and 2,3-dinor-TXB_2 in man is largely indirect and derived from the effects of low-dose aspirin on metabolite excretion. When administered to healthy subjects[45] or

***Figure 3** Effects of low-dose aspirin on TXA_2 production in vivo and ex vivo. Aspirin, 40 mg, was administered daily for 5 days to three healthy subjects. The urinary excretion of 11-dehydro-TXB_2 (TX-M) and the production of thromboxane B_2 (TXB_2) in whole blood were measured before, during, and after treatment with aspirin. Measurements are expressed as percentages of the predosing control values and reported as mean values ± SD. (Data from Ref. 36)*

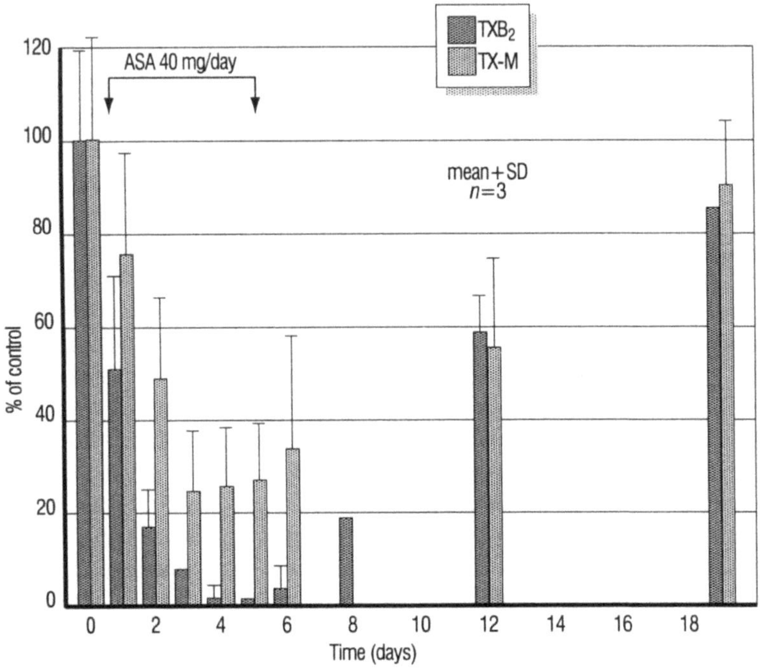

patients with persistent platelet activation[46–48], low-dose aspirin (50 mg daily) caused progressively increasing inhibition of TXB_2 metabolite excretion during the first 5–7 days, consistent with the cumulative nature of platelet COX acetylation upon repeated daily dosing[23]. Moreover, upon aspirin withdrawal, the return of TXB_2 metabolites to baseline excretion rates occurred slowly over 10–15 days, consistent with the platelet turnover-dependent recovery of cyclooxygenase activity in the systemic circulation[23]. In a study of unstable angina, however, Vejar et al.[49] reported episodic increases in 11-dehydro-TXB_2 excretion in some patients treated with low-dose aspirin, despite ex vivo evidence of virtually complete blockade of platelet cyclooxygenase activity. The discovery of COX-2 prompted us to re-examine TXA_2 biosynthesis in unstable angina as modified by two distinct cyclooxygenase inhibitors, aspirin and indobufen, differentially affecting monocyte COX-2 despite a comparable impact on platelet

COX-1 (Cipollone et al., in preparation). We randomized 20 unstable angina patients to short-term treatment with aspirin (100 mg daily) or indobufen (200 mg b.i.d.) and collected consecutive urine samples during the first 72 h after randomization. The urinary excretion of 11-dehydro-TXB_2 averaged 136±148 (mean±SD, $n=90$) pg/mg creatinine in the aspirin group and 63±63 ($n=108$) in the indobufen group ($p<0.001$). These results raise the possibility that episodes of aspirin-insensitive enhanced TXA_2 biosynthesis in unstable angina may reflect extraplatelet sources possibly expressing COX-2 in response to a local inflammatory stimulus. The clinical relevance of this finding is currently being investigated.

Acknowledgements

These studies were supported by a BIOMED grant from the European Union (BMH1-CT93-1533) and a grant from Consiglio Nazionale delle Ricerche (Progetto Finalizzato FATMA, SP8 94.00152.PF41). The expert editorial assistance of Alessandra Migliavacca is gratefully acknowledged.

References

1. DeWitt DL. Prostaglandin endoperoxide synthase: regulation of enzyme expression. Biochim Biophys Acta. 1991;1083:121–34.
2. Smith WL. Prostanoid biosynthesis and mechanisms of action. Am J Physiol. 1992;263:F181–91.
3. Simmons DL, Xie W, Chipman JG, Evett GE. Multiple cyclooxygenases: cloning of a mitogen-inducible form. In: Bailey JM, editor. Prostaglandins, Leukotrienes, Lipoxins, and PAF. New York: Plenum Press; 1991:67–78.
4. DeWitt DL, Smith WL. Primary structure of prostaglandin G/H synthase from sheep vesicular gland determined from the complementary DNA sequence. Proc Natl Acad Sci USA. 1988; 85:1412–6.
5. Kujubu DA, Fletcher BS, Varnum BC, Lim RW, Hershman HR. TIS10, a phorbol ester tumor promoter inducible mRNA from Swiss 3T3 cells, encodes a novel prostaglandin synthase/cyclo-oxygenase homologue. J Biol Chem. 1991;268:9049–54.
6. Fletcher BS, Kujubu DA, Perrin DM, Herschman HR. Structure of the mitogen-inducible TIS10 gene and demonstration that the TIS10-encoded protein is a functional prostaglandin G/H synthase. J Biol Chem. 1992;267:4338–44.
7. O'Banion MK, Winn VD, Yung DA. cDNA cloning and functional activity of a glucocorticoid-regulated inflammatory cyclooxygenase. Proc Natl Acad Sci USA. 1992;89:4888–92.
8. Lee SH, Soyoola E, Chanmugam P et al. Selective expression of mitogen-inducible cyclooxygenase in macrophages stimulated with lypopolysaccharide. J Biol Chem. 1992;25934–8.
9. O'Sullivan MG, Chilton FH, Huggins EM, McCall CE. Lipopolysaccharide priming of alveolar macrophages for enhanced synthesis of prostanoids involves induction of a novel prostaglandin H synthase. J Biol Chem. 1992;267:14547–50.
10. O'Sullivan MG, Huggins EM, Meade EA, DeWitt DL, McCall CE. Lipopolysaccharide induces prostaglandin H synthase-2 in alveolar macrophages. Biochim Biophys Res Commun. 1992; 187:1123–7.
11. Hempel SL, Monick MM, Hunninghake GW. Lypopolysaccharide induces prostaglandin H synthase-2 protein and mRNA in human alveolar macrophages and blood monocytes. J Clin Invest. 1994;93:391–6.
12. Patrignani P, Panara MR, Greco A et al. Biochemical and pharmacological characterization of the cyclooxygenase activity of human blood prostaglandin endoperoxide synthases. J Pharmacol Exp Ther. 1994;271:1705–12.

13. Vane JR. Inhibition of prostaglandins as a mechanism of action for aspirin-like drugs. Nature New Biol. 1971;231:232–5.
14. Vane JR. Towards a better aspirin. Nature. 1994;367:215–6.
15. Jones DA, Carlton DP, McIntyre TM, Zimmerman GA, Prescott SM. Molecular cloning of human prostaglandin endoperoxide synthase type II and demonstration of expression in response to cytokines. J Biol Chem. 1993;268:9049–54.
16. Meade EA, Smith WL, DeWitt DL. Differential inhibition of prostaglandin endoperoxide synthase (cyclooxygenase) isozymes by aspirin and other non-steroidal anti-inflammatory drugs. J Biol Chem. 1993;268:6610–4.
17. Laneuville O, Breuer DK, DeWitt DL, Hla T, Funk CD, Smith WL. Differential inhibition of human prostaglandin endoperoxide H synthase-1 and -2 by nonsteroidal antiinflammatory drugs. J Pharmacol Exp Ther. 1994;271:927–34.
18. Mitchell JA, Akarasereenont P, Thiemermann C, Flower RJ, Vane JR. Selectivity of nonsteroidal antiinflammatory drugs as inhibitors of constitutive and inducible cyclooxygenase. Proc Natl Acad Sci USA. 1993;90:11693–7.
19. Kutchera WA, Jones DA, Maclouf J, Zimmerman GA, McIntyre TM, Prescott SM. Regulation of expression of prostaglandin H synthase in human endothelial cells and macrophages. Circulation. 1993;88:I-621.
20. Patrono C, Ciabattoni G, Patrignani P et al. Clinical pharmacology of platelet cyclooxygenase inhibition. Circulation. 1985;72:1177–84.
21. Roth GJ, Stanford N, Majerus PW. Acetylation of prostaglandin synthase by aspirin. Proc Natl Acad Sci USA. 1975;72:3073–6.
22. Patrono C, Ciabattoni G, Pinca E et al. Low dose aspirin and inhibition of thromboxane B_2 production in healthy subjects. Thromb Res. 1980;17:317–27.
23. Patrignani P, Filabozzi P, Patrono C. Selective cumulative inhibition of platelet thromboxane production by low-dose aspirin in healthy subjects. J Clin Invest. 1982;69:1366–72.
24. Futaki N, Takahashi S, Yokoyama M, Arai I, Higuchi S, Otomo S. NS-398, a new anti-inflammatory agent, selectively inhibits prostaglandin G/H synthase/cyclooxygenase (COX-2) activity in vitro. Prostaglandins. 1994;47:55–9.
25. Masferrer JL, Zweifel BS, Manning PT et al. Selective inhibition of inducible cyclooxygenase 2 in vivo is antiinflammatory and nonulcerogenic. Proc Natl Acad Sci USA. 1994;91:3228–32.
26. Chan C-C, Gordon R, Brideau C et al. In vivo pharmacology of L-745,337: A novel non steroidal antiinflammatory agent (NSAID) with an ulcerogenic sparing effect in rat and monkey stomach. Can J Physiol Pharm. 1994;72(Suppl. 1):266.
27. Chan C-C, Boyce S, Brideau C et al. Pharmacology of a selective cyclooxygenase-2 inhibitor L-745,337: a novel non-steroidal antiinflammatory agent with an ulcerogenic sparing effect in rat and non-human primate stomach. J Pharmacol Exp Ther. 1995;274:1531–7.
28. Panara MR, Greco A, Santini G et al. Effects of the novel antiinflammatory compounds, NS-398 and L-745,337 on the cyclooxygenase activity of human blood prostaglandin endoperoxide synthase. Br J Pharmacol. 1995;116:2429–34.
29. Copeland RA, Williams JM, Giannaras J et al. Mechanism of selective inhibition of the inducible isoform of prostaglandin G/H synthase. Proc Natl Acad Sci USA. 1994;91:11202–6.
30. Morrow JD, Hill KE, Burk RF, Nanmour TM, Badr KF, Roberts LJ II. A series of prostaglandin F_2-like compounds are produced in vivo in humans by a non-cyclooxygenase, free radical-catalyzed mechanism. Proc Natl Acad Sci USA. 1990;87:9383–7.
31. Takahashi KT, Nammour TM, Fukunaga M et al. Glomerular actions of a free radical-generated novel prostaglandin, 8-epi-$PGF_{2\alpha}$ in the rat. Evidence for interactions with thromboxane A_2 receptors. J Clin Invest. 1992;90:136–41.
32. Morrow JD, Minton TA, Roberts LJ II. The F_2-isoprostane, 8-epi-prostaglandin $F_{2\alpha}$, a potent agonist of the vascular thromboxane/endoperoxide receptor, is a platelet thromboxane/endoperoxide receptor antagonist. Prostaglandins. 1992;44:155–63.
33. Praticò D, Lawson JA, FitzGerald GA. Cyclooxygenase dependent formation of the isoprostane, 8-epi-$PGF_{2\alpha}$. J Biol Chem. 1995;270:9800–8.
34. Wang Z, Ciabattoni G, Créminon C, Lawson J, FitzGerald GA, Patrono C, Maclouf J. Immunological characterization of urinary 8-epi-$PGF_{2\alpha}$ excretion in man. J Pharmacol Exp Ther. 1995;275:94–100.
35. Patrignani P, Panara MR, Cipollone F, Greco A, Ciabattoni G, Patrono C. Induction of

prostaglandin endoperoxide synthase 2 in monocytes of human whole blood is associated with cyclooxygenase-dependent isoprostane formation. J Invest Med. 1995;43:335A.
36. Cipollone C, Ganci A, Panara MR et al. Effects of nabumetone on prostanoid biosynthesis in man. Clin Pharmacol Ther. 1995;58:335–41.
37. Goudie AC, Gaster LM, Lake AW et al. 4-(6-methoxy-2-naphthyl)butan-2-one and related analogues, a novel structural class of antiinflammatory compounds. J Med Chem. 1978;21: 1260–4.
38. Blower PR. The unique pharmacological profile of nabumetone. J Rheumatol. 1992;19(suppl. 36):13–9.
39. Hyneck ML. An overview of the clinical pharmacokinetics of nabumetone. J Rheumatol. 1992;19(suppl. 36):20–4.
40. Boyle EA, Freeman PC, Mangan FR, Thomson MJ. Nabumetone (BRL 14777, 4-[6-methoxy-2-naphthyl]-butan-2-one); a new anti-inflammatory agent. J Pharm Pharmacol. 1982;34:562–9.
41. Lister BJ, Poland M, Delapp RE. Efficacy of nabumetone versus diclofenac, naproxen, ibuprofen, and piroxicam in osteoarthritis and rheumatoid arthritis. Am J Med. 1993;95(suppl. 2A):3S–9S.
42. Emery P, Clark A, Williams P et al. Nabumetone compared with naproxen in the treatment of rheumatoid arthritis: a multicenter, double blind, randomized, parallel group trial in hospital outpatients. J Rheumatol. 1992;19(suppl. 36):41–7.
43. DeWitt DL, Meade EA, Smith WL. PGH synthase isozyme selectivity: the potential for safer nonsteroidal antiinflammatory drugs. Am J Med. 1993;95(suppl. 2A):40S–4S.
44. Von Schrader HW, Busher G, Dierdorf D, Mugge H, Wolf D. Nabumetone, a novel anti-inflammatory drug: bioavailability after different dosage regimens. Int J Clin Pharmacol Ther Toxicol. 1984;22:672–6.
45. Catella F, FitzGerald GA. Paired analysis of urinary thromboxane B_2 metabolites in humans. Thromb Res. 1987;47:647–56.
46. Davì G, Catalano I, Averna M et al. Thromboxane biosynthesis and platelet function in type-II diabetes mellitus. N Engl J Med. 1990;322:1769–76.
47. Davì G, Notarbartolo A, Catalano I et al. Increased thromboxane biosynthesis in type IIa hypercholesterolemia. Circulation. 1992;85:1792–7.
48. Koudstaal PJ, Ciabattoni G, Van Gijn J et al. Increased thromboxane biosynthesis in patients with acute cerebral ischemia. Stroke. 1993;24:219–22.
49. Vejar M, Fragasso G, Lipkin DP et al. Dissociation of platelet activation and spontaneous myocardial ischemia in unstable angina. Thromb Haemostasis. 1990;63:163–8.

8 Expression and regulation of COX-2 in synovial tissues of arthritic patients

L.J. CROFFORD

Rheumatoid arthritis (RA) is a systemic illness characterized by inflammatory polyarticular synovitis. Proliferative and invasive synovial tissues lead to joint swelling, pain and erosion of cartilage and juxta-articular bone. Although the aetiology of RA is not known, the pathogenesis of the disease involves complex interactions between cells of the immune system and resident cells of the synovia. A number of mediators, including cytokines, growth factors and eicosanoids, produced by infiltrating mononuclear cells as well as by endothelial cells and fibroblast-like cells (synoviocytes), contribute to the proliferative and invasive phenotype of inflamed synovial tissues in RA.

Prostaglandins (PGs), products of the cyclooxygenase (COX, PGH synthase) pathway of arachidonic acid (AA) metabolism, are important autocrine and paracrine mediators of inflammation in RA[1,2]. PGs may also play a role in the erosion of juxta-articular bone by induction of matrix metalloproteinases[3–5]. The initial step in AA metabolism is the release of free AA from cell membrane phospholipids by phospholipase A_2 (PLA_2)[6], which exists in distinct forms: the low molecular weight secretory group II ($sPLA_2$)[7,8] and the high molecular weight cytosolic form ($cPLA_2$)[9,10]. Arachidonate is converted to PGG_2 and then to PGH_2 by the cyclooxygenase and peroxidase activities, respectively, of the COX protein, of which there are two isoforms, COX-1 and COX-2. COX-1 is constitutively expressed in a wide range of cells and tissues[11], and may undergo slow changes in levels of expression associated with cellular differentiation[12–14]. COX-2 is highly regulated in vitro in response to many extracellular stimuli. Expression of this isoform is increased dramatically by cytokines and mitogens, and decreased by glucocorticoids[15–20]. The characteristics of COX-1 and -2 expression suggest that COX-1 may be the isoform important for production of PGs mediating homeostatic functions, while COX-2 may contribute heavily to increased PG production localized to specific tissues affected by inflammatory pathology[15].

In this review, available data regarding expression and regulation of COX-2 in synovial tissues will be summarized. The potential importance of a highly regulated enzyme in the PG synthetic pathway for rapid and highly localized production of PGs will be discussed. Finally, we will speculate on the role of COX-2 in the pathogenesis of inflammatory synovitis and the potential for specific COX-2 inhibitors as treatments for chronic inflammatory arthritis.

Table 1 COX expression in joint tissues of rats[23]

	LEW/N	LEW.rnu/rnu	F344/N
SCW injected			
Day 0	–	–	–
Day 3	3+	2+	–
Day 28	4+	–	–
Adjuvant injected			
Day 0	–	–	–
Day 2	1+	ND	–
Day 4	2+	3+	–
Day 10	3+	±	–
Day 18	3+	–	–

COX EXPRESSION IN ANIMAL MODELS OF ARTHRITIS AND INFLAMMATION

Streptococcal cell wall (SCW)-derived peptidoglycan–polysaccharide injected in aqueous suspension into susceptible rat strains reproducibly induces a model of proliferative and erosive synovitis that has many features of RA. The acute phase of SCW-induced arthritis is clinically characterized by swelling and erythema, typically involving peripheral joints including ankles, wrists, metacarpophalangeal, and interphalangeal joints. The acute arthritis reaches maximum severity in about 3 days and slowly diminishes, but 14–28 days after SCW administration an exacerbation of arthritis develops that may persist for months. The chronic phase of the disease eventually results in synovial proliferation and invasive destruction of periarticular bone and cartilage in the most severely involved joints[21,22]. Chronic, erosive polyarthritis also develops in rats injected intradermally with Freund's complete adjuvant, an oil and water emulsion containing mycobacterial components. The disease is highly species specific, and develops only in susceptible rat strains. After adjuvant injection and a latent period of 10–12 days, inflammation develops abruptly in distal joints, especially the ankles, wrists, and interphalangeal joints. The arthritis peaks in severity at 20–28 days after injection[22]. Lewis (LEW) rats are highly susceptible to the induction of both arthritis models, while Fischer (F344) rats are relatively resistant. The acute phase of SCW-induced arthritis is independent of T-lymphocytes, but the chronic phase of both SCW- and adjuvant-induced arthritis are dependent on the presence of T-lymphocytes. Therefore, athymic nude Lewis (LEW.rnu/rnu) rats develop acute, but not chronic SCW-induced arthritis or adjuvant-induced arthritis.

Sano and colleagues evaluated LEW, F344, and LEW.rnu/rnu rats for expression of COX after intraperitoneal injection of SCW or intradermal injection of Freund's complete adjuvant (Table1)[23]. These animal studies were performed prior to the characterization of the COX-2 isoform, and the antisera used recognized *both* COX-1 and COX-2. Nevertheless, there was little immunostaining for COX in untreated animals, and markedly increased expression of immunoreactive COX that paralleled the development of arthritis. COX immunostaining was detected in multiple cell types within the joints and surrounding tissues, including synovial lining cells, sub-lining synovial fibroblast-like cells, vascular endothelial cells, infiltrating mononuclear inflammatory cells, chondrocytes, subchondral osteoblasts, and adjacent bone marrow. In acute SCW-induced arthritis, treatment with the synthetic glucocorticoid dexamethasone (dex) decreased COX expression in a dose-dependent manner, while treatment with progesterone had no effect. In addition, continuous infusion of dex in animals injected with adjuvant suppressed expression of COX. Finally, although immunoreactive COX expression was markedly increased, there was no increase in COX-1 mRNA measured by reverse transcription and polymerase chain reaction (RT-PCR). The RT-PCR findings and the glucocorticoid sensitivity of the COX immunostaining strongly suggest that increased expression of COX-2 was responsible for the majority of the increased in vivo COX expression detected in these animal models of arthritis.

Further support for the important role of COX-2 in inflammatory processes in vivo is provided by other models of inflammation. A model of acute inflammation is induced by injection of the seaweed-derived polysaccharide carrageenin into a subcutaneous pouch[24]. A model of acute and chronic inflammation is induced by injection of croton oil in Freund's complete adjuvant[25]. The pouch is formed by injection of air over several days, and subsequently develops a lining layer composed of macrophages and fibroblasts. Either carrageenin or croton oil is then injected into the subcutaneous pouch. After carrageenin injection, animals rapidly develop an inflammatory reaction in surrounding tissues that is accompanied by a predominantly neutrophilic cellular infiltrate in the pouch fluid. Masferrer and co-workers determined that COX-2 mRNA and protein expression were markedly increased with a time course that paralleled that of carrageenin-induced PG production[24]. Vane and colleagues demonstrated that COX activity, as well as COX-2, but not COX-1 protein, was increased in acute and chronic croton oil-induced inflammation[25]. Increased COX-2 expression paralleled COX activity in both acute and chronic inflammation. Taken together, these experiments support the notion that up-regulated COX-2 expression is responsible for increased local PG production in animal models of acute and chronic inflammation.

COX EXPRESSION IN SYNOVIA OF PATIENTS WITH RHEUMATOID ARTHRITIS AND OSTEOARTHRITIS

Using a polyclonal antibody that recognized both COX-1 and -2 and immunohistochemical staining, Sano and colleagues examined synovial tissues from patients with RA, osteoarthritis (OA) and non-arthritic patients with traumatic injury, for COX expression[23]. Synovial tissues from patients with RA exhibited intense staining of the synovial lining layer, sub-synovial synoviocytes, vascular endothelial cells and mononuclear inflammatory cells. The extent and intensity of COX immunostaining correlated with the degree of mononuclear cell infiltration that provided a measure of the synovial inflammation. COX immunostaining was less intense in patients with OA; nevertheless, we demonstrated COX expression in the synovial lining layer, vascular endothelial cells, and scattered mononuclear inflammatory cells. Little immunoreactive COX was detected in non-arthritic synovial tissues.

An antibody specific for the unique carboxyterminal peptide of human COX-2 was generated, and was used for immunostaining of rheumatoid synovial tissues[15]. Staining for COX-2 using specific antisera was far more variable than immunohistochemical staining using the polyclonal anti-COX antisera[15,23]. While there was staining in vascular endothelial cells and infiltrating mononuclear inflammatory cells, there was little staining in the synovial lining layer and sub-lining synoviocytes. In addition, levels of COX-2 were lower than COX-1 mRNA in these patients when studied by RT-PCR[15]. The lower levels of COX-2 in patients may be due to the rapid degradation of COX-2 mRNA compared with the more stable COX-1 transcript.

COX EXPRESSION AND REGULATION IN SYNOVIAL TISSUES IN VITRO

We evaluated the expression and regulation of COX-1 and -2 protein in fresh explants of rheumatoid synovia[15]. These synovial explant tissues contain macrophage-like and fibroblast-like synovial cells, as well as endothelial cells and mononuclear inflammatory cells. COX-1 and -2 were detected by immunoprecipitation of metabolically labelled proteins and/or by Western blot under basal conditions. Treatment with IL-1β or phorbol ester (PMA) markedly increased expression of COX-2, while pretreatment with dex eliminated basal and IL-1β- and PMA-stimulated COX-2 expression. These same treatments had no effect on the level of COX-1 expression.

Since fibroblast-like synovial cells (synoviocytes) are a major source of PG in rheumatoid synovial tissues, we examined expression and regulation of COX mRNA and protein expression in primary cultured rheumatoid synoviocytes[15]. COX-2 protein was not expressed at baseline, but was increased after treatment with IL-1β and PMA. IL-1β-stimulated expression was almost completely inhibited by pretreatment with dex (Figure 1). mRNA expression paralleled that of the protein (not shown). In addition, treatment with the transcription inhibitor actinomycin-D completely eliminated COX-2 mRNA expression, while treatment with cycloheximide, which inhibits translation, markedly increased COX-2 expression. These findings are consistent with the notion that COX-2 acts as an immediate early gene in these cells. COX-1 mRNA was not affected by any

***Figure 1** Northern analysis of COX-1 and -2 mRNA in rheumatoid synoviocytes cultured for 6h in media alone or in media containing IL-1β (1 ng/ml) or PMA (20 ng/ml) as indicated, with or without pretreatment with dexamethasone (10^{-6} M) for 24 h or indomethacin (2 μm). Total RNA was extracted, 20 μg was separated by gel electrophoresis, and transferred to a nylon filter. The filter was hybridized with probes for COX-2 and COX-1, and G3PDH sequentially (Reprinted from Ref. 15).*

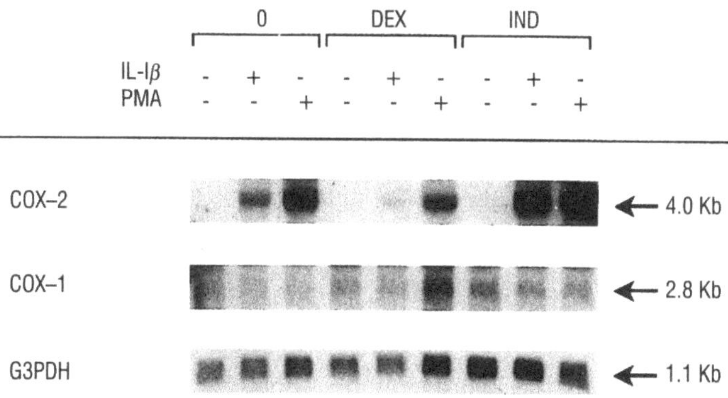

of these treatments. Hulkower and colleagues also demonstrated that COX-2 mRNA and protein levels in rheumatoid synoviocytes are increased after treatment with IL-1β[20]. In their experiments, $cPLA_2$ expression was increased after IL-1β treatment, and may also contribute to increased PGE_2 production. A recent report by Sugiyama and colleagues demonstrated that IL-2 inhibited the spontaneous production of PGE_2 in freshly isolated synovial cells[26]. In addition, IL-4 antagonized LPS- and IL-1-stimulated increases in levels of COX-2, but not COX-1, protein and mRNA.

Mehindate and co-workers examined regulation of COX-2 and $cPLA_2$ in rheumatoid synoviocytes in a system whereby synoviocytes were induced to express MHC class II by treatment with interferon (IFN)-γ, then exposed to superantigen crosslinked with antibody[5]. There was increased expression of COX-2 and $cPLA_2$, but not COX-1 or $sPLA_2$ after exposure to superantigen. Induction of these synthetic enzymes was associated with increased expression of PGE_2 and of collagenase, the matrix metalloproteinase implicated in tissue destruction in inflammatory and erosive joint diseases such as RA. Increased collagenase gene expression could be inhibited with indomethacin and arachidonyl-trifluoromethyl-ketone, an inhibitor of $cPLA_2$[5].

TRANSCRIPTIONAL AND POST-TRANSCRIPTIONAL REGULATION OF COX-2 mRNA

The promoter/enhancer of the human COX-2 gene contains a number of potential binding sites for recognized transcription factors. Several of these transcription factors are known to be stimulated by IL-1, including nuclear factor-kB (NF-kB), CCAAT/enhancer binding protein (c/EBP also known as nuclear factor for IL-6 or NF-IL-6), and the cyclic AMP responsive element binding protein (CREBP). We have found that early (30–60 min), but not late ($\geq$4 h) IL-1β-stimulated COX-2 expression is mediated through NF-kB in human rheumatoid synoviocytes (unpublished data). Hempel and co-workers demonstrated that LPS-stimulated COX-2 expression in human alveolar macrophages can be inhibited by changes in oxidant tone, a manipulation known to inhibit NF-kB[34]. In mouse 3T3 fibroblasts, the v-*src* oncogene, which acts as a protein tyrosine kinase, stimulates COX-2 expression through the CRE transcriptional response element[27]. Furthermore, in a rat granulosa cell system, Sirois and Richards showed that stimulation of COX-2 transcription by gonadotropins utilized c/EBP[28].

The COX-2 transcript contains multiple copies of the 'AUUA' mRNA instability sequence characteristic of many cytokine-responsive mRNAs with a high rate of degradation[29]. These unstable transcripts are also induced by inhibitors of translation, possibly by blocking synthesis of mRNA degradation factor(s). Studies by Rïstimaki and co-workers demonstrated a COX-2 mRNA half-life of 1 h in cells pre-treated with cycloheximide[30]. IL-1 treatment prolonged the half-life of COX-2 mRNA, and this effect was potentiated when transcription was inhibited[30].

POTENTIAL ROLE FOR COX-2 IN THE PATHOGENESIS OF RA

It is clear that acutely increased PG production plays a critical role in acute inflammatory processes. Increased COX-2 expression appears to be an important enzymatic determinant of increased PG production in acute inflammation, as demonstrated by the ability of selective COX-2 inhibitors to block carrageenin-induced inflammation when administered prior to the stimulus and to decrease significantly inflammatory indices and PG levels when administered 6 h after an acute inflammatory stimulus[26]. However, the role played by PGs in the development and maintenance of chronic inflammatory arthritis is far more complex, with some effects likely to contribute to ongoing inflammation and other effects likely to inhibit leukocyte functions. In addition, the relative importance of COX-1 and -2 in chronic inflammatory processes is less clear (Figure 2)[15,25].

The chronically inflamed synovial tissues of patients with RA display characteristics often associated with malignancies, including proliferation, angiogenesis and invasion of surrounding tissues[31,32]. However, this 'transformed

***Figure 2** Schematic representation of the roles of COX-1 and -2 in PG production. COX-1 appears to be constitutively expressed, and to function in maintaining PG production important for homeostatic functions. COX-2 is tightly regulated and appears to function to increase local production of PGs during inflammation and dysregulated growth. Increased expression of COX-2 is stimulated by pro-inflammatory cytokines, growth factors, and mitogens. COX-2 expression is inhibited by glucocorticoids and anti-inflammatory cytokines. Localized increase in PG production mediates many of the cardinal features of acute inflammation; however, sustained PG production may contribute to angiogenesis and increased expression of matrix degrading enzymes. Increased cellularity of inflamed tissues might subsequently result in elevated levels of COX-1, enhancing further the localized production of PG.*

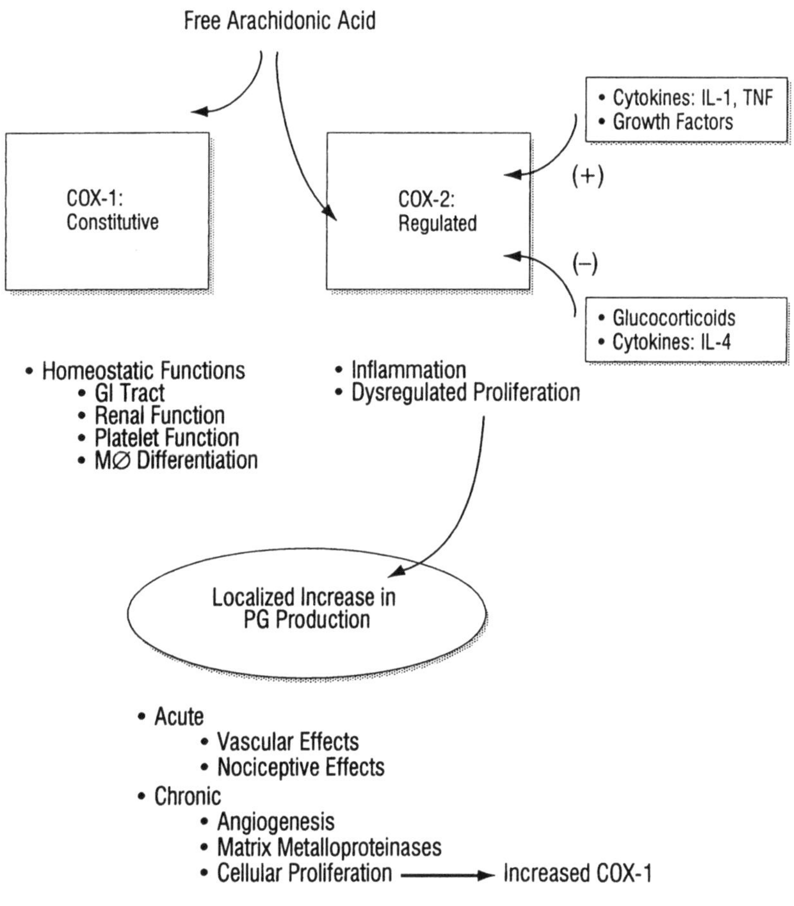

phenotype' is not constitutive, but rather appears to be mediated by locally elaborated factors, including cytokines, growth factors and eicosanoids. Interactions between resident cells of the synovia and infiltrating mononuclear inflammatory cells appear to be a key factor in the development and maintenance of this phenotype, in part by production of cytokine mediators[33]. One consequence of increased cytokine production is regulation of synoviocyte products, including PGs. In vitro evidence demonstrates that pro-inflammatory cytokines increase PG production by stimulating COX-2 expression in synoviocytes[15,20]. However, the pro-inflammatory cytokine IL-1 also increases production of COX-2 in macrophages, endothelial cells, osteoblasts and chondrocytes[30,34–37]. The in vivo effects of increased COX expression in these tissues are likely to be pleiotropic; for example, inhibition of COX exacerbates cartilage erosion, but reduces bone loss[25].

Increased COX-2 expression and PG production could play a role in the 'transformed' phenotype exhibited by rheumatoid synovial tissues. PGs are important mediators of matrix metalloproteinase expression by synoviocytes, and increased COX-2 expression has been implicated in vitro as correlating with stimulated increases in collagenase[5]. PGs have been implicated in the process of angiogenesis that supports synoviocyte proliferation. COX-2 expression is increased by pro-inflammatory cytokines in human vascular endothelial cells, making a role for COX-2 in the angiogenesis associated with rheumatoid synovia plausible[30]. However, since there is likely to be an overall increase in COX-1 levels in rheumatoid synovial tissues due to markedly increased cellularity, the relative role of COX-2 in maintaining PG levels in chronic inflammatory conditions is uncertain[15,23].

POTENTIAL ROLE OF SPECIFIC COX-2 INHIBITORS IN ARTHRITIS

Glucocorticoids exhibit selective effects on COX-2, compared with COX-1; however, glucocorticoids affect the AA metabolic pathway at multiple levels[15,38]. Glucocorticoids also have effects on multiple inflammatory processes mediated directly through the glucocorticoid receptor. The synovitis of RA is exquisitely sensitive to corticosteroids: in fact, the dramatic clinical improvement of patients with RA after glucocorticoid treatment led early investigators to hypothesize that RA developed as a consequence of adrenal insufficiency[39]. Data exist which suggest that patients with RA may have insufficient production of glucocorticoids[40–42], which could contribute to inappropriately sustained expression of COX-2. Recent reports have suggested that low-dose glucocorticoid treatment, in combination with other treatments, in patients with a disease duration of <2 years may reduce radiographic progression of disease[43]. How these findings may relate to glucocorticoid effects on COX-2 expression is not known.

The efficacy of non-steroidal selective COX-2 inhibitors in chronic inflammatory disorders has yet to be determined. Theoretical and experimental considerations suggest that specific inhibitors of COX-2 are likely to have a more favourable side effect profile than the non-steroidal anti-inflammatory drugs (NSAIDs) currently in use that inhibit both COX-1 and 2. Under normal physiological conditions, PG production depends on the availability of AA, the combined enzymatic activity of COX-1 and -2, and the activity of tissue-specific PG synthetases/isomerases. COX-2 is increased acutely after inflammatory stimuli, although its long-term expression in chronic inflammation processes is less well defined. Selective COX-2 inhibitors should decrease PG production in situations where COX-2 activity is increased, but should not alter basal PG production mediated via COX-1. This is likely to result in less pronounced effects on tissues where PGs mediate important homeostatic functions, including the gastrointestinal tract, kidney and platelets. In experiments performed by Masferrer and colleagues, NS-398, a selective COX-2 inhibitor, suppressed PG production in inflamed tissues, but did not inhibit gastric PG synthesis[24]. In addition, short term administration of NS-398 was not associated with gastric lesions. These results stand in sharp contrast to results with indomethacin, which inhibited both lesional and gastric PG production, and caused gastric lesions[24]. Preliminary studies in patients with OA by Bjarnason and colleagues, demonstrated fewer gastric erosions in patients taking a selective COX-2 inhibitor, flosulide, than in those treated with naproxen[44]. However, the efficacy of the treatment was not reported in this abstract.

References

1. Salmon JA, Higgs GA, Vane JR et al. Synthesis of arachidonate cyclo-oxygenase products by rheumatoid and nonrheumatoid synovial lining in nonproliferative organ culture. Ann Rheum Dis. 1983;42:36–9.
2. Davies P, Bailey PJ, Goldenberg MM, Ford-Hutchinson AW. The role of arachidonic acid oxygenation products in pain and inflammation. Annu Rev Immunol. 1984;2:335–57.
3. Robinson DR, Tashijian AHJ, Levine L. Prostaglandin-stimulated bone resorption by rheumatoid synovia: a possible mechanism for bone destruction in rheumatoid arthritis. J Clin Invest. 1975;56:1181–8.
4. Dayer J-M, Krane SM, Russell RGG, Robinson DR. Production of collagenase and prostaglandins by isolated adherent rheumatoid synovial cells. Proc Natl Acad Sci USA. 1976;73: 945–9.
5. Mehindate K, Al-Daccak R, Dayer J-M et al. Superantigen-induced collagenase gene expression in human IFN-γ-treated fibroblast-like synoviocytes involves prostaglandin E2. J Immunol. 1995;155:3570–7.
6. DeWitt DL. Prostaglandin endoperoxide synthase: regulation of enzyme expression. Biochem Biophys Acta. 1991;1083:121–34.
7. Lai CY, Wada K. Phospholipase A2 from human synovial fluid: purification and structural homology to the placental enzyme. Biochem Biophys Res Commun. 1988;157:488–93.
8. Kramer RM, Hession C, Johansen B et al. Structure and properties of a human non-pancreatic phospholipase A2. J Biol Chem. 1989;264:5768–75.
9. Clark JD, Milona N, Knopf JL. Purification of a 110-kilodalton cytosolic phospholipase A2 from the human monocytic cell line U937. Proc Natl Acad Sci USA. 1990;87:7708–12.
10. Kramer RM, Roberts EF, Mannetta J, Putnam JE. The Ca^{2+} sensitive cytosolic phospholipase A2 is a 100-kDa protein in human monoblast U937 cells. J Biol Chem. 1991;266:5268–72.

11. Funk CD, Funk LB, Kennedy ME, Pong AS, Fitzgerald GA. Human platelet/erythroleukemia cell prostaglandin G/H synthase: cDNA cloning, expression, and gene chromosomal assignment. FASEB J. 1991;5:2304–12.
12. Hoff T, DeWitt D, Kaever V, Resch K, Goppelt-Strueber M. Differentiation-associated expression of prostaglandin G/H synthase in monocytic cells. FEBS Lett. 1993;320:38–42.
13. Smith CJ, Morrow JD, Roberts LJ, Marnett LJ. Differentiation of monocytoid THP-1 cells with phorbol ester induces expression of prostaglandin endoperoxide synthase-1 (COX-1). Biochem Biophys Res Commun. 1993;192:787–93.
14. Murakami M, Matsumoto R, Urades Y, Austen KF, Arm JP. c-Kit ligand mediates increased expression of cytosolic phospholipase A2, prostaglandin endoperoxide synthase-1, and hematopoietic prostaglandin D2 synthase and increased IgE-dependent prostaglandin D2 generation in immature mouse mast cells. J Biol Chem. 1995;270:3239–46.
15. Crofford LJ, Wilder RL, Ristimaki AP, Remmers EF, Epps HR, Hla T. Cyclooxygenase-1 and -2 expression in rheumatoid synovial tissues: effects of interleukin-1β, phorbol ester, and corticosteroids. J Clin Invest. 1994;93:1095–101.
16. O'Banion MK, Sadowski HB, Winn V, Young DA. A serum- and glucocorticoid-regulated 4-kilobase mRNA encodes a cyclooxygenase-related protein. J Biol Chem. 1991;266:23261–7.
17. Lee SH, Soyoola E, Chanmugam P et al. Selective expression of mitogen-inducible cyclooxygenase in macrophages stimulated with lipopolysaccharide. J Biol Chem. 1992;267:25934–8.
18. Fu J-I, Masferrer JL, Seifert K, Raz A, Needleman P. The induction and suppression of prostaglandin H_2 synthase (cyclooxygenase) in human monocytes. J Biol Chem. 1990;265: 16737–40.
19. Koehler L, Hass R, DeWitt DL, Resch K, Goppelt-Struebe M. Glucocorticoid-induced reduction of prostanoid synthesis in TPA-differentiated U937 cells is mainly due to a reduced cyclooxygenase activity. Biochem Pharmacol. 1990;40:1307–16.
20. Hulkower KI, Wertheimer SJ, Levin W et al. Interleukin-1β induces cytosolic phospholipase A2 and prostaglandin H synthase in rheumatoid synovial fibroblasts. Evidence for their roles in the production of prostaglandin E2. Arthritis Rheum. 1994;37:653–61.
21. Wilder RL. Streptococcal cell wall-induced polyarthritis in rats. In: Greenwald RA, Diamond HS, editors. CRC Handbook of Animal Models for the Rheumatic Diseases. Boca Raton: CRC Press, Inc., 1988:33–40.
22. Crofford LJ, Wilder RL. Arthritis and autoimmunity in animals. In: McCarty DJ, Koopman WJ, editors. Arthritis and Allied Conditions. Philadelphia, PA: Lea & Febiger; 1993:525–39.
23. Sano H, Hla T, Maier JAM et al. In vivo cyclooxygenase expression in synovial tissues of patients with rheumatoid arthritis and osteoarthritis and rats with adjuvant and streptococcal cell wall arthritis. J Clin Invest. 1992;89:97–108.
24. Masferrer JL, Zweifel BS, Manning PT et al. Selective inhibition of inducible cyclooxygenase 2 in vivo is antiinflammatory and nonulcerogenic. Proc Natl Acad Sci USA. 1994;91:3228–32.
25. Vane JR, Mitchell JA, Appleton I et al. Inducible isoforms of cyclooxygenase and nitric-oxide synthase in inflammation. Proc Natl Acad Sci USA. 1994;91:2046–50.
26. Sugiyama E, Taki H, Kuroda A, Mino T, Hori T, Kobayashi M. Interleukin-4 inhibits prostaglandin E2 production by freshly prepared rheumatoid synovial cells via inhibition of biosynthesis and gene expression of cyclooxygenase II but not those of cyclooxygenase I. Arthritis Rheum. 1995;38(suppl):S352.
27. Xie W, Fletcher BS, Andersen RD, Herschman HR. v-*src* induction of the TIS10/PGS2 prostaglandin synthase gene is mediated by an ATF/CRE transcription response element. Mol Cell Biol. 1994;14:6531–9.
28. Sirois J, Richards JS. Transcription regulation of the rat prostaglandin endoperoxide synthase 2 gene in granulosa cells: Evidence for the role of a *cis*-acting C/EBPβ promoter element. J Biol Chem. 1993;268:21931–8.
29. Shaw G, Kamen R. A conserved AU sequence from the 3′ untranslated region of GM-CSF mRNA mediates selective mRNA degradation. Cell. 1986;29:659–67.
30. Rïstimaki A, Garfinkel S, Wessendorf J, Maciag T, Hla T. Induction of cyclooxygenase-2 by interleukin-1 alpha. Evidence for post-transcriptional regulation. J Biol Chem. 1994;269: 11769–75.
31. Brinckerhoff DR, Harris ED Jr. Survival of rheumatoid synovium implanted into nude mice. Am J Pathol. 1981;103:411–8.

32. Lafyatis R, Remmers EF, Roberts AB, Yocum DE, Sporn MB, Wilder RL. Anchorage-independent growth of synoviocytes from arthritis and normal joints: Stimulation by exogenous platelet derived growth factor and inhibition by transforming growth factor-beta and retinoids. J Clin Invest. 1989;83:1267–76.
33. Arend WP, Dayer J-M. Cytokines and cytokine inhibitors or antagonists in rheumatoid arthritis. Arthritis Rheum. 1990;33:305–15.
34. Hempel SL, Monick MM, He B, Yano T, Hunninghake GW. Synthesis of prostaglandin H synthase-2 by human alveolar macrophages in response to lipopolysaccharide is inhibited by decreased cell oxidant tone. J Biol Chem. 1994;269:32979–84.
35. Wilborn J, DeWitt DL, Peters-Golden M. Expression and role of cyclooxygenase isoforms in alveolar and peritoneal macrophages. Am J Physiol. 1995;268:L294–301.
36. de Brum-Fernandes AJ, Laporte S, Heroux M et al. Expression of prostaglandin endoperoxide synthase-1 and prostaglandin endoperoxide synthase-2 in human osteoblasts. Biochem Biophys Res Commun. 1994;198:955–60.
37. Morrisset S, Lora M, Leduc R, de Brum-Fernandes AJ. Regulation of the expression of cyclooxygenase-1 and cyclooxygenase-2 in bovine chondroblasts in culture. Arthritis Rheum. 1995;39(suppl.):S389.
38. Abramson SB, Weissman G. The mechanisms of action of nonsteroidal antiinflammatory drugs. Arthritis Rheum. 1989;32:1–9.
39. Hench PS, Kendall EC, Slocumb LH, Polley HF. The effect of a hormone of the adrenal cortex (17-hydroxy-11-dehydrocorticosterone: compound E) and of pituitary adrenocorticotropic hormone on rheumatoid arthritis. Proc Mayo Clin. 1949;24:181–97.
40. Neeck G, Federlin K, Graef V, Rusch D, Schmidt KL. Adrenal secretion of cortisol in patients with rheumatoid arthritis. J Rheumatol. 1989;17:24–9.
41. Cash JM, Crofford LJ, Gallucci WT et al. Pituitary-adrenal responsiveness to ovine corticotropin releasing hormone in patients with rheumatoid arthritis treated with lose dose prednisone. J Rheumatol. 1992;19:1692–6.
42. Chikanza IC, Petrou P, Kingsley G, Chrousos G, Panayi GS. Defective hypothalamic response to immune and inflammatory stimuli in patients with rheumatoid arthritis. Arthritis Rheum. 1991;35:1281–8
43. Kirwan JR. The effect of glucocorticoids on joint destruction in rheumatoid arthritis. N Engl J Med. 1995;333:142–6.
44. Bjarnason I, Macpherson A, Schupp J, Hayllar J. A randomised, double blind, crossover comparative endoscopy study on the tolerability of flosulide, a selective cyclo-oxygenase-2 inhibitor, and naproxen. Arthritis Rheum. 1995;38(suppl.):S280.

9 An inhibitor of injury-induced COX-2 transcriptional activation elicits neuroprotection in a brain damage model

N.G. BAZAN, G. ALLAN and V.L. MARCHESELLI

The quest to understand the molecular changes in brain injury is providing new ideas that might lead to more effective therapeutic approaches. Early molecular events in brain injury, such as the hydrolysis of membrane phospholipids, can trigger cascades of events which may constitute decision pathways leading to neuronal damage or cell death, or conversely to repair and regeneration. The fundamental problems are to identify which second messengers accumulate, the signals that trigger their production and the pathways that, in turn, they affect in the damaged regions of the brain. In the design of more discriminating pharmacological approaches it is important to understand how intervention at a single point in a signalling pathway will affect the complex web of cellular communications between neurones, and between the neurone, glia and cerebral microvasculature. While the short term survival of the subject in the acute phase of stroke, head injury or epilepsy is obviously of paramount importance, an understanding of the mechanisms which lead to the alterations in synaptic circuitry involved in delayed neurobehavioural disorders such as post-traumatic epilepsy, delayed amnesia, psychosis and dementia could help in designing therapies which promote better long-term recovery.

In this chapter, we discuss the mechanisms by which lipid second messengers accumulate during brain injury, show how one of these second messengers, platelet-activating factor (PAF), is involved in the induction of the inducible cyclooxygenase (COX-2), and present ideas for pharmacological intervention in brain injury by specific modulation of this form of COX.

PHOSPHOLIPASE ACTIVATION AND ARACHIDONIC ACID RELEASE

The accumulation of biologically active lipid second messengers is an early event in brain injury[1]. Many of these changes are the result of phospholipase activation following an increased calcium influx and/or intracellular calcium mobilization in the cell[2]. While phospholipid metabolism in excitable membranes is very sensitive to brain injury[3–6], the detailed events involved in the activation of neural phospholipases under pathophysiological conditions are still not fully understood. Under normal conditions, the metabolism of arachidonoyl phos-pholipids in the CNS, regulated through phospholipase A_2 (PLA_2) and acyltransferase, favours cellular retention and maintenance of very low levels of free arachidonic acid (20:4)[7]. During brain injury there is membrane depolarization and calcium influx[8], followed by the massive release of free 20:4[9-11]. While the main release of free 20:4 occurs after a lag during which cellular conditions become favourable for phospholipase activation, in cerebral ischaemia 20:4 accumulates gradually as brain ATP levels drop, but before membrane depolarization. This suggests that in addition to phospholipase activation, accumulation of free 20:4 also involves a down-regulation of energy-dependent reacylation into membrane phospholipids[8].

Two enzymatic pathways have been suggested as contributors to 20:4 release during the rapid early phase of free fatty acid (FFA) accumulation: PLA_2-mediated deacylation of phospholipids and the sequential degradation of inositol lipids by phospholipase C-diacylglycerol (DAG) and monoacylglycerol lipases[7,12]. An additional mechanism may be the activation of a phospholipase D (PLD) that hydrolyses phosphatidylcholine to release phosphatidic acid; this, in turn, is acted upon by phosphatidate phosphohydrolase[12,13] to yield DAG.

Elevated PLA_2 activity in brain has been reported during ischaemia and head injury[14-16]. However, the generation of free 20:4 through the PLC–DAG lipase pathway during ischaemia and seizures is supported by the observation that accumulation of free 20:4 coincides with the release of 20:4–DAG through the phosphodiesteratic degradation of polyphosphoinositides[4,17-19]. However, dissociation between 20:4 accumulation and DAG release was observed in the anoxic immature murine brain, where free 20:4 accumulates after a prolonged lag period with no accompanying release of 20:4–DAG[20]. It is likely that more than one phospholipase is responsible for 20:4 release during brain trauma. Questions regarding the timing and sequence of phospholipase activation, and the phospholipid pools from which individual membrane-derived lipid second messengers are derived, remain to be answered. Analysis of the kinetics of inositol phospholipid degradation and accumulation of free 20:4 and 20:4–DAG in rat brain following a single electroconvulsive shock (ECS) suggests that activation of the individual phospholipases is time-dependent and that different phospholipid pools are involved[19,21]. During the tonic phase of the seizure, the fall in 20:4 content in PPI is accounted for by the increase of 20:4 in free fatty acids and DAG. Later, during the clonic phase, degradation of other 20:4-containing phospholipids contributes to the increased 20:4 content in the free fatty acid pool. The tonic-phase accumulation of PPI-derived second messengers appears to involve activation of both PLC and PLA_2, as treatment of rats with *Ginkgo biloba* extract prior to ECS blocks the release of 20:4–DAG in the hippocampus without affecting free 20:4 accumulation[22]. The sequential contribution of the PLC/DAG lipase pathway, followed by PLA_2, to the accumulation of free 20:4 in the mouse brain after post-decapitation ischaemia has also been reported[23,24]. During global ischaemia of the rat brain, the inositol phospholipid pool is the main contributor to free fatty acid release via the PLC/DAG-lipase pathway. After longer times of ischaemia (2–4 min), the calcium-dependent PLA_2 pathway prevails, releasing fatty acids from phosphatidylcholine (PC) and phosphatidylethanolamine (PE)[25].

Several mechanisms may contribute to phospholipase activation during brain trauma. The primary mechanism is thought to be an elevated cytosolic concentration of Ca^{2+} triggered either by IP_3-mediated calcium mobilization from intracellular stores or by influx of extracellular calcium through plasma membrane channels[2,13,26]. Perhaps the most significant means by which intracellular calcium concentrations are raised during brain trauma is through activation of the NMDA receptor calcium channel. The massive release of glutamate under these conditions leads to an overload of intracellular Ca^{2+} and the stimulation of Ca^{2+}-dependent lipases, protease and nucleases, resulting in glutamate neurotoxicity. PLA_2-mediated release of 20:4 is triggered by NMDA receptor activation in primary cultures of striatal neurones and cerebellar granule cells[27,28], and in hippocampal slices[29], and is blocked by PLA_2 inhibitors[30]. The main PLA_2 responsible for 20:4 release in the CNS could be a high molecular weight cytosolic PLA_2 that undergoes membrane translocation upon an increase in intracellular Ca^{2+} [16,31], and which has a substrate specificity for 20:4-containing phospholipids[32,33].

Agonist interaction with receptor–G protein complexes provides another mechanism of PLA_2 stimulation. Dissociation of the heterotrimeric G proteins in α and $\beta\gamma$ subunits mediates the activation of phospholipases: the α subunit stimulates PLC while the $\beta\gamma$ subunits have been shown to activate PLA_2 in retinal rod outer segments[34,35]. The high homology between PLA_2 activating protein (PLAP) and β-transducin[36] implicates the G protein signalling pathway in the direct activation of PLA_2.

The release of 20:4 may also be modulated by lipocortins (annexins), a family of calcium and phospholipid binding proteins that inhibit PLA_2. While, as discussed later in this chapter, glucocorticoids are known to inhibit induction of the inducible prostaglandin synthase, their anti-inflammatory properties have also been linked to their ability to induce lipocortin synthesis[37]. Steroid-inducible lipocortin-1 is present in neuronal and glial cells, especially in the hippocampus[38], where it is thought to be an endogenous neuroprotective agent[39]. When administered intraventricularly to rats, the protein significantly reduces infarct size and oedema induced by cerebral ischaemia[40] and attenuates excitotoxic damage mediated by NMDA receptors[41].

ROLES OF ARACHIDONIC ACID IN NEURONAL PHYSIOLOGY AND PATHOPHYSIOLOGY

Release of 20:4 plays a central role in the development of brain injury. Eicosanoids synthesized from free 20:4 are potent mediators of inflammation, increasing vascular permeability and promoting the development of brain oedema[42]. It should not be forgotten, however, that the free fatty acid itself is a significant modulator of neuronal activity, acting on a variety of functional membrane proteins, including receptors, ion channels and enzymes[43–45].

The NMDA receptor-stimulated release of 20:4 results in perturbations of ionic homeostasis and alterations in neuronal excitability. Arachidonic acid-mediated activation of potassium channels leads to neuronal hyperpolarization and synaptic depression[43]. However, neuronal excitability is promoted by inhibition of glutamate uptake[46,47], stimulation of glutamate release[48,49], activation of A_1-adenosine receptors[50], and increasing the open-channel probability of the NMDA receptor[51]. While it is not always possible to distinguish which of these effects are due to the direct action of the fatty acid, analysis of the NMDA receptor amino acid sequence shows a domain homologous to fatty acid-binding proteins[52] and thus supports a direct interaction of free 20:4 with the NMDA receptor. Arachidonic acid may also stimulate glutamatergic neurotransmission, probably acting as a retrograde messenger at the presynaptic level, stimulating further release of glutamate. These pre- and post-synaptic effects may contribute to long lasting changes in glutamate synaptic efficacy or long term potentiation (LTP), a form of synaptic plasticity essential to the process of memory and learning in the brain[53]. This is discussed in more detail below.

PROSTAGLANDIN SYNTHESIS IN BRAIN DAMAGE

In the early stages of brain damage, the release of 20:4 is the rate-limiting step in the synthesis of prostaglandins, potent modulators of neuronal function[42,54]. The molecular mechanism of ischaemia/reperfusion-induced neuronal injury involves the release of 20:4 during the ischaemic phase and its conversion to prostaglandins[55,56] and leukotrienes[57,58] during reperfusion (Figure 1). These metabolites can elicit a variety of effects, not only in neural cells but also in the microvasculature: prostaglandins affect cerebral blood flow[59] and leukotrienes increase blood–brain barrier permeability[60,61].

The entry point of free 20:4 into the prostaglandin synthesis pathway is the cyclooxygenation of 20:4 to PGG_2 followed by its hydroperoxidation to PGH_2, catalysed by prostaglandin synthase (COX, cyclooxygenase endoperoxide synthase, PGH synthase, EC 1.14.99.1). For a long time it was thought that there was only a single, constitutive COX, and that the increased synthesis of prostaglandins in pathophysiological situations simply reflected the increased availability of substrate. There is now known to be two forms of COX, a typically constitutive enzyme (COX-1) insensitive to glucocorticoids, and an inducible enzyme (COX-2), expressed in response to mitogen stimulation and sensitive to glucocorticoid inhibition[62,63]. COX-2 was originally cloned as one of a series of primary response genes induced in Swiss 3T3 cells by tetradecanoyl phorbol acetate (TPA) known as TPA-induced sequences (TIS genes)[64], and as a mitogen-

Figure 1 ***Free arachidonic acid release, eicosanoid formation and lipid peroxidation during brain injury, as illustrated by ischaemia–reperfusion. Under physiological conditions there is a low level of receptor-mediated PAF and eicosanoid synthesis. During the ischaemic phase, there is an overactivation of phospholipase A2 and an accumulation of free arachidonic acid. The lowering of oxygen tension and metabolic energy impairs synthesis of eicosanoids and the re-esterification of arachidonic acid into membrane phospholipids. Reperfusion leads to a rise in oxygen tension and a massive burst of oxidative metabolism and synthesis of eicosanoids. A by-product of oxidative metabolism is superoxide and other oxygen radicals. Their accumulation under these conditions can exceed the capacity of the cellular free radical scavenging and antioxidant mechanisms, leading to lipid peroxidation and other manifestations of oxidative stress***

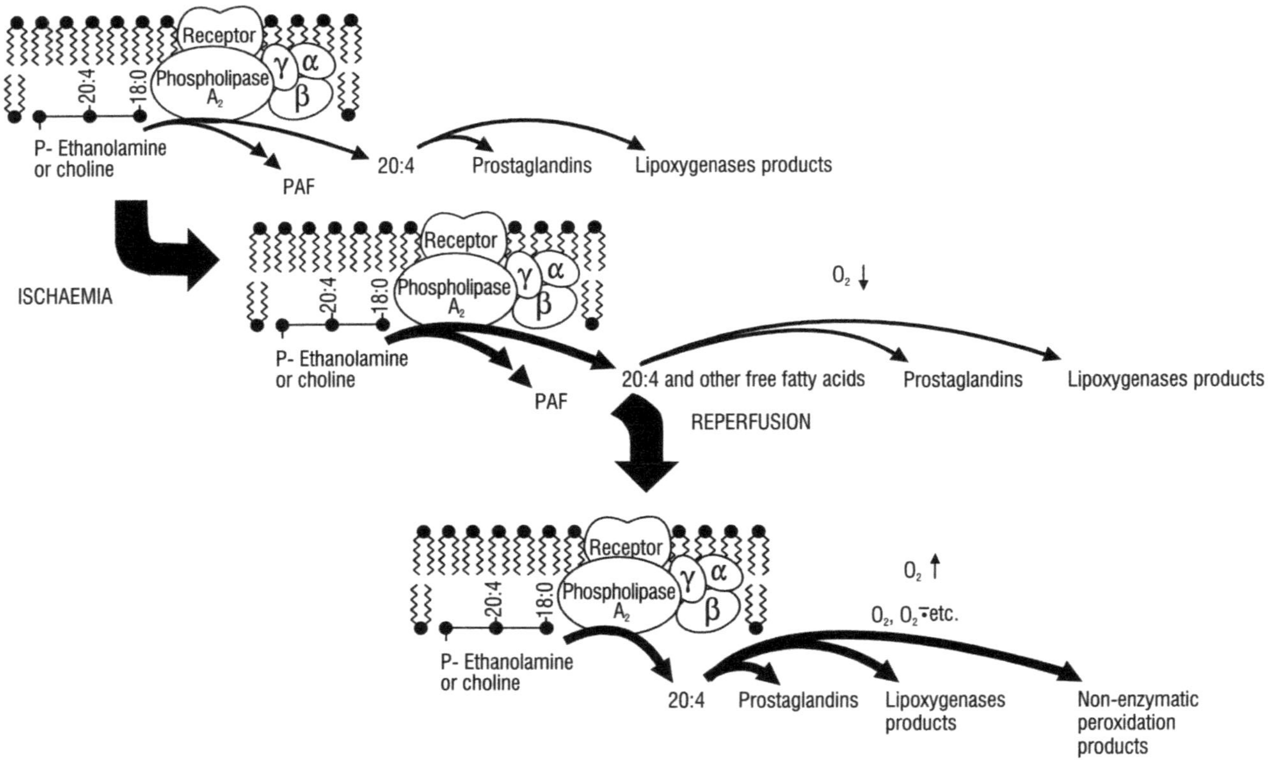

inducible gene in chick embryo fibroblasts[65]. In the brain, COX-2 is expressed mainly in cortical and limbic neurones but not in glia or vascular endothelium[66,67]. NMDA-dependent synaptic activity implicated in memory and learning processes as well as in excitotoxic neuronal damage has been shown to regulate the expression of the COX-2 gene[66]. Antibodies against COX-2 stain primarily dendrites and cell bodies[67], implying post-synaptic localization. This suggests that prostaglandins may play a role in NMDA-mediated neuronal plasticity and, under pathological conditions (i.e. ischaemia, stroke), in neural cell injury and death.

PLATELET-ACTIVATING FACTOR AND BRAIN

PAF (1-*O*-alkyl-2-acetyl-glycero-3-phosphocholine) is an acetylated alkyl ether phospholipid originally described as a mediator released by leukocytes which induces the aggregation and activation of rabbit platelets[68,69]. It is now known to have much broader functions as a mediator of inflammatory and immune responses, and as a second messenger involved in intracellular communication[70–72]. PAF is found in the central nervous system, including in brain and retina[73–75]. It is rapidly produced in brain in response to ischaemia and seizures[73,76] and in neuronal cell cultures in response to neurotransmitters[77]. PAF can accumulate in the brain in the absence of inflammatory cells, which implies that some or all of the endogenous cell types in the CNS are capable of synthesizing PAF.

A small, but metabolically active pool of 1-*O*-alkyl-2-arachidonoyl-glycero-3-phosphocholine (alkylacyl-GPC), is an important phospholipid component of excitable membranes. Its hydrolysis, catalysed by PLA_2, yields both 20:4, the precursor of eicosanoids, and lyso-PAF, a direct precursor of PAF. Alkylacyl-GPC is a substrate for a cytosolic PLA_2 that is present in the brain and is activated and translocated to the membrane following an increase in intracellular calcium levels[16,31]. As a result, lyso-PAF becomes available for transacetylation by acetyl CoA:lyso-PAF acetyltransferase to yield biologically active PAF. This route of PAF synthesis is known as the remodelling pathway (Figure 2). There are at least two alternative pathways by which PAF can be generated: the de novo synthesis route and a CoA-independent transacylase. The de novo synthesis pathway involves the synthesis of 1-*O*-alkyl-2-acetylglycerol, which is then converted to PAF by the cholinephosphotransferase-catalysed transfer of a choline moiety from CDP-choline. The other pathway consists of an alternative route for the generation of lyso-PAF via the CoA-independent transacylation of 20:4 acid from alkylarachidonoyl-GPC to an acceptor lysophospholipid. The contribution of these pathways to PAF synthesis during neuronal stimulation has yet to be fully evaluated, although the full complement of enzymes required for all pathways are present in brain[78,79]. Acetylcholine and dopamine stimulate PAF synthesis in developing retina via the de novo pathway[75], and the brain has high

Figure 2 ***The PAF cycle. The membrane phospholipid precursor of PAF, alkylacyl-GPC, is cycled through lyso-PAF, PAF, and after inactivation by PAF acetylhydrolase is reincorporated into the membrane phospholipid pool. The de novo pathway (top right) is independent of this cycle, but there can be input into the lyso-PAF pool from alkylacyl-GPC which has undergone lipid peroxidation and fragmentation of the polyunsaturated acyl chain. The resulting PAF-like molecule is then a substrate for PAF acetylhydrolase. Not shown here is the transacylase pathway, in which transacylation of the arachidonoyl chain of alkylacyl-GPC to an acceptor lysophospholipid leads to formation of lyso-PAF***

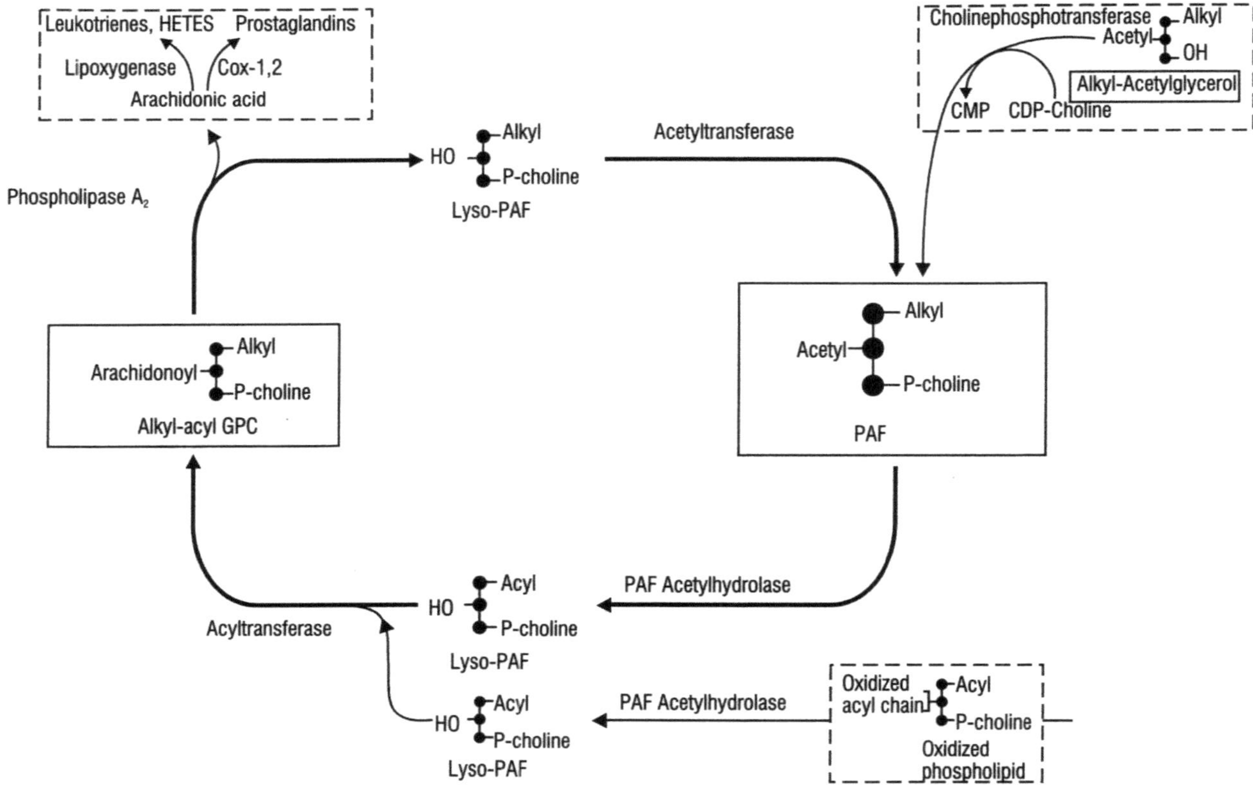

levels of 1-*O*-alkyl-glycero-3-phosphate:acetyl CoA acetyltransferase, which catalyses the synthesis of 1-*O*-alkyl-2-acetylglycerol (the direct precursor of PAF in the de novo pathway)[80]. However, the rise in intracellular calcium which accompanies activation of many receptors, including the NMDA class of glutamate receptors, and the disruption of ion homeostasis in cerebral trauma[81] inhibits the phosphocholine transferase required in the de novo pathway[82].

High-affinity PAF binding sites are found in synaptosomal and microsomal membrane subcellular fractions of rat cortical homogenates[83]. The two sites differ in the kinetics of [^{3}H]PAF binding: the microsomal membranes in fact display cold-ligand displacement kinetics characteristic of two binding sites. They also show differential sensitivity to PAF receptor antagonists. The most experimentally useful of these drugs are BN 52021, a terpenoid extracted from the leaf of the *Ginkgo biloba* tree which binds preferentially to the synaptosomal site[83], and the hetrazepine BN 50730, which shows complete specificity for the microsomal sites. The synaptosomal site appears to correspond to the cloned PAF receptor[84–86], which is a member, along with receptors for other lipid mediators such as prostacyclin[87], of the seven membrane-spanning domain, G protein-coupled receptor superfamily. Of the two transcripts produced from this gene (1 and 2), only type 1 is expressed in brain[88]. Multiple signal transduction pathways can be stimulated by activation of the PAF receptor (Figure 2). PAF treatment of hippocampal neurones in culture elicits intracellular calcium fluxes, the dynamics of which are characteristic of release from intracellular stores rather than gating of extracellular calcium[89]. This correlates with evidence that the primary mode of signal transduction for the cell surface PAF receptor is via a G protein-activated phospholipase C[90,91]. PAF is also reported to down-regulate adenyl cyclase via a pertussis toxin-sensitive mechanism[92] in some cells, to induce extracellular calcium influx[93] and to activate the microtubule-associated protein kinase (MAP kinase) and other protein kinase cascades[92,94]. The identity of the BN 50730-sensitive receptors(s) remains unclear, as does their cellular origin (neurones, glia or microvascular endothelium). It is apparent, however, that the two classes of receptor differ in the signal transduction mechanisms to which they are coupled.

There is evidence to suggest that PAF is a mediator of signal transcription coupling that may, in turn, be involved in neuronal plasticity, remodelling of synaptic circuitry and epileptogenesis. PAF rapidly and transiently augments levels of the c-*fos* and c-*jun* transcription factor mRNAs in a neuronal cell line[95]. Phorbol esters and PAF synergistically stimulate c-*fos* expression, suggesting that the transcriptional effects of PAF are not mediated by protein kinase C. The effect of PAF is at the transcriptional level, as opposed to increasing the stability of the mRNA 5′ deletion; mutagenesis studies of the c-*fos* promoter show that the calcium-response element is necessary for the PAF-induced response. There are other examples of PAF-induced gene expression in neuronal and non-neuronal cells, including the heparin-binding epidermal growth factor in monocytes[96], c-

fos and *egr-2* in lymphoblastoid cell lines[97], the transcription factor NF-κB and immunoglobulins[98] in human B cell lines, c-*fos* and zif/268 in rat astroglia[99], and c-*fos* and TIS 1 in A-431 epidermoid carcinoma cells[100]. There are also reports that PAF is able to autoregulate gene expression of its own cell surface receptor[101,102].

PAF ENHANCES COX-2 PROMOTER ACTIVITY IN VITRO

COX-1 and COX-2 are encoded for by distinct, but evolutionarily related, genes. The human and mouse COX-1 genes contain 11 exons and 10 introns, and span about 22 kb of DNA[103,104]. The human, mouse and chicken COX-2 genes contain 10 exons and 9 introns[105–107] and span only 8–9 kb of DNA. Exons 1–9 of COX-2 are homologous to exons 2–10 of COX-1, and thus both enzymes include haem ligand sites, glycosylation sites, aspirin acetylation sequence, and an epidermal growth factor homology region. The COX-2 gene, however, lacks the exon present in the COX-1 gene that encodes a hydrophobic N-terminal region. The 3′ exon of COX-2 encodes an additional 18 amino acid region in the C-terminal region of COX-2, and a significantly longer 3′-untranslated region in the mRNA which includes several AUUUA sequences characteristic of short-lived messages.

The COX-2 promoters from human[108], rat[109], mouse[105] and chicken[106] have been cloned and analysed. There are some species differences in the organization of promoter elements, but, in the mouse promoter, a number of responsive elements for different inducers of COX-2 expression have been tentatively identified, including v-*src*[106], gonadotrophic hormone[109] and, most significantly in the context of this chapter, PAF[110].

PAF can induce mouse COX-2 promoter activity when constructs are transfected into neuronal (NG108-15 neuroblastoma×glioma hybrid) and non-neuronal (NIH-3T3) cells. When constructs containing the proximal 371 bases (−371 to −1) of the mouse COX-2 promoter are transfected into cells using the calcium phosphate co-precipitation procedure, in the presence of retinoic acid (100 nM), there is dose-dependent (1–50 nM) PAF-induced expression of the luciferase reporter gene. When the vector is transfected into the cells using cationic liposomes (lipofection), reporter gene expression can be induced by PAF alone. There is also activity from constructs containing the proximal 963 bases of the mouse COX-2 promoter, although this is less, suggesting the presence of inhibitory sequences upstream from −371. The effect is rapid, with some activity after as little as 15 or 45 min of incubation with the ligands. This is not sufficient time for de novo protein synthesis, indicating that COX-2 promoter activation in this system involves the modulation of pre-existing transcription factors. Preincubation of the cells with the intracellular PAF antagonist BN 50730 inhibits the PAF/RA induction of luciferase reporter gene expression, which supports this effect as being a specific receptor-mediated phenomenon, and indicates that it is mediated through the intracellular PAF receptor. The use of constructs with 5′ deletions of this promoter in similar transfection experiments narrows down the region of the promoter containing the 'PAF-responsive' element to between −371 and −300; deletion of this region lowers PAF induction from 31 times to 4.1 times control levels. More detailed mapping of this region and the identification of the transcription factors responsible for the PAF regulation of COX-2 are the subjects of ongoing research.

EXPERIMENTAL SEIZURES PROMOTE SUSTAINED TRANSCRIPTIONAL ACTIVATION OF COX-2 IN HIPPOCAMPUS

The PAF antagonist BN 50730 inhibits COX-2 gene expression in the brains of rats subjected to two types of experimental seizures, a single ECS which elicits a single, generalized tonic-clonic seizure or seizures induced by kainic acid (KA), a conformationally rigid analogue of glutamic acid which is an agonist of the AMPA-kainate subclass of glutamate receptors. Injection of KA, either parenterally or intracerebrally, induces limbic seizures similar to the complex partial seizures seen in human temporal lobe epilepsy. In addition, there is a loss of pyramidal cells and damage to the CA3 region of the hippocampus which results in sprouting of mossy fibres from the dentate gyrus. The brain damage produced is similar to that which occurs in the human epileptogenic condition of Ammon's horn sclerosis[111].

A single pretreatment of the animals by intracerebroventricular injection with BN 50730 is sufficient to block most of the COX-2 mRNA accumulation in both seizures models (Marcheselli VL and Bazan NG, submitted for publication), and is a more effective inhibitor of COX-2 induction than the glucocorticoid dexamethasone. This implies that PAF accumulation and activation of the intracellular PAF receptor leads to the majority of the induced prostaglandin synthesis under these conditions. Interestingly, the level of induction of COX-2 and other immediate early genes is much greater and more prolonged in the KA than in the ECS model. This may be reflected in the more profound long-term effects of the KA treatment.

The consequences of inhibiting COX-2 and other PAF-mediated effects on the progression of KA-induced brain lesions is the subject of ongoing research. There is, however, another model of brain injury, cryogenically induced vasogenic cerebral ischaemia, in which inhibition of COX-2 expression correlates with an abrogation of the oedema.

VASOGENIC CEREBRAL OEDEMA INDUCES COX-2

Application of a liquid nitrogen-cooled metal probe to the exposed skull of an experimental animal produces a localized lesion in the parietal cortex, and oedema in the ipsilateral, and to a lesser degree in the contralateral, cerebral hemisphere[112]. The oedema results from the increased permeability of the cerebral microvasculature and the accumulation of fluid in brain tissue. Within the closed, rigid structure of the skull, the resultant swelling leads to increased hydrostatic pressure on the brain, and provides an animal model of the life-threatening consequences of brain oedema seen in humans with closed head injury.

In the cryogenic injury model, the lesion results in the transient accumulation of COX-2 mRNA and protein in the ipsilateral cerebral hemisphere (Marcheselli VL and Bazan NG, submitted for publication). Up-regulation of COX-2 mRNA and protein expression following the insult is strongly inhibited by pretreatment of the animals with a single intracerebroventricular injection of BN 50730, and to a less, but still significant extent, by treatment with dexamethasone. Drug treatment also drastically reduces the brain oedema, and the relative efficacy of the PAF antagonist and the glucocorticoid correlates with their ability to inhibit COX-2 induction. These findings provide a correlation between PAF receptor activation in the brain, induction of COX-2 expression, and increased permeability of the cerebral microvasculature. This suggests that either PAF antagonists or COX-2 inhibitors might be useful drugs in protecting against the formation of cerebral oedema within 24h or so following head injury. It may, however, be the case that accumulation of PAF and/or prostaglandins has a role in the long term survival of neurones and retention of normal synaptic pathways following this type of brain trauma. In this case, the use of either PAF antagonists or COX-2 inhibitors might alleviate the oedema, but may also potentiate long term neuronal damage. Alternatively, while the PAF/COX-2 pathway might be involved in oedema, other pathways may contribute to neuronal damage and pathophysiological synaptic plasticity. If this were so, then adjuvant therapy with other drugs might be needed to combat both the cerebral ischaemia and the neuronal damage in individuals with head injury.

PAF INDUCES COX-2 EXPRESSION IN CORNEAL EPITHELIUM

PAF has been shown to induce COX-2 gene expression in a non-neuronal tissue, the corneal epithelium. The cornea provides a transparent aperture through which light can reach the retina, and provides much of the eye's refractive power. As the integrity of the cornea is obviously essentially for normal vision, it is acutely sensitive to traumatic and irritative insults. Although avascular, the cornea is the most richly innervated tissue in the whole body. The outer few layers of cells comprise the corneal epithelium. This responds very rapidly to damage, initially by cells migrating and spreading to cover the wound, followed by cell division to re-form the stratified epithelium.

PAF accumulates in the rabbit cornea in response to alkali burn, the amount accumulated being dependent on the severity of injury[112]. In the rabbit isolated cornea, treatment with a calcium ionophore elicits PAF synthesis, and the primary PC species from which arachidonic acid is released upon wound healing is the PAF precursor alkylacyl-GPC[113]. This implicates the remodelling pathway in wound-induced PAF release.

Endogenous PAF administered to rabbit corneas in organ cultures induces the BN 50730-sensitive expression of the immediate early genes c-*fos*, c-*jun*, urokinase plasminogen activator (uPA), and COX-2[114–116], and of the secondary response genes matrix metalloproteinases (MMP) 1 (type 1 collagenase) and 9 (gelatinase)[114,117]. Levels of COX-2 protein are elevated 4h after PAF exposure and remain elevated after 16h. Expression of matrix MMP is an important step in wound healing, as modifications of the extracellular matrix are involved in cellular migration. Although the wound can close within 24h, levels of MMP activity remain elevated for many days[118]. In addition, excessive activity of proteinases is thought to be responsible for the destruction of the extracellular matrix involved in corneal ulceration.

Prostaglandins are important regulators of MMP expression in a range of cell and tissue types, up-regulating MMP expression in osteosarcoma cells[119] and monocytes[120], but down-regulating expression in rabbit chondrocytes[121] and synoviocytes[122]. PAF-induced COX-2 expression and prostaglandin synthesis could therefore play a role in the regulation of MMP expression during corneal wound healing, and could conceivably be involved in other pathophysiological manifestations of collagen metabolism such as certain forms of arthritis.

PAF IS A MODULATOR OF NEURONAL PLASTICITY

In experimental models, PAF enhances glutamate release in hippocampal neurons in vitro[123], possibly acts as a presynaptic modulator (retrograde messenger) in hippocampal LTP[124] and is involved in the formation of certain types of memory in the limbic system[125,126] and in the caudate nucleus (Packard MG, Teather L, Bazan NG, submitted for publication). Each of these effects is inhibited by the synaptic PAF receptor antagonist BN 52021. LTP is a phenomenon in which a sustained high-frequency presynaptic stimulation of excitatory amino acid neuronal pathways results in a prolonged enhanced postsynaptic response. LTP, as a use-dependent strengthening of synaptic connections, is considered to be a simple model of the neurophysiological processes underlying memory[53]. As there is some evidence that LTP may underlie hippocampal-based learning[127], the role of PAF in LTP and learning models could be accounted for by the activity of PAF on glutamate release from the presynaptic terminal.

While these activities of PAF models appear to be independent of changes in gene expression, they nevertheless require glutamate release from the presynaptic axonal terminal to result in the accumulation of PAF in the postsynaptic dendritic terminal and cell body. Thus, under conditions of prolonged stimulation or massive glutamate release, there is the potential to greatly enhance PAF accumulation in these cellular structures, and hence the potential for activation of the intracellular PAF receptor and induction of gene expression (Figure 3).

CONCLUSIONS

PAF, produced rapidly after brain injury, is involved in the delayed (~3–4h post-injury) and prolonged (24h post-injury) up-regulation of COX-2 expression and synthesis of prostaglandins. In seizures and ischaemia this correlates with vulnerable parts of the brain e.g. hippocampus. COX-2 expression is inhibited by the intracellular PAF antagonist BN 50730 and by the glucocorticoid dexamethasone in ECS and KA-induced seizures. Inhibition by the PAF antagonist and dexamethasone correlates with inhibition of brain oedema in a cryogenically-induced vasogenic oedema model. Protection by PAF antagonists in cerebral ischaemia also correlates with release of lipid second messengers.

What aspects of COX-2 activation, if any, cause pathophysiological effects? Increased production of PGE_2 has been suggested to be neuroprotective in some models. However, the burst of oxidative metabolism that occurs with reperfusion following ischaemia is accompanied by an increased generation of reactive oxygen species and other free radicals. The peroxidase activity of PG synthase has been shown to catalyse the generation of reactive oxygen species from a number of substrates. Thus, overexpression of COX-2 could contribute to oxidative stress.

The identification of distinct pathways by which COX-2 expression can be modulated, and the development of novel COX-2 enzyme inhibitors, provides us with several new strategies for targeting inducible cyclooxygenase activation in neuroprotection (Figure 4). COX-2 overexpression during brain injury may be an important link between the acute effects of neuronal and/or cerebrovascular damage, and long-term deficits in brain function (Figure 5). Further research in this field holds promise for the treatment of brain damage and neurodegenerative diseases.

ACKNOWLEDGEMENTS

This work was sponsored by the DAMD17-93-V-3-QT3. This does not necessarily reflect the position or the policy of the US Government and no official endorsement should be inferred.

References

1. Bazan NG. Effects of ischemia and electroconvulsive shock on free fatty acid pool in the brain. Biochim Biophys Acta. 1970;218:1–10.
2. Nicotera P, Bellomo G, Orrenius S. Calcium-mediated mechanisms in chemically induced cell death. Annu Rev Pharmacol Toxicol. 1992;32:449–70.
3. Siesjö BK, Ingvar M, Westerberg Z. The influence of bicuculline-induced seizures on free fatty acid concentration in cerebral cortex, hippocampus and cerebellum. J Neurochem. 1992;39: 796–802.
4. Yoshida S, Harik S, Busto R, Santiso M, Martinez E, Ginsberg MD. Free fatty acids and energy metabolites in ischemic cerebral cortex with noradrenaline depletion. J Neurochem. 1984;42: 711–7.

Figure 3 ***Coupling between short term neuronal signalling signals and longer-term changes in cellular physiology. Receptor-mediated synthesis of PAF in the postsynaptic terminal or cell body leads to activation of the intracellular PAF receptor. Through signalling mechanisms involving MAP and possibly other kinases, endogenous nuclear transcription factors are activated and promote the expression of immediate early genes (IEG). IEG transcription factors modulate the transcription of other genes, the expression of which can in turn lead to the expression of further sets of genes. These gene cascades are a mechanism by which expression of a small number of IEG can be amplified into profound long term changes in neuronal phenotype. Also shown is COX-2 ($PGHS_2$) which may be activated by distinct transcription factors. COX-2 expression augments prostaglandin synthesis and promotes the inflammatory response***

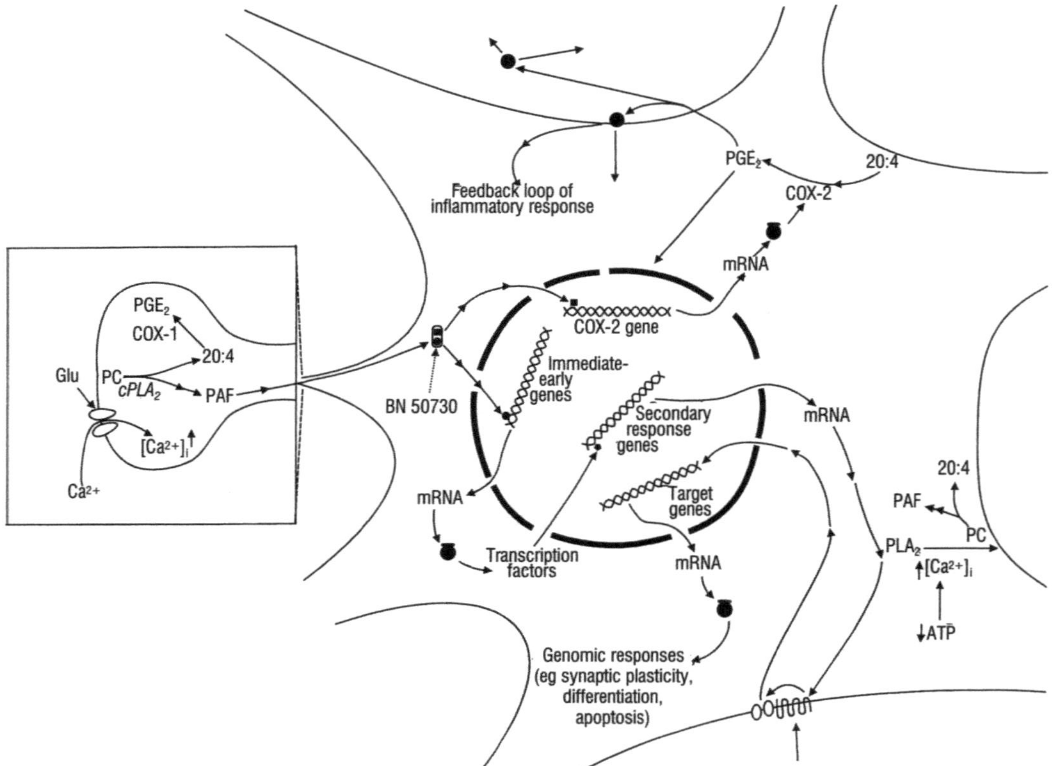

***Figure 4** Sites of regulation of PAF-induced COX-2 expression and prostaglandin synthesis. PLA_2 activation generates lyso-PAF, which is then transacetylated to form PAF. PAF has a short biological half-life. It is quickly deacetylated by PAF acetylhydrolase and only under stimulated conditions does sufficient PAF accumulate to activate the intracellular PAF receptor, the target for the PAF antagonist BN 50730. Receptor activation triggers a series of events which allows one or more transcription factors to bind to the 'PAF-responsive' domain on the COX-2 gene promoter. Glucocorticoids, bound to their nuclear receptor, may inhibit COX-2 gene induction by sterically hindering binding of the PAF-induced transcription factor. Immediate early gene mRNAs are inherently unstable, containing 3′ sequences which direct their rapid degradation. COX-2 induction is longer-lived than, for instance, induction of transcription factor immediate-early genes such as c-fos; nevertheless, post-transcriptional regulation of COX-2 expression via proteins which bind to the mRNA is being investigated. Finally, the development of cyclooxygenase inhibitors specific for the inducible enzyme enables this pool of prostaglandin synthesis to be targeted in experimental and therapeutic approaches*

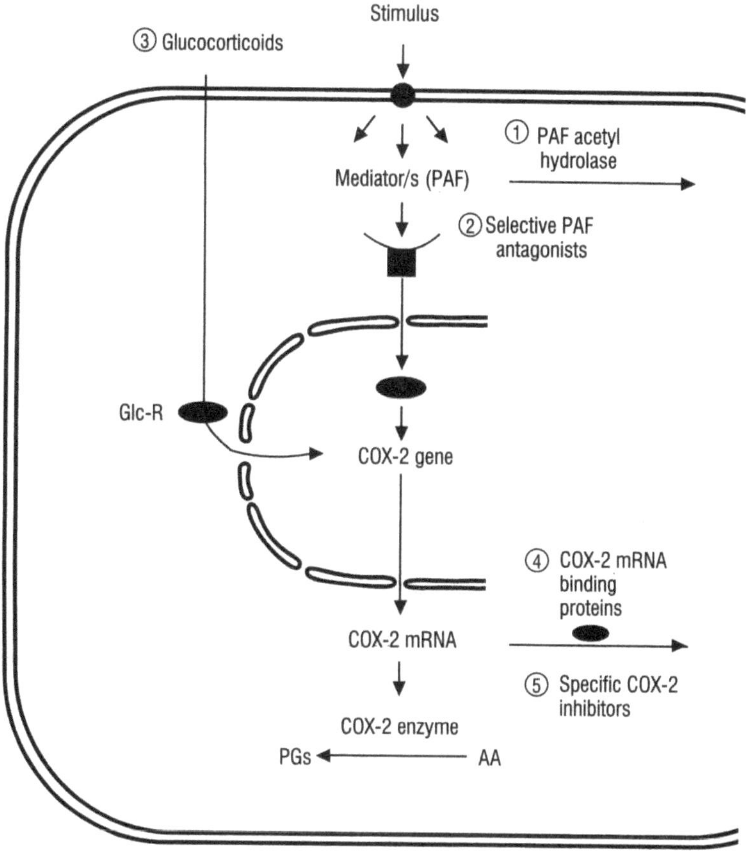

Figure 5 ***PAF, COX-2 and the vicious cycle of brain pathology. Many factors contribute to the acute and long term effects of brain injury and neurodegenerative diseases. The aim of this figure is to pick out the strand in these many complex processes that involves PAF and COX-2 activation, and to show that therapeutic approaches involving these steps can potentially have profound effects not only on the immediate effects of neuronal cell damage and death, but also in the delayed neurological deficits such as aberrant synaptic plasticity and epileptogenesis which lead to a spiral in the normal functioning of the brain***

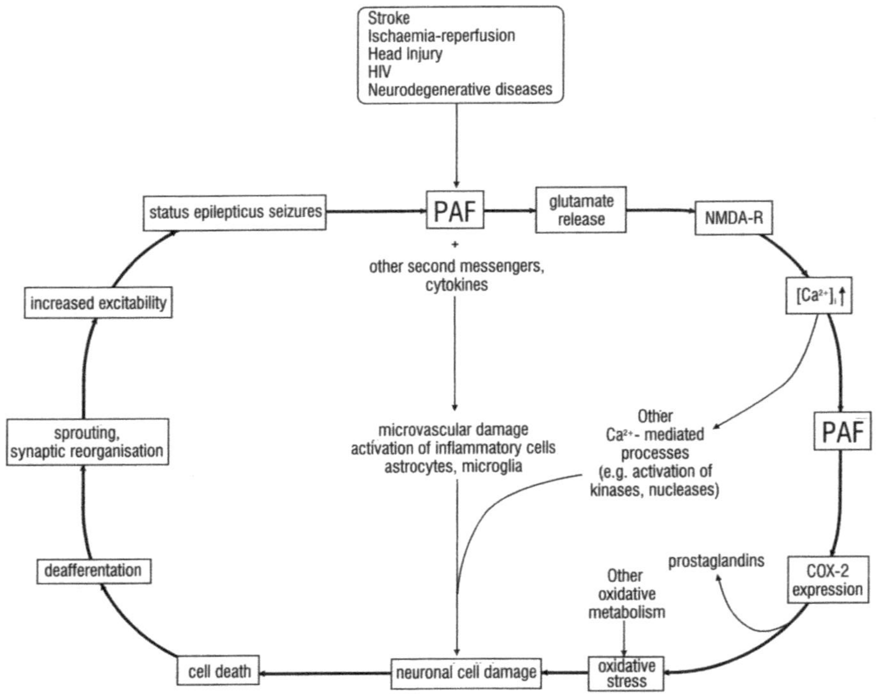

5. Birkle DL, Bazan NG. Effect of bicuculline-induced status epilepticus on prostaglandins and hydroxyeicosatetraenoic acids in rat brain subcellular fractions. J Neurochem. 1987;48:1768–78.
6. Huang SF-L, Sun GY. Acidic phospholipids, diacylglycerols, and free fatty acids in gerbil brain: a comparison of ischemic changes resulting from carotid ligation and decapitation. J Neurosci Res. 1987;17:162–7.
7. Bazan NG. Arachidonic acid (AA) in the modulation of excitable membrane function and at the onset of brain damage. Ann NY Acad Sci. 1989;559:1–16.
8. Katsura K, Rodriguez de Turco EB, Folbergrova J, Bazan NG, Siesjö BK. Coupling among energy failure, loss of ion homeostasis, and phospholipase A2 and C activation during ischemia. J Neurochem. 1993;61:1677–84.
9. Pediconi MF, Rodriguez de Turco EB. Free fatty acid content and release kinetics as manifestations of cerebral lateralization in mouse brain. J Neurochem. 1984;43:1–7.
10. Yasuda H, Kishiro K, Izumi N, Nakanishi M. Biphasic liberation of arachidonic and stearic acids during cerebral ischemia. J Neurochem. 1985;45:168–72.
11. Katayama Y, Kawamata T, Maeda T, Ishikdawa K, Tsubokawa T. Inhibition of the early phase of free fatty acid liberation during cerebral ischemia by excitatory amino acid antagonist administered by microdialysis. Brain Res. 1994;635:331–4.
12. Farooqui AA, Hirashima Y, Horrocks LA. Brain phospholipases and their role in signal transduction. Adv Exp Med Biol. 1992;318:11–25.
13. Nishizuka Y. Intracellular signaling by hydrolysis of phospholipids and activation of protein kinase C. Science. 1992;258:607–14.
14. Shohami E, Shapira Y, Reisfeld N, Yedgar S. Brain phospholipase A_2 is activated after experimental closed head injury in the rat. J Neurochem. 1989;53:1541–6.
15. Rordorf G, Uemura Y, Bonventre JV. Characterization of phospholipase A2 (PLA2) activity in gerbil brain: enhanced activities of cytosolic, mitochondrial, and microsomal forms after ischemia and reperfusion. J Neurosci. 1991;11:1829–36.
16. Bonventre JV, Koroshetz WJ. Phospholipase A_2 (PLA_2) activity in gerbil brain: characterization of cytosolic and membrane-associated forms and effects of ischemia and reperfusion on enzymatic activity. J Lipid Mediat. 1993;6:457–71.
17. Aveldaño MI, Bazan NG. Rapid production of diacylglycerols enriched in 20:4 and stearate during early brain ischemia. J Neurochem. 1975;25:919–20.
18. Ikeda M, Yoshida S, Busto R, Santiso M, Ginsberg MD. Polyphosphoinositides as a probable source of brain free fatty acids accumulated at the onset of ischemia. J Neurochem. 1986;47:123–32.
19. Reddy TS, Bazan NG. Arachidonic acid, stearic acid and diacylglycerol accumulation correlates with the loss of phosphatidylinositol 4,5-bisphosphate in cerebrum 2 seconds after electroconvulsive shock. Complete reversion of changes 5 minutes after stimulation. J Neurosci Res. 1987;18:449–55.
20. Rodriguez de Turco EB, Bazan NG. Changes in free fatty acids and diglycerides in mouse brain at birth and during anoxia. J Neurochem. 1983;41:794–800.
21. Bazan NG, Allan G, Rodriguez de Turco EB. Role of phospholipase A_2 and membrane-derived lipid second messengers in excitable membrane function and transcriptional activation of genes: Implications in cerebral ischemia and neuronal excitability. Prog Brain Res. 1993;96:247–57.
22. Rodriguez de Turco EB, Droy-Lefaix MT, Bazan NG. Decreased electroconvulsive shock-induced diacylglycerols and free fatty acid accumulation in the rat brain by *Ginkgo biloba* extracts (EGB 761): Selective effect in hippocampus as compared with cerebral cortex. J Neurochem. 1993;61:1438–44.
23. Sun GY. Contributions to arachidonic acid release in mouse cerebrum by the phosphoinositide-phospholipase C and phospholipase A2 pathways. Adv Exp Med Biol. 1992;318:103–14.
24. Sun GY, Lu FL, Lin SE, Ko MR. Decapitation ischemia-induced release of free fatty acids in mouse brain. Relationship with diacylglycerols and lysophospholipids. Mol Chem Neuropathol. 1992;17:39–50.
25. Umemura A, Mabe H, Nagai H, Sugino F. Action of phospholipase A_2 and C on free fatty acid release during complete ischemia in rat cortex. Effect of phospholipase C inhibitor and *N*-methyl-D-aspartate antagonist. J Neurosurg. 1992;76:648–51.
26. Berridge MJ. Inositol trisphosphate and calcium signalling. Nature. 1993;361:315–25.
27. Dumuis A, Sebben M, Haynes J-P, Bockaert J. NMDA receptors activate the arachidonic acid cascade system in striatal neurons. Nature. 1988;336:68–70.

28. Lazarewicz JW, Wroblewski JT, Palmer ME, Costa E. Activation of *N*-methyl-D-aspartate-sensitive glutamate receptors stimulates arachidonic acid release in primary cultures of cerebellar granule cells. Neuropharmacology. 1988;27:765–9.
29. Pellerin L, Wolfe LS. Release of arachidonic acid by NMDA-receptor activation in the rat hippocampus. Neurochem Res. 1991;16:983–9.
30. Sanfeliu C, Hunt A, Patel AJ. Exposure to *N*-methyl-D-aspartate increases release of arachidonic acid in primary cultures of rat hippocampal neurons and not in astrocytes. Brain Res. 1990;256:241.
31. Yoshijara Y, Watanabe Y. Translocation of phospholipase A_2 from cytosol to membranes in rat brain induced by calcium ions. Biochem Biophys Res Commun. 1990;170:484–90.
32. Fujimori Y, Murakami M, Kim DK et al. Immunochemical detection of arachidonoyl-preferential phospholipase A2. J Biochem (Tokyo). 1992;111:54–60.
33. Kudo I, Murakami M, Hara S, Inoue K. Mammalian non-pancreatic phospholipases A2. Biochem Biophys Acta. 1993;1170:217–31.
34. Axelrod J, Burch RM, Jelsema CL. Receptor-mediated activation of phospholipase A_2 via GTP-binding proteins: Arachidonic acid and its metabolites as second messengers. Trends Neurochem Sci. 1988;11:117–23.
35. Jelsema CL, Axelrod J. Stimulation of phospholipase A_2 activity in bovine rod outer segment by the β gamma subunits of transducin and its inhibition by the α subunit. Proc Natl Acad Sci USA. 1987;84:3623–7.
36. Peitsch MC, Borner C, Tschopp J. Sequence similarity of phospholipase A2 activating protein and the G protein beta-subunits: a new concept of effector protein activation in signal transduction? Trends Biochem Sci. 1993;18:292–3.
37. Flower RJ. Lipocortin and the mechanism of action of the glucocorticoids. Br J Pharmacol. 1988;79:987–1015.
38. Strijbos PJLM, Tilders FJN, Carey F, Forder RA, Rothwell NJ. Localization of immunoreactive lipocortin-1 in the brain and pituitary gland of the rat. Brain Res. 1991;553:249–60.
39. Rothwell NJ, Relton JK. Involvement of interleukin-1 and lipocortin-1 in ischaemic brain damage. Cerebrovasc Brain Metab Rev. 1993;5:178–98.
40. Relton JK, Strijbos PJLM, O'Shaughnessey CT et al. Lipocortin-1 is an endogenous inhibitor of ischemic damage in the rat brain. J Exp Med. 1991;174:305–10.
41. Black MD, Carey F, Crosman AR, Relton JK, Rothwell N. Lipocortin-1 inhibits NMDA receptor-mediated neuronal damage in the striatum of the rat. Brain Res. 1992;585:135–40.
42. Shimizu T, Wolfe LS. Arachidonic acid cascade and signal transduction. J Neurochem. 1990;55: 1–15.
43. Volterra A, Trotti D, Cassutti P et al. A role for the arachidonic acid cascade in fast synaptic modulation: ion channels and transmitter uptake systems as target proteins. Adv Exp Med Biol. 1992;318:147–58.
44. Ordway RW, Singer JJ, Walsh JV Jr. Direct regulation of ion channels by fatty acids. Trends Neurosci. 1991;14:96.
45. Bazan NG. Involvement of arachidonic acid and platelet-activating factor in the response of the nervous system to ischemia and convulsions. In: Bazan NG, editor. Lipid Mediators in Ischemic Brain Damage and Experimental Epilepsy. New Trends in Lipid Mediators. Basel: Karger; 1990:241–52.
46. Yu ACH, Chan PH, Fishman RA. Effects of arachidonic acid on glutamate and gamma-aminobutyric acid uptake in primary culture of rat cerebral cortical astrocytes and neurons. J Neurochem. 1986;47:1181–9.
47. Barbour B, Szatkowski M, Ingledew N, Attwell D. Arachidonic acid induces a prolonged inhibition of glutamate uptake into glial cells. Nature. 1989;342:918–20.
48. Dorman RV, Hamm TF, Damron DS, Freeman EJ. Modulation of glutamate release from hippocampal mossy fiber nerve endings by arachidonic acid and eicosanoids. Adv Exp Med Biol. 1992;318:121–36.
49. Zhange L, Dorman RV. Synergistic potentiation of glutamate release by arachidonic acid and oleoyl-acetyl-glycerol. Brain Res Bull. 1993;32:437–41.
50. Domanska-Janik K. Unsaturated fatty acids induce inhibition of the A1-adenosine receptor in rat brain membranes. Neuro Report. 1992;4:451–53.
51. Miller B, Sarantis M, Traynelis SF, Attwell D. Potentiation of NMDA receptor currents by arachidonic acid. Nature. 1992;355:722–5.

52. Petrou S, Ordway RW, Singer JJ, Walsh JV Jr. A putative fatty acid-binding domain of the NMDA receptor. Trends Biochem Sci. 1993;18:41–2.
53. Bliss TV, Collingridge GL. A synaptic model of memory: long-term potentiation in the hippocampus. Nature. 1993;361:31–9.
54. Piomelli D. Eicosanoids in synaptic transmission. Crit Rev Neurobiol. 1994;8:65–83.
55. Gaudet RJ, Alam I, Levine L. Accumulation of cyclooxygenase products of arachidonic acid metabolism in gerbil brain during reperfusion after bilateral common carotid artery occlusion. J Neurochem. 1981;35:653.
56. Kempski O, Shohami E, von Lubitz D, Hallenbeck JM, Feuerstein G. Postischemic production of eicosanoids in gerbil stroke. Stroke. 1987;18:111–9.
57. Moskowitz MA, Kiwak KJ, Hekiman K, Levine L. Synthesis of compounds with properties of leukotrienes C_4 and D_4 in gerbil brains after ischemia and reperfusion. Science. 1984;224:886.
58. Dempsey RJ, row MW, Meyer K, Cowen DE, Tai HH. Development of cyclooxygenase and lipoxygenase metabolites of arachidonic acid after transient cerebral ischemia. J Neurosurg. 1986;64:118–24.
59. Moncada S, Vane JR. Pharmacology and endogenous roles of prostaglandin endoperoxides, thromboxane A_2 and prostacyclin. Pharmacol Rev. 1979;30:293–331.
60. Unterberg A, Wahl M, Hammerson F, Baethman A. Permeability and vasomotor response of cerebral vessels during exposure to arachidonic acids. Acta Neuropathol (Berl). 1987;73: 209–11.
61. Baba T, Black KL, Ikezaki K, Chen KN, Becker DP. Intracarotid infusion of leukotriene C4 selectively increases blood–brain barrier permeability after focal ischemia in rats. J Cerebr Blood Flow Metab. 1991;11:638–43.
62. Herschman HR. Regulation of prostaglandin synthase-1 and prostaglandin synthase-2. Cancer Metastatis Rev. 1994;13:241–56.
63. Vane JR, Botting RM. A better understanding of anti-inflammatory drugs based on isoforms of cyclooxygenase (COX-1 and COX-2). Adv Prost Thromb Leuk Res. 1995;23:41–8.
64. Kujubu DA, Fletcher BS, Varnum BC, Lim RW, Herschman HR. TIS10, a phorbol ester tumor promoter-inducible mRNA from Swiss 3T3 cells, encodes a novel prostaglandin synthase/cyclooxygenase homologue. J Biol Chem. 1991;266:12866–72.
65. Xie W, Chipman JG, Robertson DL, Erikson RL, Simmons DL. Expression of a mitogen-responsive gene encoding prostaglandin synthase is regulated by mRNA splicing. Proc Natl Acad Sci USA. 1991;88:2692–6.
66. Yamagata K, Andreasson KI, Kaufmann WE, Barnes CA, Worley PF. Expression of a mitogen-inducible cyclooxygenase in brain neurons: Regulation by synaptic activity and glucocorticoids. Neuron. 1993;11:371–86.
67. Breder CD, Dewitt D, Kraig RP. Characterization of inducible cyclooxygenase in rat brain. J Comp Neurol. 1995;355:296–315.
68. Henson PM. Release of vasoactive amines from rabbit platelets induced by antiplatelet antibody in the presence and absence of complement. J Immunol. 1970;104:934.
69. Benveniste J, Henson PM, Cochrane CG. Leukocyte-dependent histamine release from rabbit platelets. The role of IgE, basophils, and platelet-activating factor. J Exp Med. 1972;136: 1356–77.
70. Braquet P, Touqui L, Shen TY, Vargaftig BB. Perspectives in platelet-activating factor research. Pharmacol Rev. 1987;39:97–145.
71. Prescott SM, Zimmerman GA, McIntyre TM. Platelet-activating factor. J Biol Chem. 1990; 265:17381–4.
72. Bussolino F, Soldi R, Arese M, Jaranowska A, Sogos V, Gremo F. Multiple roles of platelet-activating factor in the nervous system. Neurochem Int. 1995;26:425 33.
73. Kumar R, Harvey S, Kester N, Hanahan D, Olsen M. Production and effects of platelet-activating factor in the rat brain. Biochim Biophys Acta. 1988;963:375–83.
74. Tiberghein C, Laurent L, Junier MP, Dray F. A competitive receptor binding assay for platelet-activating factor (PAF): quantification of PAF in rat brain. J Lipid Mediat. 1991;3:249 66.
75. Bussolino F, Torelli S, Stefanini E, Gremo F. Platelet-activating factor production occurs through stimulation of cholinergic and dopaminergic receptors in the chick retina. J Lipid Mediat. 1989;1:283–8.
76. Panetta T, Marcheselli VL, Braquet P, Spinnewyn B, Bazan NG. Effects of a platelet-activating

factor antagonist (BN 52021) on free fatty acids, diacylglycerols, polyphosphoinositides and blood flow in the gerbil brain. Inhibition of ischemia-reperfusion induced cerebral injury. Biochem Biophys Res Commun. 1987;149:580–7.
77. Sogos V, Bussolino F, Pilia E, Torelli S, Gremo F. Acetylcholine-induced production of platelet-activating factor by human fetal brain cells in culture. J Neurosci Res. 1990;27:706–11.
78. Goracci G, Francesangeli E. Properties of PAF-synthesizing phosphocholinetransferase and evidence for lysoPAF acetyltransferase activity in brain. Lipids. 1991;26:986–91.
79. Blank ML, Smith ZL, Fitzgerald V, Snyder F. The CoA-independent transacylase in PAF biosynthesis: tissue distribution and molecular species selectivity. Biochim Biophys Acta. 1995; 1254:295–301.
80. Lee T-C, Malone B, Snyder F. Formation of 1-alkyl-2-acetyl-sn-glycerols via the de novo biosynthetic pathway for platelet-activating factor. J Biol Chem. 1988;263:1755–60.
81. Deshpande JK, Siesjö BK, Wieloch T. Calcium accumulation and neuronal damage in the rat hippocampus following cerebral ischemia. J Cerebr Blood Flow Metab. 1987;7:89–95.
82. Francescangeli E, Goracci G. The de novo biosynthesis of platelet-activating factor in rat brain. Biochem Biophys Res Commun. 1989;161:107–12.
83. Marcheselli VL, Rossowska M, Domingo MT, Braquet P, Bazan NG. Distinct platelet-activating factor binding sites in synaptic endings and in intracellular membranes of rat cerebral cortex. J Biol Chem. 1990;265:9140–5.
84. Honda Z, Nakamura M, Miki I et al. Cloning by functional expression of platelet-activating factor receptor from guinea-pig lung. Nature. 1991;394:342–6.
85. Kunz D, Gerard NP, Gerard C. The human leukocyte PAF receptor. cDNA cloning, cell surface expression and construction of a novel epitope-bearing analog. J Biol Chem. 1992;267:9101–6.
86. Sugimoto T, Tsuchimochi H, McGregor CG, Mutoh H, Shimizu T, Kurachi Y. Molecular cloning and characterization of the platelet-activating factor receptor from human heart. Biochem Biophys Res Commun. 1992;189:617–24.
87. Sasaki Y, Usui T, Tanaka I et al. Cloning and expression of a cDNA for rat prostacyclin receptor. Biochim Biophys Acta. 1994;1224:601–5.
88. Mutoh H, Bito H, Minami M et al. Two different promoters direct expression of two distinct forms of mRNA of human platelet-activating factor receptor. FEBS Lett. 1993;322:129–34.
89. Bito H, Nakamura M, Honda Z et al. Platelet-activating factor (PAF) receptor in rat brain: PAF mobilizes intracellular Ca^{2+} in hippocampal neurons. Neuron. 1992;9:285–94.
90. Ali H, Richardson RM, Tomhave ED, DuBose RA, Haribabu B, Snyderman R. Regulation of stably transfected platelet activating factor receptor in RBL-2H3 cells. Role of multiple G proteins and receptor phosphorylation. J Biol Chem. 1994;269:24557–63.
91. Honda Z, Takano T, Hirose N et al. Gq pathway desensitizes chemotactic receptor-induced calcium signaling via inositol trisphosphate receptor down-regulation. J Biol Chem. 1995; 270:4840–4.
92. Honda Z, Takano T, Gotoh Y, Nishida E, Ito K, Shimizu T. Transfected platelet-activating factor receptor activates mitogen-activated protein (MAP) kinase and MAP kinase in Chinese hamster ovary cells. J Biol Chem. 1994;269:2307–15.
93. Kornecki E, Ehrlich YH. Neuroregulatory and neuropathological actions of the ether-phospholipid platelet-activating factor. Science. 1988;240:1792–4.
94. Kuruvilla A, Pielop C, Shearer WT. Platelet-activating factor induces the tyrosine phosphorylation and activation of phospholipase C-$\gamma 1$, fyn and lyn kinases, and phosphatidylinositol 3-kinase in a human B cell line. J Immunol. 1994;153:5433–42.
95. Squinto SP, Block AL, Braquet P, Bazan NG. Platelet-activating factor stimulates a Fos/Jun/AP-1 transcriptional signaling system in human neuroblastoma cells. J Neurosci Res. 1989;24: 558–66.
96. Pan Z, Kravchenko VV, Ye RD. Platelet activating factor stimulates transcription of the heparin-binding epidermal growth factor-like growth factor in monocytes. Correlation with an increased kappa B binding activity. J Biol Chem. 1995;270:7787–90.
97. Mazer B, Domenico J, Sawami H, Gelfand EW. Platelet-activating factor induces an increase in intracellular calcium and expression of regularity genes in human B lymphoblastoma cells. J Immunol. 1994;146:1914–20.
98. Smith CS, Shearer WT. Activation of NF-kappa B and immunoglobulin expression in response to platelet-activating factor in a human B cell line. Cell Immunol. 1994;155:292–303.

99. Dell'Albani P, Condorelli DF, Mudo G, Amico C, Bindoni M, Belluardo N. Platelet-activating factor and its methoxy analogue ET-18-OCH3 stimulate immediate-early gene expression in rat astroglial cultures. Neurochem Int. 1993;22:567–74.
100. Tripathi Y, Kandala J, Guntaka R, Lim R, Shukla S. Platelet-activating factor induces expression of early response genes *c-fos* and TIS-1 in human epidermoid carcinoma-432 cells. Life Sci. 1991;49:1761–7.
101. Mutoh H, Ishii S, Izumi T, Kato S, Shimizu T. Platelet-activating factor (PAF) positively autoregulates the expression of human PAF receptor transcript 1 (leukocyte-type) through NF-kappa B. Biochem Biophys Res Commun. 1994;205:1137–42.
102. Shirasaki H, Adcock IM, Kwon OJ, Nishikawa M, Mak JC, Barnes PJ. Agonist-induced upregulation of platelet-activating factor receptor messenger RNA in human monocytes. Eur J Pharmacol. 1994;268:263–6.
103. Yokoyama C, Tanabe T. Cloning of the human gene encoding prostaglandin endoperoxide synthase and primary structure of the enzyme. Biochem Biophys Res Commun. 1989;165: 888–94.
104. Kraemer SA, Meade EA, DeWitt DL. Prostaglandin endoperoxide synthase gene structure: identification of the transcriptional start site and 5′-flanking regulatory sequences. Arch Biochem Biophys. 1992;293:391–400.
105. Fletcher BS, Kujubu DA, Perrin DM, Herschman HR. Structure of the mitogen-inducible TIS10 gene and demonstration that the encode protein is a functional prostaglandin synthase. J Biol Chem. 1992;267:4338–44.
106. Xie W, Merril JR, Bradshaw WS, Simmons DL. Structural determination and promoter analysis of the chicken mitogen-inducible prostaglandin G/H synthase gene and genetic mapping of the murine homolog. Arch Biochem Biophys. 1994;300:247–52.
107. Appleby SB, Ristimaki A, Neilson K, Narko K, Hla T. Structure of the human cyclo-oxygenase-2 gene. Biochem J. 1994;302:723–7.
108. Tazawa R, Xu XM, Wu KK, Wang LH. Characterization of the genomic structure, chromosomal location and promoter of human prostaglandin H synthase-2 gene. Biochem Biophys Res Commun. 1994;203:190–9.
109. Sirois J, Richards JS. Transcriptional regulation of the rat prostaglandin endoperoxide synthase 2 gene in granulosa cells. Evidence for the role of a cis-acting C/EBP beta promoter element. J Biol Chem. 1993;268:21913–8.
110. Bazan NG, Fletcher BS, Herschman HR, Mukherjee PK. Platelet-activating factor and retinoic acid synergistically activate the inducible prostaglandin synthase gene. Proc Natl Acad Sci USA. 1994;91:5252–6.
111. Babb TL, Leib JP, Brown WJ, Pretorius J, Crandell PH. Distribution of pyramidal cell density and hyperexcitability in the epileptic human hippocampal formation. Epilepsia. 1984;25:71–9.
112. Bazan NG, Politi E, Rodriguez de Turco EB. Endogenous pools of arachidonic acid-enriched membrane lipids in cryogenic brain injury. In: Go KG, Baethmann A, editors. Recent Progress in the Study and Therapy of Brain Edema. New York: Plenum; 1984:203–12.
113. Hurst JS, Bazan HE. The platelet-activating factor precursor of the injured cornea is selectively implicated in arachidonate and eicosanoid release. Curr Eye Res. 1993;12:655–63.
114. Bazan HEP, Tao Y, Bazan NG. Platelet activating factor induces collagenase expression in corneal epithelium cells. Proc Natl Acad Sci USA. 1993;90:8672–82.
115. Tao Y, Bazan HEP, Bazan NG. Platelet-activating factor (PAF) induces expression of the urokinase type, but not the tissue type plasminogen activator in the corneal epithelium. Invest Ophthalmol Vis Sci. 1994;35(Suppl.):S1457.
116. Tao Y, Bazan HEP, Bazan NG. Platelet-activating factor (PAF) increases prostaglandin synthase-2 (COX-2) gene expression in corneal epithelium. Invest Ophthalmol Vis Sci. 1995: 36:S573.
117. Tao Y, Bazan HEP, Bazan NG. Platelet-activating factor induces the metalloproteinase-1 and -9 but not -2 or -3, in the corneal epithelium. Invest Ophthalmol Vis Sci. 1995;36:345–54.
118. Fini ME, Girard MT, Matsubara M. Collagenolytic/gelatinolytic enzymes in cornea wound healing. Acta Ophthalmol. 1992;202(Suppl.):26–33.
119. Clohisy JC, Connolly TJ, Bergman KD, Quinn CO, Partridge NC. Prostanoid-induced expression of matrix metalloproteinase-1 mRNA in rat osteosarcoma cells. Endocrinology. 1994; 135:1447–54.

120. Mertz PM, DeWitt DL, Stetler-Stevenson WG, Wahl LM. Interleukin 10 suppression of monocyte prostaglandin H synthase-2. Mechanisms of inhibition of prostaglandin-dependent matrix metalloproteinase production. J Biol Chem. 1994;269:21322–29.
121. Ito A, Nose T, Takahashi S, Mori Y. Cyclooxygenase inhibitors augment the production of pro-matrix metalloproteinase-9 (progelatinase B) in rabbit articular chondrocytes. FEBS Lett. 1995;360:75–9.
122. Salvatori R, Guidon PT Jr, Rapuano BE, Bockman RS. Prostaglandin E1 inhibits collagenase gene expression in rabbit synoviocytes and human fibroblasts. Endocrinology. 1992;131:21–8.
123. Clark GD, Happel LT, Zorumski CF, Bazan NG. Enhancement of hippocampal excitatory synaptic transmission by platelet-activating factor. Neuron. 1992;9:1211–6.
124. Kato K, Clark GD, Bazan NG, Zorumski CF. Platelet-activating factor as a potential retrograde messenger in CA1 hippocampal long-term potentiation. Nature. 1994;367:179–82.
125. Izquierdo I, Fin C, Schmitz PK et al. Memory enhancement by intrahippocampal, intra-amygdala, or intraentorhinal infusion of platelet-activating factor measured in an inhibitory avoidance task. Proc Natl Acad Sci USA. 1995;92:5047–51.
126. Jerusalinsky D, Quillfeldt JA, Walz R, Da Silva R, Medina JH, Izquierdo I. Post-training intrahippocampal infusion of protein kinase C inhibitors causes amnesia in rats. Behav Neurol Biol. 1994;61:107–9.
127. Korol DL, Abel TW, Church LT, Barnes CA, McNaughton BL. Hippocampal synaptic enhancement and spatial learning in the Morris swim task. Hippocampus. 1993;3:127–32.

10 COX-2 expression in labour

P. BENNETT and D. SLATER

THE INITIATION OF LABOUR

The biochemical mechanisms of the initiation of human labour are not yet understood. Much of the work in this field has been done in animals, but there are fundamental differences in placentation, the anatomy of pregnancy and the ways in which parturition is controlled. Thus it is not always possible to draw parallel conclusions between these animals and man.

In the sheep, near to term, stimulation of the fetal anterior pituitary by neuropeptides causes increased ACTH release. During the last 20–25 days of gestation there is a progressive increase in output of cortisol from the fetal adrenals and a rise in fetal plasma glucocorticoid levels[1]. This increases the expression of the P450 17α-hydroxylase gene and, therefore, increases placental 17α-hydroxylase activity[2]. Placental metabolism of C21 to C19 steroids is increased. Progesterone is not a good substrate for placental 17α-hydroxylase: instead metabolism is via the delta-5 pathway from pregnenolone to 17-hydroxypregnenolone, through dihydroepiandrosterone and aromatization to oestrogen[3]. Placental aromatase activity is also increased by cortisol. In consequence there is a decrease in placental progesterone output and an increase in output of oestrogen. These changes are reflected in the maternal plasma as a decrease in peripheral progesterone concentrations followed by an increase in oestrogen concentrations. Similar changes can be induced by administration of exogenous cortisol or by inhibitors of the 3β-hydroxysteroid dehydrogenase which converts pregnenolone to progesterone[3,4].

It is now generally accepted that an increase in prostaglandin synthesis within the uterus is an essential component of the parturition process[5]. A large volume of work has been published in the past 20 years demonstrating the interrelationship between prostaglandin synthesis and labour. Prostaglandin levels in the circulation rise in association with labour. Several groups have measured serum levels of prostaglandins during pregnancy and labour. This has generally been done by measurement of prostaglandin metabolites rather than of the prostaglandin itself since the natural prostaglandins have a very short half life in the circulation. There is general agreement that plasma levels of prostaglandin $F_{2\alpha}$ ($PGF_{2\alpha}$) do not vary significantly throughout pregnancy, but are elevated during spontaneous labour at term[6–8]. Similar changes in prostaglandin levels in amniotic fluid have been reported[9]. Amniotic fluid levels of prostaglandins and arachidonic acid have been shown to increase significantly during labour, the increase being in proportion to the degree of cervical dilatation[10,11]. Fetal membranes obtained after spontaneous labour contain significantly less arachidonic acid than membranes obtained at Caesarean section prior to labour. It has been calculated that the difference in arachidonic acid levels is easily sufficient to account for the increased levels of arachidonic acid, prostaglandins and their metabolites in the amniotic fluid and maternal urine. Instillation of arachidonic acid into the amniotic fluid of women requesting termination of their pregnancy has been shown to induce labour[11] whereas instillation of oleic acid, a similar fatty acid which is not a prostaglandin precursor, has no effect.

$PGF_{2\alpha}$ is known to be a potent oxytocic agent, and its metabolite 13,14-dihydro-$PGF_{2\alpha}$ has a similar effect. The duration of action of $PGF_{2\alpha}$ is considerably longer than its persistence in the circulation. It has been suggested that this may be due to the actions of its metabolites[12]. The increase in myometrial contractility caused by $PGF_{2\alpha}$ has also been demonstrated in vitro using isolated strips of myometrium, with equally potent effects upon lower and upper segment muscle.

Prostaglandin E_2 (PGE_2) does not appear to be as potent an oxytocic as $PGF_{2\alpha}$. Although Gordon-Wright[13] was unable to demonstrate any increase in lower segment myometrial contractility in vitro, in similar experiments Karim and Hillier[14] found that PGE_2 stimulated upper segment myometrium whilst causing relaxation of the lower segment and cervix. It is a common obstetrical experience that intravaginal PGE_2 causes an increase in uterine activity, and an increase in uterine tone has been reported following intravenous administration of PGE_2[15].

Artificial rupture of the membranes or vaginal examination at term causes a release of prostaglandins. Turnbull[16] found higher levels of PGE_2 and $PGF_{2\alpha}$ in amniotic fluid following amniotomy compared with that obtained by amniocentesis. Circulating prostaglandin levels have also been shown to rise within 5 min of vaginal examination or amniotomy at term and to remain elevated for at least 30 min[17]. Prostaglandins are now widely used either for prior ripening of the cervix or as the sole agent for induction of labour.

ARACHIDONIC ACID METABOLISM WITHIN THE UTERUS DURING LABOUR

The amnion

Prior to labour arachidonic acid metabolism in the amnion is principally via the lipoxygenase and epoxygenase enzyme pathways with little metabolism via the cyclooxygenase (COX) pathway to prostaglandins[18-20]. Following labour there is an increase in total arachidonic acid metabolism with a great increase in COX metabolism to PGE_2. Although there is also a small increase in lipoxygenase metabolism COX metabolism becomes predominant[19,21] (Figure 1). The overall increase in arachidonic acid metabolism implies an increase in the activity of phospholipases. Amnion in vivo is an avascular tissue and therefore has no

***Figure 1** Metabolism of endogenous, radiolabelled arachidonic acid in amnion cells in monolayer culture obtained by caesarean section prior to labour, or after spontaneous labour and delivery at term. Arachidonic acid metabolites were separated by HPLC. Mean values ± SD (n = 10). *p < 0.05, **p < 0.01, Tr = retention time (min), M = metabolites*

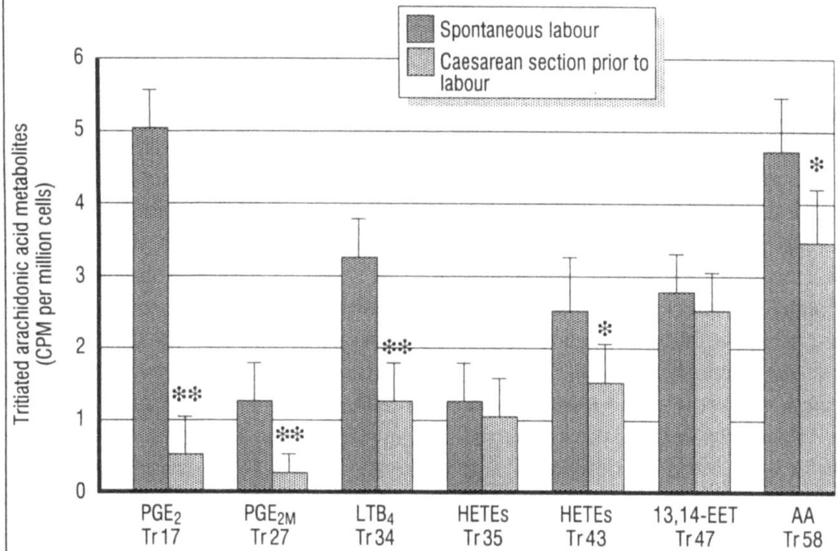

source of extracellular arachidonic acid, other than the amniotic fluid itself. The change from principally lipoxygenase to COX metabolism also suggests that there are changes in the activities of these two enzymes. Amnion cells established in culture following elective caesarean section do not synthesize prostaglandins from endogenous arachidonic acid, but will produce prostaglandins if supplied with an exogenous source of substrate[21]. It is possible that endogenous and exogenous arachidonic acid are metabolized at different sites within the amnion cell, or that arachidonic acid itself increases expression of COX.

In early studies, it was postulated that an initiating event in the process leading to human parturition was an increase in PGE_2 synthesis in amnion. It has been suggested that amniotic fluid may contain inhibitors of arachidonic acid metabolism during pregnancy, and that these are withdrawn near to term. Saeed *et al.*[22] found that the ability of amniotic fluid to inhibit prostaglandin biosynthesis in amnion cells in culture fell by 25% between early pregnancy and term. Amniotic fluid collected at term prior to labour exhibited more than double the inhibitory power of that collected after spontaneous onset of labour. It is not clear whether this is an effect of withdrawal of inhibition or the addition of stimulatory substances. Experiments performed by Strickland *et al.*[23] suggest that near to term the fetus may excrete substances into the amniotic cavity which stimulate prostaglandin biosynthesis in the amnion. Urines collected at first voiding from neonates delivered at elective caesarean section, or following spontaneous vaginal delivery, both stimulated PGE_2 biosynthesis in cultured amnion cells, but the effect was significantly greater following spontaneous delivery.

More recently two compounds, platelet activating factor (PAF)[24] and interleukin 1 (IL-1)[25] have become specific candidates for the fetal signal which increases prostaglandin synthesis in amnion and initiates labour. Both of these are found in increased concentration in the amniotic fluid in association with labour, and both stimulate prostaglandin production in amnion cells in vitro. PAF is a particularly strong candidate since its secretion by the fetus into the amniotic fluid is related to fetal lung maturity. An alternative hypothesis for the stimulus to prostaglandin synthesis with parturition implicates corticotrophin-releasing hormone (CRH) production within the placenta and fetal membranes[26]. CRH concentration in placenta, membranes, amniotic fluid and maternal serum increases with labour, and there is a concomitant decrease in CRH binding protein concentrations such that free CRH rises sharply from 36 weeks[27]. CRH stimulates prostaglandin production by amnion cells. This mechanism is closer in evolutionary terms to the known mechanism in sheep and it may be that changes in local PAF and interleukin concentrations are a consequence rather than a cause of parturition, or that they may play a more important role in the genesis of preterm rather than term labour, especially where infection is involved.

Chorion and the transfer of prostaglandins from amnion across the fetal membranes

A major objection to the hypothesis that the initiation of prostaglandin synthesis with labour begins in amnion is the chorionic barrier between it and the decidua, cervix and myometrium. Chorion is rich in prostaglandin dehydrogenases and may inactivate any prostaglandins produced by the amnion[8,21]. The transfer of prostaglandins across fetal membranes has been studied by using radiolabelled compounds and membranes collected following delivery. Studies by Nakla *et al.*[29] and Bennett *et al.*[30] have demonstrated that prostaglandins may cross the chorion and that while some is metabolized in the process, a large proportion remains intact and active. Roseblade *et al.*[31] have performed similar studies and argue that this transfer is artifactual. However $PGF_{2\alpha}$ concentrations increase in amniotic fluid in parallel with those of PGE_2. Since amnion is not a source of $PGF_{2\alpha}$ this presumably represents diffusion from decidua and myometrium. Since PGE_2 and $PGF_{2\alpha}$ have very similar lipid solubilities[18] it seems likely that prostaglandin E_2 should be able to diffuse in the opposite direction.

The cellular localization of prostaglandin dehydrogenases in the fetal membranes has been extensively studied by Challis *et al.*[26]. Using immuno-histochemistry they found that, at term, prostaglandin dehydrogenase activity was absent from the amnion and the cellular and reticular layers of the chorion but was found extensively in the trophoblast layer of the chorion. However, only about 50% of chorionic trophoblast cells were positively stained for prostaglandin dehydrogenase. This observation suggests that although the chorion contains significant prostaglandin dehydrogenase activity, there are both intra- and extracellular routes by which prostaglandins might pass from the amnion to the decidua without being inactivated. They identified a subset of patients in preterm labour who appeared to have unusually low prostaglandin dehydrogenase activity. This suggests that disorders of prostaglandin dehydrogenase function may underlie some cases of preterm labour. It remains possible that changes in dehydrogenase activity in the chorion may parallel increased prostaglandin synthesis in the amnion or that amnion prostaglandin synthesis at term is sufficient to overwhelm metabolism in the chorion.

Whether or not amnion is involved in the onset of term labour, it is clear that the presence of a functioning amnion epithelium is not essential for the onset of preterm labour since chorioamnionitis may be associated with complete destruction of the amnion and yet labour will still ensue.

Decidua

Decidua has been shown to be a source of both PGE_2 and $PGF_{2\alpha}$. Its synthesis of both of these prostaglandins appears to increase following the onset of labour at term[21]. Decidua consists of macrophages and T lymphocytes, which may represent up to 20% of the cell population at term, as well as decidual stromal cells. The latter appear to be the principle source of prostaglandins within the decidua[32]. The extent to which decidual prostaglandin synthesis apparently increases with labour varies from study to study. Skinner and Challis[21] measured prostaglandin production from dispersed cells and reported an increase in PGE_2 and $PGF_{2\alpha}$ synthesis of approximately 2- to 3-fold. Khan *et al.*[32], however, separated decidual stromal cells from the other cell types and reported an increase in PGE_2 synthesis of 60-fold. Decidua is also a site of prostaglandin dehydrogenase activity, although not to the same extent as chorion[26]. The possibility that $PGF_{2\alpha}$ is produced in the decidua from PGE_2, which itself may have been synthesized by either amnion or chorion, has been explored by Cheung and Challis[28]. Their experiments, in which dispersed chorion cells were incubated with exogenous PGE_2 showed that interconversion of PGE_2 to $PGF_{2\alpha}$ via the 9-keto reductase enzyme does not occur to any great extent in the chorion.

Myometrium

Unlike the fetal membranes, myometrium synthesizes large amounts of prostacyclin[33]. This compound acts to effect uterine quiescence. No studies have been performed relating arachidonic acid metabolism in myometrium to parturition, possibly because it is ethically difficult to obtain tissue for study. Glucocorticoids appear to suppress prostaglandin metabolism in myometrial cultures obtained at hysterectomy but have no effect upon metabolism in cells from the amnion or decidua[34]. Glucocorticoids generally suppress arachidonic acid metabolism, probably by stimulation of lipocortin activity. It is possible that the increased plasma levels of cortisol during labour inhibit prostacyclin biosynthesis in the myometrium whereas the immunity of the amnion and decidua may allow accelerated production of those prostaglandins promoting myometrial activity.

Lipoxygenase metabolites of arachidonic acid

The role of the lipoxygenase metabolites of arachidonic acid in the initiation of labour is not yet understood. Since arachidonic acid metabolism in amnion before labour yields a greater proportion of these it would be tempting to suggest that they act as suppressors of labour. This appears not to be the case. Studies of most of the leukotriene and other hydroxyfatty acid metabolites of arachidonic acid have found no effect upon contractility of pregnant myometrium[35]. 5-HETE, however, appears to stimulate pregnant myometrium to contract but its effect is 10-fold less than that of $PGF_{2\alpha}$[35,36]. Studies in monkeys have shown that prelabour contractions are associated with an elevation of amniotic fluid 5-HETE levels whereas labour is associated with an increase in prostaglandin concentrations[37]. It is possible that 5-HETE may mediate Braxton Hicks contractions in humans.

POSSIBLE CELLULAR MECHANISMS FOR THE ONSET OF LABOUR IN HUMANS

It is now accepted that the process of human labour begins several days or weeks before the onset of clinical labour, with changes in the cervix uteri. PGE_2 can be used clinically to bring about these changes, and in vitro it appears to cause relaxation of the lower uterine segment and may increase the activity of upper segment myometrium. $PGF_{2\alpha}$ does not have a significant effect upon the cervix but causes a marked increase in myometrial activity. It seems likely that PGE_2 has a major role in the initiation of labour, while $PGE_{2\alpha}$ is subsequently important in stimulating contractions.

The role of oxytocin in early labour is disputed; the importance of prostaglandins is universally agreed. It was thought for many years that human labour was initiated by increased release of oxytocin from the maternal posterior pituitary. However in 1961 Fitzpatrick measured human plasma oxytocic activity by bioassay during pregnancy and labour and was only able to demonstrate a significant rise during the second stage of labour. More recent work using a sensitive and specific radioimmunoassay[38] has demonstrated that oxytocin levels are not significantly different in males, non-pregnant females, and pregnant females prior to labour. During labour there is no correlation between oxytocin levels and intrauterine pressure and oxytocin levels only rise during delivery of the fetal head and prior to and during breast feeding. Oxytocin may therefore be more important during the expulsive phase of labour than in its initiation and it is possible that the most important roles of oxytocin are during lactation and in the prevention of post-partum haemorrhage. There is not total agreement, however. Fuchs argues that oxytocin is released in pulses and that the levels needed to initiate myometrial contractions at term are low; the failure of other investigators to demonstrate changes may therefore be due to infrequent sampling and insensitive assays. Furthermore, although large rises in oxytocin levels near to term cannot be demonstrated the number and sensitivity of oxytocin receptors has been shown to increase dramatically[39,40]. It has been suggested by Lye that the oxytocin receptor, together with other genes including myometrial gap junction proteins such as connexin 43, may form a 'cassette' of genes whose expression increases with advancing gestational age as a pre-requisite to labour. the success of oxytocin antagonists in suppressing preterm contractions shows that oxytocin must play at least a facilitatory role in parturition but it is doubtful whether it controls the timing of labour.

It is highly likely that in humans, as in certain animals, the switching on of prostaglandin synthesis is central to the initiation of labour. The level at which prostaglandin synthesis is controlled and in which tissue the process begins has not been clearly established. There is no shortage of the precursor arachidonic acid, but it is sequestered in phospholipid pools. Phospholipase activity is therefore essential for prostaglandin synthesis. Since amnion and trophoblast will both synthesize large amounts of prostaglandins if provided with exogenous arachidonic acid, it seems likely that the activity of the phospholipase enzyme plays a major part in the control of arachidonic acid metabolism. The change in the ratio of arachidonic acid metabolism between COX and lipoxygenase products in association with labour suggests that there are also changes in the activity of these enzymes.

Central to this theory is the increase in phospholipase activity in the fetal membranes preceding the onset of labour. There is definite evidence for such an increase in association with labour. In addition to those studies described above which have shown increases in prostaglandin metabolism in fetal membranes following labour, Sbarra *et al.*[41] have demonstrated increased activity of lysosomal enzymes in association with parturition. They assessed lysosomal activity by measurement of *N*-acetylglucosaminidase activity and demonstrated increased activity in fetal membranes collected following spontaneous labour when compared with those collected following elective caesarean section. Furthermore they were able to stimulate activity in post-elective caesarean section samples by incubation with latex particles, but were unable to further increase the activity in post-parturition samples.

One way in which phospholipase activity within the uterus might be controlled is through the action of lipocortins. Wilson *et al.*[42] have identified a lipocortin-like protein produced by chorion. This protein appears to be inactivated in association with labour and has many properties consistent with its having a role in the control of parturition. It is produced by the decidua, a fetal tissue, but in its active form can inhibit prostaglandin synthesis in a maternal tissue, the decidua or myometrium. Since the activities of lipocortins are regulated by phosphorylation, protein kinase C activity may play an additional regulatory role.

PHOSPHOLIPASE REGULATION

The presence of phospholipase activity in the fetal membranes has been long established[43]. At labour there is a significant loss of arachidonic acid from phospholipid substrates in the amnion[44,45]. Several pathways may be involved with the liberation of arachidonic acid from membrane phospholipids[46], including the phospholipase A_2 and the phospholipase C enzymes. Release of arachidonic acid by phospholipase A_2 is direct, while the release of arachidonic acid by phospholipase C requires the further action of a diacylglycerase. Phospholipase C activity has been measured in amnion but does not appear to show any changes in association with labour[47]. Phospholipase A_2 activity has been found in all intrauterine tissues and increases with gestational age[48,49].

Aitken *et al.*[50] have suggested that increased expression of the secretory type II PLA_2 gene is associated with increased prostaglandin release from the fetal membranes. Using Northern analysis we found expression of $sPLA_2$ in fetal membranes and placenta. High levels of $sPLA_2$ expression were found in placenta, while expression was much lower in amnion and chorion-decidua. No significant differences in the expression of these genes in these tissues were associated with labour[51] (Figure 2).

Recently a novel, high molecular weight cytosolic phospholipase A_2 ($cPLA_2$) has been described[52]. Whereas $sPLA_2$ has no substrate preference, $cPLA_2$ shows a substrate preference for sn-2 arachidonyl-containing phospholipids[53]. Using RT-PCR we have found that $cPLA_2$ mRNA is expressed in amnion and in placenta, but placental expression was approximately 8- to 16-fold lower than in amnion. The enzyme activity of $cPLA_2$ measured using a specific assay, was similarly higher in the amnion. In addition, $cPLA_2$ activity increased with the onset of labour whereas $sPLA_2$ activity was unchanged[54]. Lopez-Bernal *et al.*[49] measured placental phospholipase enzyme activity and found no increased activity in association with labour at term. However, they did observe an increased phospholipase activity in placental tissue at preterm labour.

Recently immunohistochemical localization of both $sPLA_2$ and $cPLA_2$ in term human fetal membranes and in amnion-derived (WISH) cells has been demonstrated. In the fetal membrane, $sPLA_2$ was seen in amnion epithelial cells

Figure 2 Expression of the $sPLA_2$ gene in human fetal membranes before and after labour

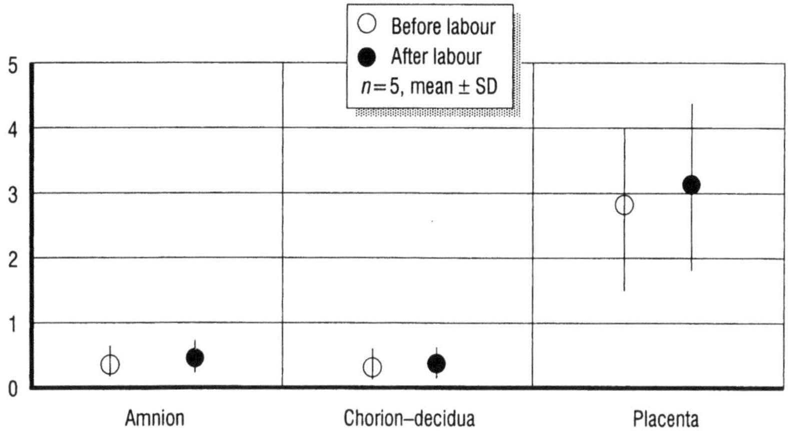

and chorionic cytotrophoblast cells. Whilst $cPLA_2$ immunostaining was also found in the amnion epithelial and chorionic cytotrophoblast cells, it appeared more diffuse. In the WISH cells both secretory and cytosolic isoforms were identified: $sPLA_2$ appeared to be localized around the nucleus, possibly associated with the endoplasmic reticulum, in intracellular secretory vesicles. However, the $cPLA_2$ was distributed throughout the cell cytoplasm with a more intense immunostain associated with the cell membrane. Treatment of the WISH cells with IL-1β resulted in the $cPLA_2$ becoming further associated with the cell membrane, i.e. it appeared to translocate to the cell membrane[55]. This suggests that while $sPLA_2$ may regulate substrate release in placenta $cPLA_2$ plays a more important role in the fetal membranes and in the onset of labour.

The phosphorylation of $cPLA_2$ results in a rapid increase in enzyme activation, while de novo synthesis of $cPLA_2$ protein is less likely to be such a rapid response. We have found that bacterial endotoxins, which stimulate prostaglandin synthesis in fetal membranes, induce the $cPLA_2$ gene in a delayed fashion characteristic of a secondary effect, perhaps due to cytokine stimulation[56]. We have not, however, been able to demonstrate an acute change in $cPLA_2$ gene expression with labour. One hypothesis for the regulation of $cPLA_2$ associated with labour could be that at some time prior to the onset of labour there is an increase in the de novo synthesis of $cPLA_2$ protein as part of a 'labour-associated cassette'. Nearer to the actual onset of labour there may be increased phosphorylation of the $cPLA_2$ enzyme which elicits a rapid increase in activity and results in the large increase in the synthesis of PGE_2 seen at labour.

There is considerable evidence for regulation of $cPLA_2$ activity by site specific phosphorylation. In rat mesangial cells and Chinese hamster ovary (CHO) cells $cPLA_2$ activity is coupled to hormonal regulation of arachidonic acid release and subsequent prostaglandin production[57,58]. In CHO cells, phosphorylation of $cPLA_2$ at serine-505 by another kinase, p-43 mitogen activated protein (MAP) kinase, resulted in a greater increase in enzyme activity than did phosphorylation with protein kinase C alone[59].

The phospholipase inhibitory proteins, lipocortins, may also be a substrate for protein kinase C[60]. The lipocortins may be possible inhibitors of phospholipase activity in amnion. Phosphorylation of lipocortins results in their decreased binding to phospholipid substrates. We and others[61] have also shown, using Northern analysis, that the expression of lipocortin I mRNA decreases in fetal membranes but not the placenta after labour (Figure 3). There is an associated decrease in protein concentrations[62]. In human amnion at labour the inositol and ethanolamine phospholipids are preferentially hydrolysed, resulting in increased arachidonic acid release[45]. Lipocortin I has been shown to bind with high affinity these two phospholipid substrates[63].

COX REGULATION

Until recently phospholipase activity was thought to be the limiting factor in prostaglandin production in the fetal membranes. However, any stimulus to prostaglandin production must also increase the activity of COX since this has a short half life and is destroyed after a limited number of reactions[64]. Our evidence that amnion produces only lipoxygenase metabolites of arachidonic acid before labour, and the change in the ratio of COX lipoxygenase metabolism with labour suggests that the activities of the two enzymes, COX and phospholipase, must be independently controlled[18,65].

De Witt has suggested that COX activity is regulated in two ways; by controlling the rate of enzyme turnover, and/or by a general increase in level of production of the enzyme. The first is characteristic of fibroblasts and endothelial cells and involves the regulation of steady state levels of prostaglandin synthesis. In these cell types a 1- to 3-fold increase of COX protein may result in a 15- to 20-fold increase in prostaglandin output. The second type of regulation appears to involve the rapid synthesis of new enzyme where a 15-fold increase in the COX protein levels may lead to a 50- to 100-fold increase in prostaglandin output. This type of regulation was suggested by DeWitt to be characteristic of both pro-monocyte cell lines and reproductive tissues[66].

The enzyme kinetics studies of Smieja *et al.*[67] suggest that the increase in COX activity in amnion with the onset of labour is due entirely to an increase in the synthesis of the COX enzyme. We and others (Myatt, personal communication) have attempted to use Western blot analysis to demonstrate an increase in COX protein but this work was complicated by cross-reactivity between specific COX antibodies and other proteins, including albumin.

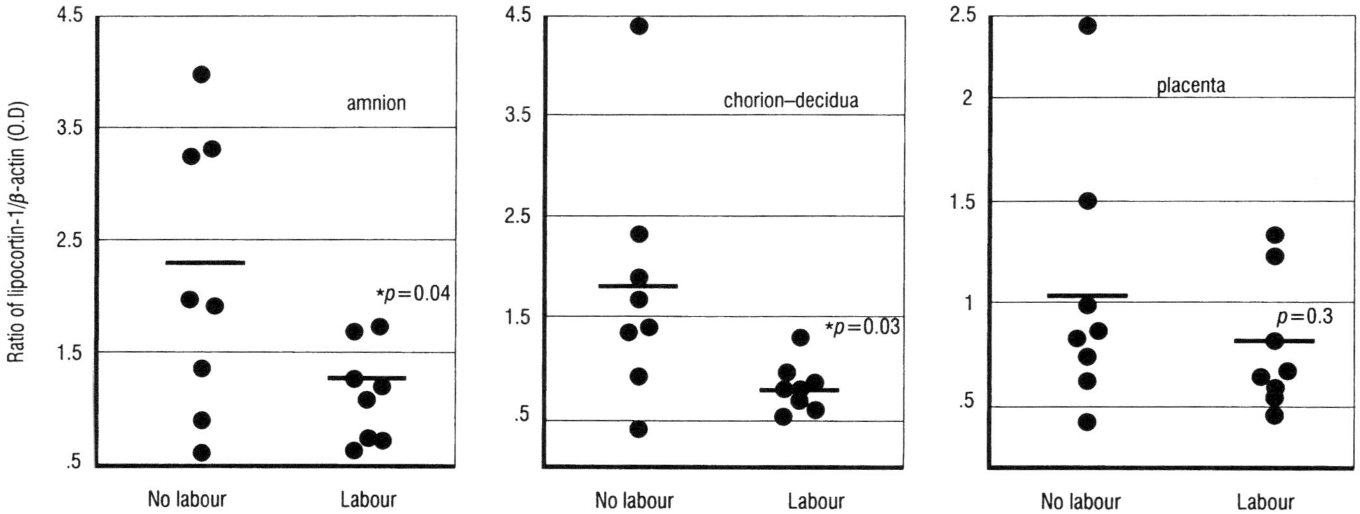

***Figure 3** Measurement of lipocortin-1 mRNA by Northern analysis in human amnion, chorion, decidua and placenta. Mean and individual ratio of signal density values (lipocortin/β-actin) from placenta collected at elective caesarean section prior to the onset of labour ($n = 8$) or following the spontaneous onset of labour ($n = 8$)*

Figure 4 Intron–exon arrangements of COX-1 and COX-2 genes. Above: exon sizes; below: intron sizes

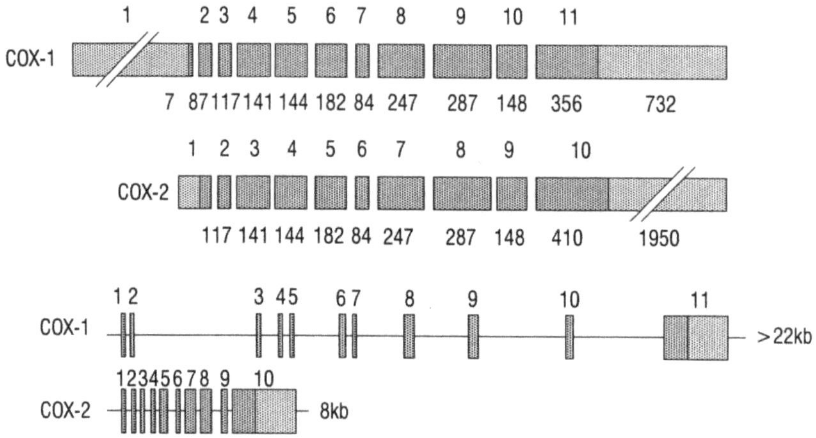

A COX gene which produces a mRNA transcript of 2.8 kb was reported in human and other species in 1988 and 1989[68]. In 1991 a second COX gene whose expression is induced by mitogens and inhibited by glucocorticoids was reported[69]. This gene usually encodes an mRNA of >4 kb. The difference in transcript size between the type 1 and type 2 COX enzymes is accounted for by a long 5′ untranslated region in the type 2 mRNA. Although not identical, the type 1 and type 2 proteins are of similar molecular size and show a high degree of homology. The COX-1 and COX-2 genes are on different chromosomes but have a similar intron/exon arrangement (Figure 4). The COX-1 gene spans over 22 kb of genomic DNA whilst the COX-2 gene spans only 8 kb. The long 3′ untranslated portion of COX-2 contains 17 copies of the Shaw–Kamen sequence (AUUUA) which is a feature of early response genes whose mRNA is degraded rapidly. COX-2 has been demonstrated to act as an immediate early response gene in various cell types. The COX-2 message is rapidly induced in vitro by various cytokines and growth factors[70].

We used Northern blot analysis to demonstrate an increase in COX expression in the fetal membranes with the onset of labour. These experiments used a sheep COX-1 cDNA probe and we wrongly interpreted them as showing increased expression of COX-1[65]. Using gene-specific oligonucleotide probes for in situ hybridization we found that COX-1 was expressed diffusely in amnion, chorion and decidua, but not especially in the amnion epithelium. Levels were so low that autoradiograph exposures of the order of several weeks were required for detection. COX-2, however, was expressed specifically within the amnion epithelium and decidua, and at much higher levels. We therefore developed a reverse transcriptase polymerase chain reaction assay (RT-PCR) which allows the expression of the two genes to be independently studied. Initial experiments were performed to determine the correct number of cycles to maintain a linear relationship between initial mRNA concentration and final product concentration. Final product concentration was assessed by densitometry after Southern blotting and hybridization to radiolabelled probes or by scintillation counting. We found that, both before and after labour, the COX-2 mRNA has over 100-fold greater abundance than the COX-1 mRNA in the amnion[71]. We also found a significant increase in the expression of COX-2 mRNA within the amnion of patients delivered following labour when compared with those delivered by elective caesarean section[72] (Figure 5). Although the increase was significant there was a large experimental variation in COX-2 expression levels. One of the difficulties with using elective caesarean section patients as a control for absence of labour arises from the assessment of how close to the onset of labour the patient was at the time of specimen collection; such variability may reduce any differences observed between sample groups. It is not known at what rate the translation of the COX-2 mRNA is increased. A doubling of the mRNA could result in a higher fold increase in the levels of protein and subsequent enzyme activity, as suggested by DeWitt. This may then result in the greatly increased levels of PGE_2 associated with the onset of labour. No significant difference was observed in the levels of COX-2 expression between pre- and post labour tissue and levels were 100-fold lower than those of COX-2 in all amnion samples analysed, whether before or after labour. These data suggest that the levels of COX-1 expression in amnion at term are not affected by labour onset and probably only contribute a minor proportion of the total COX activity. In the myometrium, whose principle prostaglandin product is prostacyclin, Moore *et al.*[73] have studied expression of COX-1 and COX-2 using our RT-PCR methodology. They found that COX-1 and COX-2 mRNA levels at term are similar. It is possible that myometrial prostacyclin synthesis is COX-1 mediated while synthesis of oxytocic prostaglandins is COX-2 mediated.

In experiments using an immortalized amnion cell line (WISH), both IL-1β and the phorbol ester tumour promoting agent TPA caused an induction of COX-2 expression (Figure 6). Similarly, lipopolysaccharide (LPS) stimulation of human fetal membranes, in a model of infection, causes a biphasic increase in COX-2 expression, with peaks at 30 min and 4 h, probably due to an initial direct effect on transcription followed by a secondary effect through cytokine induction (Figure 7). This suggests that COX-2 expression may mediate the onset of preterm labour associated with infection.

Bailey and Verma[74] have shown that, in vascular smooth muscle cells, dexamethasone suppression of prostaglandin synthesis is mediated by synthesis of a protein, possibly lipocortin-1, which binds to cyclooxygenase mRNA and prevents its transcription. They showed that in aspirin-inactivated vascular

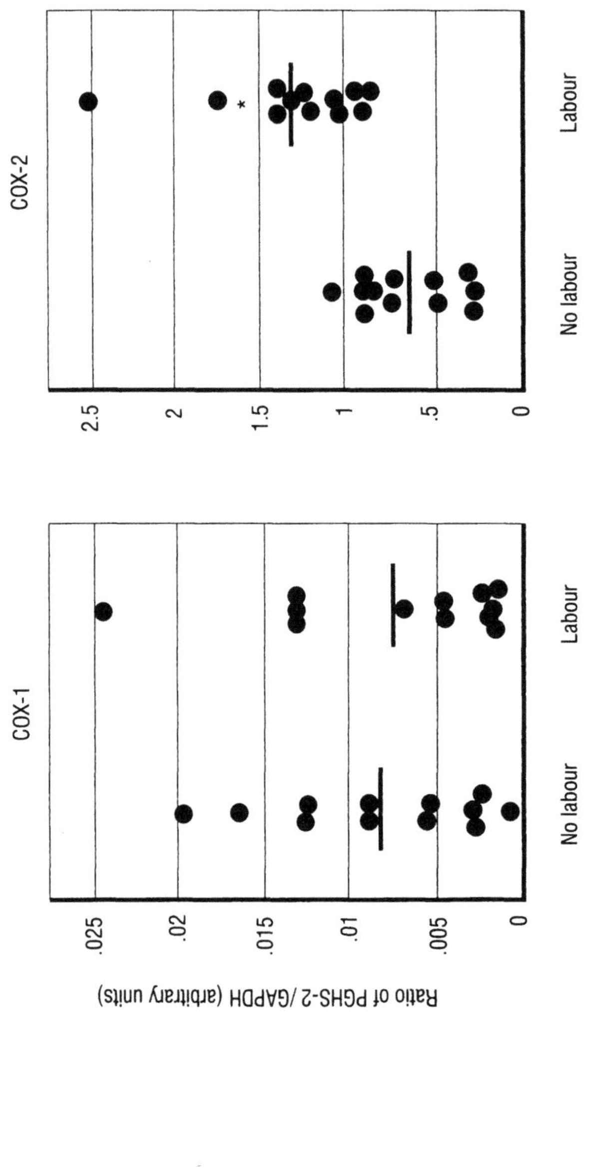

***Figure 5** Measurement of COX mRNA in human amnion. Mean and individual ratio of signal density values (COX-2/GAPDH) from amnion collected at elective caesarean section prior to the onset of labour or following the spontaneous onset of labour (n = 12). *p < 0.005*

***Figure 6** Time course of expression of COX-2 in WISH cells stimulated with IL-1β or TPA. COX-2 expression was measured by RT-PCR and expressed as a ratio relative to the expression of GAPDH*

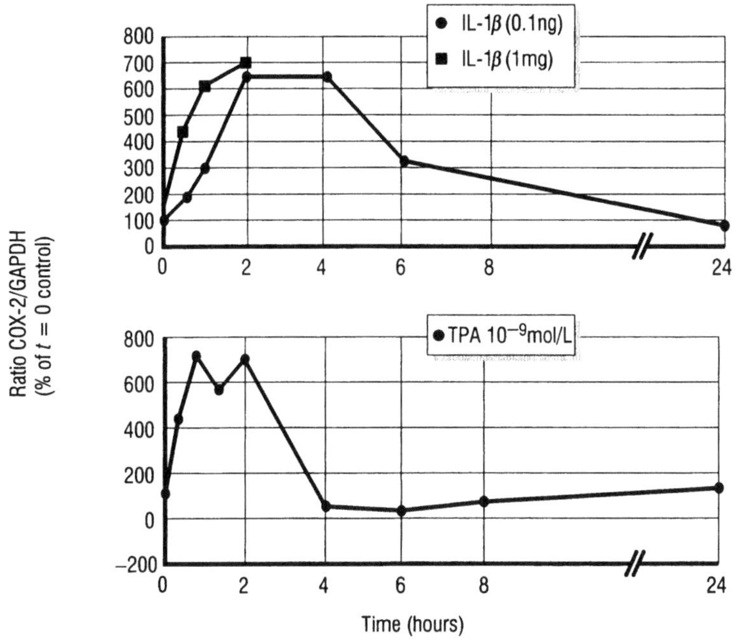

***Figure 7** Biphasic COX-2 expression in amnion stimulated with LPS. COX-2 was measured by RT-PCR and expressed as a ratio relative to the expression of GAPDH*

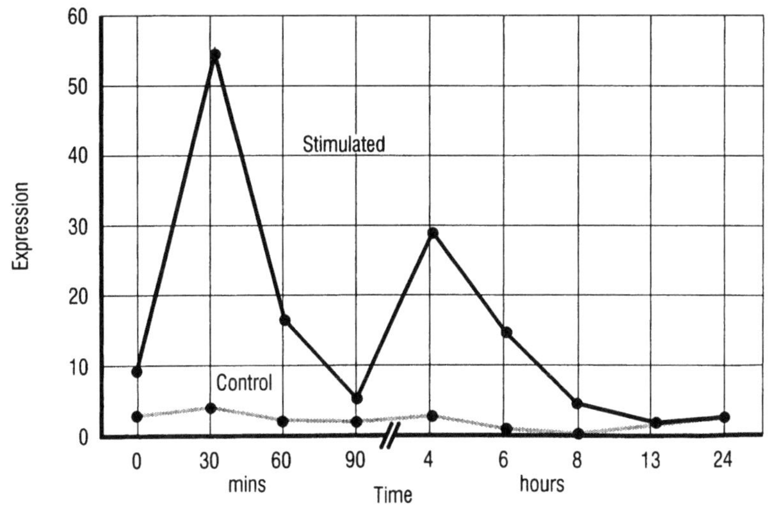

smooth muscle cells, the recovery of COX activity was dependent on the addition of epidermal growth factor (EGF), transforming growth factor-β (TGF-β) or fresh serum to the media. This EGF-dependent recovery could be inhibited by the translational inhibitor cycloheximide but not by the transcriptional inhibitor actinomycin D. The EGF-dependent recovery of COX synthesis was also blocked by the synthetic glucocorticoid, dexamethasone, suggesting that dexamethasone was inhibiting the translation of COX. Northern analysis demonstrated that the addition of dexamethasone results in the levels of hybridizable COX mRNA being reduced by $>90\%$[75]. Bailey[76] suggested that the mRNA was being converted into a non-translated form, by the binding of a glucocorticoid-induced protein. Investigation of this phenomenon, used two differential RNA extraction techniques to optimize the isolation of either the bound non-translational (glucocorticoid-suppressed) mRNA or the isolation of normal unbound translatable 'free' mRNA[74]. It has recently been shown that COX mRNA contains an extensive 3′ untranslated terminal region (UTR) that appears to be highly conserved between species. It is possible that this highly conserved 3′UTR may also serve as a binding site for various regulatory proteins[77].

To determine whether the changes in COX expression seen in amnion associated with labour onset are controlled by the binding of an inhibitory protein to the COX mRNA, we used the differential mRNA isolation methods described by Bailey and Verma[74,76]. Reverse transcriptase polymerase chain reaction (RT-PCR) was then employed to quantify levels of COX-2 and COX-1 expression from amnion collected before and after the spontaneous onset of labour. Before labour there was no difference in the relative levels of expression of COX-2 in the amnion detected between the two methods, i.e. the amount of unbound translatable 'free' mRNA was equal to the amount of 'free+bound' mRNA. However, after labour an overall increase in COX-2 mRNA was found, and use of these differential RNA isolation techniques enabled us to show that this was due to message apparently bound with protein rather than simply an increase in the free (unbound) mRNA[77]. This is in marked contrast to the mechanism of dexamethasone induced down-regulation of COX seen in vascular smooth muscle cells[74]. There did not appear to be a protein bound form associated with the COX-1 mRNA.

COX EXPRESSION THROUGHOUT PREGNANCY

Using RT-PCR we have studied the expression of both COX-1 and COX-2 throughout pregnancy in the fetal membranes and placenta. Tissues were obtained in the first and second trimesters following surgical termination of pregnancy. In the early third trimester, tissues were collected following caesarean section for indications such as pre-eclampsia and growth retardation without the onset of labour. COX-1 expression was higher in placenta in the first trimester. COX-2 expression was low in all three trimesters in fetal membranes and placenta but increased markedly towards the end of the third trimester, before labour, and again with the onset of labour. This suggests that there is a significant increase in COX protein within the fetal membranes several weeks prior to the onset of labour and that COX-2 may also be a member of the 'cassette' of genes which is a prerequisite for labour, but that there is a second stimulus of COX-2 expression associated with labour itself. There are two ways in which this might be controlled. First a circulating signal such as CRH may up-regulate COX-2 expression together with the other 'cassette' genes with a second acute fetal stimulus such as PAF or IL-1β to labour itself. Alternately COX-2 expression may be up-regulated slowly between 36 weeks and term, with the products of each of the cassette genes up-regulating the other (e.g. oxytocin up-regulating COX while prostaglandins up-regulate oxytocin receptor), allowing a gradual increase in prostaglandin synthesis until a threshold is reached at which prostaglandin synthesis accelerates and labour ensues as the result of a positive feed-ward system from which the only escape is delivery (a concept proposed by Challis[26]).

FETAL COX EXPRESSION AND ANTI-PROSTAGLANDINS FOR TOCOLYSIS

Indomethacin, a cyclooxygenase inhibitor is highly effective in preventing the contractions of preterm labour and more effective in prolongation of pregnancy than the more commonly used β-sympathomimetics. β-Sympathomimetics cause significant maternal cardiovascular, respiratory and metabolic side effects; however the use of indomethacin is limited by fetal side effects. Indomethacin causes reduced fetal urine output leading to oligohydramnios, presumably through changes in fetal renal flow, or through a direct effect upon the fetal kidney[78,79]. There is an increased risk of constriction or closure of the ductus arteriosus in fetuses whose mothers have received high dose indomethacin therapy, presumably caused by suppression of the synthesis of vasodilatory prostaglandins produced by the ductus arteriosus[80]. Antenatal use of indomethacin is also a risk factor for neonatal cerebral haemorrhage and for necrotizing enterocolitis[81]. Each of these side effects is presumably due to inhibition of constitutively produced prostaglandins, which would therefore be products of COX-1. It may therefore be predicted that the therapeutic use of COX inhibitors which are specific for the COX-2, such as nimesulide or flosulide should effectively suppress the contractions of preterm labour without causing the fetal side effects seen with indomethacin. In support of this hypothesis we have shown, using RT-PCR, that expression of COX-1 is greater than that of COX-2 in fetal heart, lung, kidney and brain and that COX-2 expression in these tissues is some 1000-fold less than in the fetal membranes at term[82]. The COX-2 specific inhibitors nimesulide and flosulide are equally effective in inhibiting both basal and IL-1β stimulated prostaglandin synthesis in fetal membranes, and

***Figure 8** Effect of nimesulide on prostaglandin synthesis in IL-1β-treated whole fetal membranes (n = 4; mean ± SD)*

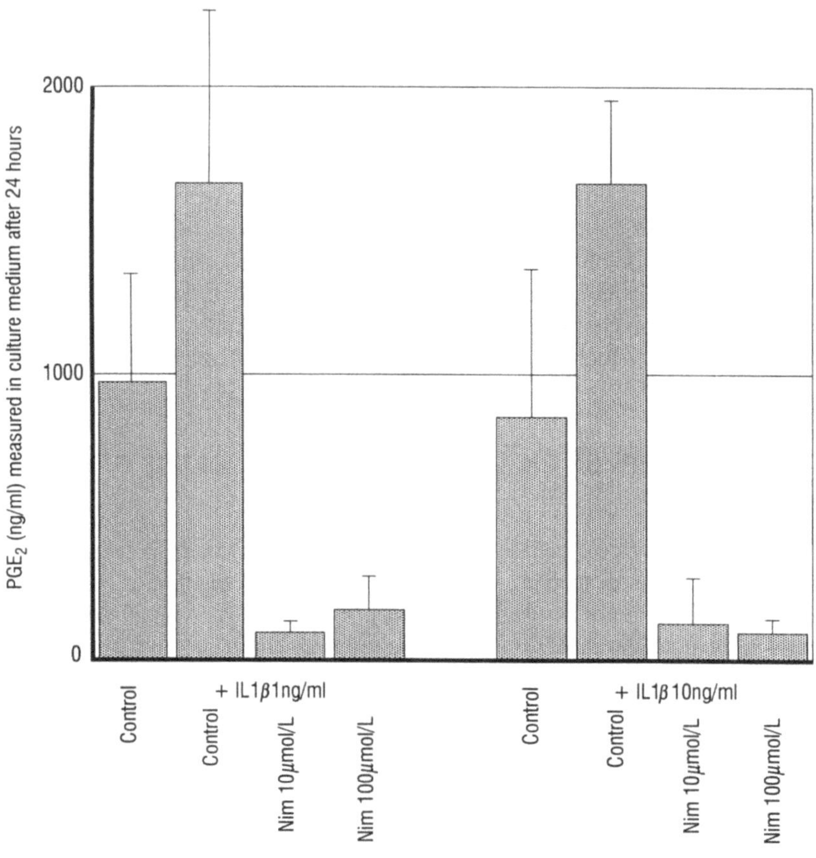

several orders of magnitude more effective than aspirin (Sawdy *et al.*, 1995; unpublished observations) (Figure 8). These findings should provide the basis for clinical trials of COX-2 specific inhibitors in preterm labour.

References

1. Challis JRG, Brookes AN. Maturation and activation of hypothalamic–pituitary function in fetal sheep. Endocr Rev. 1989;10:182–204.
2. Tangelakis K, Coghlan JP, Connell J. Tissue distribution and levels of gene expression of three steroid hydroxylases in ovine fetal adrenal gland. Acta Endocrinol. 1989;120:225–32.
3. Mason JL, France JT, Magness RR, Murrey BA, Rosenfeld CR. Ovine placental steroidogenesis in dexamethasone induced and normal parturition. J Endocrinol. 1989;122:351.

4. Jenkin G, Thorburn GD. Inhibition of progesterone secretion by a hydroxy-dehydrogenase inhibitor in late pregnancy sheep. Can J Physiol Pharmacol. 1985;63:136–41.
5. Bennett PR, Elder MG. Extreme prematurity; the aetiology of preterm delivery. Br Med Bull. 1988;44:850–60.
6. Mitchell MD, Bibby J, Hicks BR, Redan CWG, Anderson ABM, Turnbull AC. Thromboxane B and human parturition. Concentrations in the plasma and production in vitro. J Endocrinol. 1978;78:435–41.
7. Sellers S, Mitchell MD, Bibby J, Anderson ABM, Turnbull AC. Comparison of plasma concentrations of prostaglandin levels in term and preterm labour. Br J Obstet Gynaecol. 1981; 88:362–66.
8. Fuchs AR, Fuchs F, Husslien P, Soloff MF, Fernstrom MJ. Oxytocin receptors and human parturition. Science. 1982;215:1396–8.
9. Keirse MJNC, Flint AP, Turnbull AC. F prostaglandin in amniotic fluid during late pregnancy and labour. J Obstet Gynecol Br Commun. 1974;81:131–5.
10. Keirse MJNC, Hicks BR, Mitchell MD, Turnbull AC. Increase in prostaglandin precursor arachidonic acid in amniotic fluid during spontaneous labour. Br J Obstet Gynaecol. 1977;84:937–40.
11. Macdonald PC, Schultz FM, Duenhoelter JH. Mechanism of action of arachidonic acid. Obstet Gynecol. 1974;44:629–36.
12. Granstrom E. On the metabolism of prostaglandin F in female subjects. Eur J Biochem. 1972;27:462–9.
13. Gordon-Wright AP, Elder MG. Effects of prostaglandin E_2 and $F_{2\alpha}$ metabolites on lower segment myometrium in vitro. Eur J Obstet Gynecol Reprod Biol. 1992;10:297–302.
14. Karim SMM, Hillier K. The role of prostaglandins in myometrial contractions. In Josimovitch JB, ed. Uterine contractions – a side effect of steroidal contraceptives. Wiley Publications; 1973.
15. Bygdeman M, Bremme K, Gillespie A, Lundström V. Effects of the prostaglandins on the uterus. Acta Obstet Gynecol Scand (Suppl.) 1979;87:33.
16. Turnbull AC. The fetus and birth. London: Elsevier; 1977.
17. Sellers S, Mitchell MD, Bibby J, Anderson ABM, Turnbull AC. Prostaglandin serum levels following vaginal examination of artificial rupture of membranes. Br J Obstet Gynaecol. 1980; 87:43–6.
18. Bennett PR, Rose M, Myatt L, Elder MG. Preterm labor; Stimulation of arachidonic acid metabolism in human amnion cells by bacterial products. Am J Obstet Gynecol. 1987;156: 649–55.
19. Bennett PR, Slater D, Moore GE. Expression of a common cellular phospholipase A2 by human intrauterine tissues. Prostaglandins. 1993;45:121–7.
20. Rose MP, Elder MG, Myatt L. Arachidonic acid metabolism in the human placenta. Troph Res. 1987;2:71–83.
21. Skinner KA, Challis JRG. Changes in synthesis and metabolism of prostaglandins by human fetal membranes and decidua at labor. Am J Obstet Gynecol. 1985;151:519–23.
22. Saeed SA, Strickland DM, Young DC, Dang A, Mitchell MD. Inhibition of prostaglandin synthesis by human amniotic fluid: Acute reduction in labor. J Clin Endocrinol Metab. 1982; 55:801–3.
23. Strickland DM, Saeed SA, Casey ML, Mitchell MD. Stimulation of prostaglandin synthesis by urine of human fetus may serve as a trigger for human parturition. Science. 1983;220:521–2.
24. Hoffman DR, Romero R, Johnston JM. Detection of platelet activating factor in amniotic fluid of complicated pregnancies. Am J Obstet Gynecol. 1990;162:525–8.
25. Romero R, Parvizi ST, Oyarzun E, *et al.* Amniotic fluid interleukin-1 in spontaneous labor at term. J Reprod Med. 1990;35:235–8.
26. Challis J, Riley SC, Yang K. Endocrinology of labour. Fetal Med Rev. 1991;3:47–66.
27. McLean M, Bissetts A, Davies J, Woods R, Lowery P, Smith R. A placental clock controlling the length of gestation. Nature Med. 1995;18:234–6.
28. Cheung PYC, Challis JRG. Prostaglandin E2 metabolism in the human fetal membranes. Am J Obstet Gynecol. 1989;16:1580–5.
29. Nakla S, Skinner K, Mitchell BF, Challis JRG. Changes in prostaglandin transfer across human fetal membranes obtained following spontaneous labour. Am J Obstet Gynecol. 1986;155: 1337–41.
30. Bennett PR, Chamberlain GVP, Patel L, Elder MG, Myatt L. Mechanisms of parturition; the

transfer of prostaglandin E2 and 5-HETE across fetal membranes. Am J Obstet Gynecol. 1990;162:683-7.
31. Roseblade CK, Sullivan MF, Khan H, Lumb MR, Elder MG. Limited transfer of prostaglandin E2 across fetal membranes before and after labour. Acta Obstet Gynecol Scand. 1990;69: 399-403.
32. Khan H, Ishihara O, Sullivan MHF, Elder MG. A comparison of two populations of decidual cells by immunocytochemistry and prostaglandin production. Histochemistry. 1991;96:149-52.
33. Bamford DS, Jogee M, Williams K. Prostacyclin formation by the human pregnant myometrium. Br J Obstet Gynaecol. 1980;87:215-18.
34. Casey LM, McDonald PC, Mitchell MD. Despite a massive increase in cortisol secretion in women during parturition there is an equally massive increase in prostaglandin synthesis: A paradox? J Clin Invest. 1985;75:1852-7.
35. Bennett PR, Elder MG, Myatt L. The effects of lipoxygenase metabolites of arachidonic acid upon contractility of human pregnant myometrium in vitro. Prostaglandins. 1988;33:837-44.
36. Bryman I, Hammerstromm S, Linblomm B, Norstrom A, Wickland M, Wiquest N. Leukotrienes and myometrial activity in the term pregnancy uterus. Prostaglandins. 1985;30:907-13.
37. Walsh SW. 5-Hydroxyeicosatetraenoic acid, leukotriene C4 and prostaglandin F2α in amniotic fluid before and during term and preterm labor. Am J Obstet Gynecol. 1989;161:1352-60.
38. Leak RD, Wiesman RE, Glatz TH, Fisher DA. Stimulation of oxytocin secretion in the human. Clin Res. 1979;27:99A.
39. Fuchs AR, Goeschen K, Husslien P, Fuchs F. Oxytocin and the initiation of human parturition; Concentrations of oxytocin and prostaglandin F in spontaneous and oxytocin induced labor at term. Am J Obstet Gynecol. 1983;147:497-502.
40. Dawood MY. Neurohypophysial hormones. In: Fuchs F, Klopper A, eds. Endocrinology of pregnancy. New York: Harper and Row; 1983:204-88.
41. Sbarra AJ, Selvaraj RJ, Cetrulo CL, Thomas G, Louis F, Kennison R. Phagocytosis and the onset of human labor. Am J Obstet Gynecol. 1983;146:622-9.
42. Wilson T, Liggins GC, Aimer GP, Skinner SJ. Partial purification and characterisation of two compounds from amniotic fluid which inhibit phospolipase activity in human endometrial cells. Biochem Biophys Res Commun. 1985;131:22-9.
43. Grieves SA, Liggins GC. Phospholipase A activity in human and ovine uterine tissues. Prostaglandins. 1976;12:229-41.
44. Bleasdale JE, Johnston JM. Prostaglandins and human parturition: regulation of arachidonic acid mobilisation. Rev Perinatal Med. 1984;5:157-91.
45. Okita JR, MacDonald PC, Johnston JM. Mobilization of arachidonic acid from specific glycerophospholipids of human fetal membranes during early labour. J Biol Chem. 1982; 257:14029-34.
46. Dennis EA. Regulation of eicosanoid production: Role of phospholipases and inhibitors. Biotechnology. 1987;5:1294-301.
47. Di Renzo GC, Johnston JM, Okazaki T, Okita JR, MacDonald PC, Bleasedale JE. Phosphatidylinositol specific phospholipase C in fetal membranes and uterine decidua. J Clin Invest. 1981;67:847-51.
48. Okazaki T, Sagawa N, Bleasedale JE, Okita JR, MacDonald PC, Johnston JM. Initiation of human parturition. XIII. Phospholipase C, phospholipase A_2 and diacylglycerol lipase activities in fetal membranes and decidua vera tissues from early and late gestation. Biol Reprod. 1981; 25:103-8.
49. Lopez Bernal A, Newman GE, Phizackerley PJR, Bryant-Greenwood G, Keeling JW. Human placental phospholipase A_2 activity in term and preterm labour. Eur J Obstet Gynaecol Reprod Biol. 1992;43:185-92.
50. Aitken MA, Rice GE, Brennecke SP. Gestational tissue phospholipase A2 mRNA content and the onset of spontaneous labour in humans. Reprod Fert Dev. 1992;2:575-80.
51. Bennett PR, Slater D, Moore GE. Expression of common cellular phospholipase A_2 by human intrauterine tissues. Prostaglandins. 1993;45:121-7.
52. Clark JD, Milona N, Knopf JL. Purification of a 110-kilodalton cytosolic phospholipase A_2 from human monocytic cell line U937. Proc Natl Acad Sci USA. 1990;87:7708-12.
53. Mayer RJ, Marshall LA. New insights on mammalian phospholipase A_2(s); comparison of arachidonyl-selective and -nonselective enzymes. FASEB J. 1993;7:339-48.

54. Slater D, Berger L, Sullivan M, Bennett PR. Differential expression of phospholipases A2 in placenta and fetal membranes and changes in expression with the onset of labour. Am J Obstet Gynecol. [in press].
55. Xue S, Myatt L. Abstract. Chicago: The Society for Gynaecological Investigations; 1994.
56. Rajasingam D, Slater D, Sullivan M, Elder MG, Bennett PR. Changes in phospholipase expression induced by LPS treatment of fetal membranes. Am J Obstet Gynecol [in press].
57. Lin L, Lin AY, Knopf JL. Cytosolic phospholipase A_2 is coupled to hormonally regulated release of arachidonic acid. Proc Natl Acad Sci USA. 1992;89:6147–51.
58. Nemenoff RA, Winitz S, Qian NX, van Putten V, Johnson GL, Heasley LE. Phosphorylation and activation of a high molecular weight form of phospholipase A_2 by p42 microtubule-associated protein 2 kinase and protein kinase C. J Biol Chem. 1993;268:1960–4.
59. Lin L, Wartmann M, Lin AY, Knopf JL, Seth A, Davis RJ. $cPLA_2$ is phosphorylated and activated by MAP kinase. Cell. 1993;72:269–78.
60. Schlaepfer DD, Haigler HT. Characterisation of Ca_{2+}-dependent phospholipid binding and phosphorylation of lipocortin I. J Biol Chem. 1987;262:6931–7.
61. Lynch-Salamon DI, Everson WV, Myatt L. Decrease in annexin I messenger ribonucleic acid expression in human amnion with labour. Am J Obstet Gynecol. 1992;167:1657–63.
62. Myatt L, Hirth J, Everson WV. Changes in annexin (lipocortin) content in human amnion and chorion at parturition. J Cell Biochem. 1992;50:363–73.
63. Blackwood RA, Ernst JD. Characterisation of Ca^{2+}-dependent phospholipid binding, vesicle aggregation and membrane fusion between enzyme and inhibitor. J Biol Chem. 1990;266:195–200.
64. Marshall PJ, Kulmacz RJ, Lands WEM. Constraints on prostaglandin synthesis in tissues. J Biol Chem. 1987;262:3510–7.
65. Bennett PR, Henderson DJ, Moore GE. Changes in the expression of cyclo-oxygenase in human fetal membranes and placenta with labour. Am J Obstet Gynecol. 1992;167:212–6.
66. DeWitt DL, Smith WL. Primary structure of prostaglandin G/H synthase from sheep vesicular gland determined from the complimentary DNA sequence. Proc Natl Acad Sci USA. 1988; 85:1412–6.
67. Smieja Z, Zakar T, Waton JC, Olson DM. Prostaglandin endoperoxide synthase kinetics in human amnion before and after labour at term and following preterm labour. Placenta. 1993;14:163–75.
68. Smith WL, Marnett LN. Prostaglandin endoperoxide synthase: structure and catalysis. Biochim Biophys Acta. 1991;1083:1–17.
69. O'Baion MK, Sadowski HB, Winn W, Young DA. A serum and glucocorticoid regulated 4kb mRNA encodes a cyclo-oxygenase related protein. J Biol Chem. 1991;266:23261–7.
70. Jones DA, Carlton DP, McIntyre TM, Zimmerman GA, Prescott SM. Molecular cloning of human prostaglandin endoperoxide synthase type II and demonstration of expression in response to cytokines. J Biol Chem. 1993;268:9049–54.
71. Slater DM, Berger L, Newton R, Moore GE, Bennett PR. The relative abundance of type 1 to type 2 cyclo-oxygenase mRNA in human amnion at term. Biochem Biophys Res Commun. 1994;198:304–8.
72. Slater DM, Berger L, Newton R, Moore GE, Bennett PR. Changes in the expression of types 1 and 2 cyclo-oxygenase in human fetal membranes at term. Am J Obstet Gynecol. 1995;172: 77–82.
73. Moore S, Burke S, Slater D, Myatt L. Expression of prostaglandin-H synthase isoforms in human myometrium at parturition. Am J Obstet Gynecol. [in press].
74. Bailey JM, Verma M. Analytical procedures for a cryptic mRNA which mediates translational control of prostaglandin synthesis by glucocorticoids. Ann Biochem. 1991;196:11–8.
75. Pash JM, Bailey JM. Inhibition by corticosteroids of epidermal factor-induced recovery of cyclooxygenase after aspirin inactivation. FASEB J. 1988;2:2613–8.
76. Bailey JM. Mini review: New mechanisms for effects of anti-inflammatory glucocorticoids. Biofactors. 1991;3:97–102.
77. Bailey JM, Verma M. Identification of a highly conserved 3'UTR in the translational regulated mRNA for prostaglandin synthase. Prostaglandins. 1990;40:585–90.
78. Norton ME, Merrill J, Cooper BA, *et al.* Neonatal complications after administration of indomethacin for preterm labour. N Engl J Med. 1993;329:1602–7.
79. Kirshon B, Moise KJ, Mari G, Willis R. Long term indomethacin therapy decreases fetal urine output and causes oligohydramnios. Am J Perinatol. 1991;8:86.

80. Moise KJ. Effect of advancing gestational age on the frequency of fetal ductal constriction in association with maternal indomethacin usage. Am J Obstet Gynecol. 1983;168:1350–53.
81. Enkin MW, Keirse MJNC, Renfrew MJ, Nielson JP, eds. The pregnancy & childbirth module. Chochrane Database of Systematic Reviews, Cochrane Collaboration; 1995.
82. Slater D, Bennett PR. Changes in expression of cyclooxygenase types I and II throughout pregnancy. Am J Obstet Gynecol [in press].

11 Re-evaluation of gut toxicity of NSAIDs

D.N. BATEMAN

The adverse effects on the gut of drugs that inhibit cyclooxygenase (COX) have been documented for nearly 50 years[1]. In the 1980s the toxicity profile of gastrointestinal (GI) haemorrhage and perforation associated with non-steroid anti-inflammatory drugs (NSAIDs) became very clear. All of the NSAIDs currently in clinical use cause upper gastrointestinal tract toxicity in animal models. Factors that need to be considered when evaluating the toxicity of individual drugs in humans include the relative potency of the drug as an inhibitor of COX in the gut, the potential local irritant effect of a particular pharmaceutical preparation on the gut lining, the extent and variability of first-pass metabolism of the parent compound in the gut wall and liver, the effect of disease states or age on clearance and the potential biological activity of metabolites.

Although it is possible to study the toxic effects of NSAIDs experimentally in volunteers by examining blood loss or endoscopic changes, these studies are often performed on populations who would not normally be receiving the drug for therapeutic reasons. In addition, it is at present unclear how the results of these types of investigations relate to the adverse effects of the drugs in clinical practice.

It is often tempting for a pharmaceutical company to try and gain a commercial advantage by claiming that its product has a low gut toxicity profile. During the early stages of marketing this may be commercially hazardous: it may induce physicians to prescribe the product for patients who they perceive to be at greater risk of GI toxicity. A spate of adverse reaction reports in such patients may then inappropriately raise the question of whether the product is less safe than has been claimed. Such claims are also based on the assumption that patients participating in clinical trials are likely to show the same biological characteristics as those to whom the drug would be given in the market place. This is, of course, frequently not the case. Data on the toxicity of any pharmaceutical can be gained from a variety of sources, of which there are three main types. These are data from spontaneous reporting schemes, cohort studies and case-control studies. The most precise of these is the case-control study. In this paper I will attempt to illustrate the information that has been obtained from these sources, and then discuss particular problems for the future assessment of anti-inflammatory compounds and their toxic effects on the upper GI tract.

***Table 1** Serious upper GI and other common NSAID reactions (liver, kidney, skin and blood) expressed per million prescriptions during the first 5 years of marketing*

	Serious GI reactions	*Other serious reactions*	*Total serious reactions*
Ibuprofen	6.6 (0.5)	6.6 (0.2)	13.2 (0.7)
Diclofenac	20.9 (2.8)	18.5 (0.3)	39.4 (3.1)
Sulindac	23.9 (3.6)	30.4 (1.4)	54.3 (5.1)
Flurbiprofen	27.4 (2.1)	8.4 (1.2)	35.8 (3.3)
Fenoprofen	32.3 (4.2)	11.4 (2.4)	43.7 (6.6)
Naproxen	32.8 (4.1)	8.4 (1.5)	41.1 (5.6)
Ketoprofen	33.2 (1.6)	5.3 (0)	38.6 (1.6)
Diflunisal	33.5 (2.6)	13.7 (1)	47.2 (3.5)
Fenbufen	35.7 (1.9)	33.8 (2.5)	69.4 (4.5)
Tolmetin	41.7 (0)	25.0 (0)	66.7 (0)
Piroxicam	58.7 (5.2)	9.4 (1)	68.1 (6.2)
Azapropazone	67.0 (7.7)	20.9 (2.2)	87.9 (9.9)

Data from Ref. 2. Numbers in brackets refer to deaths

SPONTANEOUS REPORTING SCHEMES – YELLOW CARD SYSTEM

One of the simplest approaches to monitoring adverse drug reactions is the use of spontaneous reporting schemes, of which an excellent example is the UK 'Yellow Card' system. The system was originally established in 1964, but sales data only became available to the Committee on the Safety of Medicines (CSM) from the Prescription Pricing Authority in 1968. Data from this scheme were used to draw the attention of the medical profession in the UK to toxic effects of NSAIDs in 1986[2]. At that time data on the adverse effects of aspirin, phenylbutazone, oxyphenbutazone, mefenamic acid and conventional preparations of indomethacin could not be related to sales, since they have been marketed before the yellow card system became established. Nevertheless, a clear ranking of toxicity for serious adverse reactions involving the gut (upper GI haemorrhage and perforation) and other major organs (bone marrow, liver, kidney and skin) was possible (Table 1). These data suggested that ibuprofen was the safest NSAID, whereas reactions to piroxicam and azapropazone were considerably more common than for most other agents. Since this list was published the CSM has continued to monitor the toxicity of these drugs. In addition, three new agents have been marketed in the UK, etodolac, nabumetone and fenoxicam. The 1986 publication[2] concentrated on the first 5 years of marketing, since it was during this period that adverse reaction reporting is most frequent.

In order to take into account the effects of changes in reporting with time, and the higher adverse reaction rates that occur during the early years of marketing, an alternative approach can be adopted to these data. This excludes the first 2 years of marketing for all drugs, and then relates the subsequent numbers of adverse reactions to prescription volume. A correction factor is applied to take

***Table 2** GI adverse reactions to NSAIDs detected by the UK yellow card system, excluding the first 2 complete years of marketing, expressed per 100 000 prescriptions corrected for temporal reporting trends and expressed as a ratio to ibuprofen*

Drug	*Reporting frequency (RF)*	*Corrected frequency (cRF)*	*Ratio of individual cRF to cRF for ibuprofen*
Azapropazone	8.5	22.5	13.9
Diclofenac	1.8	4.9	3.0
Diflunisal	1.3	3.2	2.0
Etodolac	1.0	2.3	1.4
Fenbufen	2.2	6.4	4.0
Fenoprofen	1.1	3.1	1.9
Flurbiprofen	2.0	5.0	3.1
Ibuprofen	0.6	1.6	1.0
Indomethacin	1.8	5.0	3.1
Ketoprofen	3.0	8.0	5.0
Mefenamic acid	0.3	0.9	0.6
Nabumetone	1.4	4.8	3.0
Naproxen	1.8	4.6	2.9
Phenylbutazone	0.3	0.8	0.5
Piroxicam	4.6	12.9	8.0
Sulindac	1.3	3.4	2.1
Tenoxicam	1.0	3.2	2.0
Tiaprofenic acid	3.2	8.9	5.5
Tolmetin	7.7	21.3	13.2
Total	1.8	4.8	

account of the change in overall reporting, which increases with time. This approach has been summarized by the CSM[3], and is shown in more detail in Table 2. Using this method, ibuprofen continues to be seen as the least toxic compound, with piroxicam and azapropazone remaining at the toxic end of the rank order. It does, however, demonstrate that nabumetone appears to have middle ranking toxicity. This approach, together with data from the epidemiological studies discussed below, was used to review the regulatory position in 1994 and resulted in restrictions on the licensed indications for azapropazone[3]. Nabumetone was marketed in 1988 and Table 3 shows the numbers of serious adverse reaction reports to principal organ systems implicated with NSAIDs received by the CSM involving nabumetone in its first 5 years of marketing. During this period over 800 000 prescriptions for the drug were written in the UK. Nabumetone was introduced into the market at a time when doctors were far more aware of the likely toxicity of NSAIDs than they had been in the 1970s and this may have contributed to the greater rate of reporting. The

Table 3 Adverse reactions to CSM implicating nabumetone in the UK in the first 5 years of marketing

Year	*All GI**	*Liver, kidney skin + blood*	*Total serious*
1988	30 (1)	24 (0)	104 (3)
1989	26 (1)	22 (0)	60 (2)
1990	11 (0)	17 (0)	42 (0)
1991	7 (0)	8 (0)	19 (0)
1992	2 (0)	6 (0)	15 (0)
Total	74 (2)	77 (0)	240 (5)

*Includes lower GI adverse reactions. Numbers in brackets are deaths.

second issue is that the rate of reporting by the yellow card system has risen regularly since its inception: the total number of reports received per annum in the 1990s is approximately twice that of 20 years ago. If the data presented in Table 3 had been analysed in the same way as the initial publication from the CSM in 1986[2] nabumetone would have been implicated in 79.8 serious GI reactions per million prescriptions, with 2.4 deaths per million prescriptions, and 91.6 other serious reactions per million prescriptions with no deaths. This contrasts with the more recent analysis.

From a practical point of view, it is clear that the spontaneous adverse reaction reporting systems allow comparison of the toxicity of individual products. Since the rate of reporting of even serious reactions to the Committee on Safety of Medicines is of the order of $\leq 10\%$ of the actual rate[4], this system cannot be used to assess directly the individual risk for a particular drug. It is also dependent on market penetration, and subject to distortions that occur during the first 2 years of marketing, when black triangle status is likely to increase reporting rates. It is also possible that marketing strategies may affect spontaneous reporting: a claim of relative gut safety in advertising may stimulate doctors to report gut toxicity.

COHORT STUDIES

Patients in cohort studies may be recruited in a variety of ways. In the UK three principle techniques can be applied. The first uses the Prescription Pricing Authority to identify patients receiving a prescription for a named drug, a system operated in Prescription Event Monitoring. One of the largest comparative studies was reported in the 1980s[5], when five NSAIDs (benoxaprofen, fenbufen, zomepirac, piroxicam and indomethacin as 'Osmosin') were compared. A total of 55 642 patients were evaluable, and age data were available for between 5058 on fenbufen and 12 709 on benoxaprofen. The data from this study were reported in two ways, first by comparing rates of events per 1000 patient–years of exposure, and second by comparing event rates per 1000 events on and off treatment (Table 4).

Table 4 Overall events and GI events (GI% of overall rate) associated with 5 NSAIDs during Prescription Event Monitoring

	Events per 1000 patient years			*GI events/1000 events 'on' prescription*	*GI events/1000 events 'off' prescription*
	GI	*Overall*	*GI% of overall*		
Benoxaprofen	192	909	21	211	165
Fenbufen	148	654	23	227	173
Zomepirac	187	779	24	240	155
Piroxicam	135	645	21	209	152
Osmosin	447	1325	34	337	217

Since no data from a specific control group were reported it is difficult to know from this publication what the background expected event rate would be in a comparative population. However, there did seem to be an excess of dyspepsia, gastritis, nausea, vomiting and peptic ulceration following administration of Osmosin. The total GI event rates are shown in Table 4: for Osmosin 22 of the GI events per 1000 patient-years were in this category. This study also identified an excess of photosensitivity reactions and onycholysis with benoxaprofen, and the total skin reaction rates per 1000 patient-years were 248 for benoxaprofen, 97 for fenbufen, 80 for zomepirac, 69 for piroxicam and 93 for Osmosin. Rates of GI symptoms per 1000 events on treatment and off treatment tended to show that the overall rate of GI events was somewhat lower off treatment. The rates for Osmosin, however, were higher both on and off treatment when dyspepsia and nausea and vomiting were considered. Thus the rate of dyspepsia on treatment per 1000 events in patients receiving fenbufen was 83 on treatment and 41 off, for piroxicam 52 on treatment and 26 off, whereas for Osmosin it was 110 on treatment and 64 off. This raises questions about the patient selection for therapy, or persistence of an adverse effect in patients who had received Osmosin. Cohorts of the size studied in Prescription Event Monitoring do not seem able to differentiate clearly the relative toxicity of individual NSAIDs, and certainly no clear rank order for GI toxicity could be drawn from the data presented.

An alternative approach is to use computerized patient data collection systems, and two such systems are available. In Tayside the Medicines Evaluation and Monitoring Group (MEMO) collects data on the same patient from hospital and primary care and links them[6]. This system is capable of detecting an excess of GI events, as demonstrated by a record link study of 57715 prescriptions for five NSAIDs (ibuprofen, indomethacin, naproxen, Osmosin and piroxicam) to 25959 patients between March and October 1983. In the published report no attempt was made to compare the individual drugs, but there was a clear excess of events documented in drug takers as opposed to their matched controls. The relative risk was calculated for GI events or diagnosis of perforation or GI haemorrhage, and both methods give relative risks significantly in excess of controls in NSAID takers [relative risk for overall events: 1.54 (95% CI 1.45–1.63): perforation and haemorrhage relative risk: males, 2.11 (95% CI 1.57–2.84), females, 2.05 (95% CI 1.63–2.50)]. The MEMO system also allowed an assessment of events per 1000 drug takers and controls before and during treatment, and showed an increased relative risk of 1.86 (95% CI 1.47–2.36) after treatment compared with before treatment. This technique is therefore applicable, but optimally depends on an adequate penetration of the new compound, and either a relatively long study period or excellent market penetration to generate sufficient numbers for a useful statistical analysis.

A much larger cohort can be collected using general practitioner computer systems. Garcia Rodriguez and Jick used the VAMP database[7] to compare the relative toxicity of individual NSAIDs in this population using a retrospective case-control approach. Since all data are collected retrospectively this can be considered as a form of cohort study. From the database, of approximately 4000000 patients, those with diagnoses of upper GI bleeding were identified. After exclusion of patients with previous known disease likely to contribute to such an event (e.g. alcoholism, cirrhosis) 3714 patients were identified from the computer system and their notes manually reviewed. Following this review 1457 patients were regarded as having had an episode of upper GI bleeding or perforation. Of the 1457 patients identified, 241 were currently receiving one or more NSAIDs, 44 had recent past use and 66 any past use. A cohort of 10000 patients was selected as controls. Comparison with this control group showed an excess risk of GI bleeding in current users and recent past users. The risk was significantly greater in the 47 multiple users than in the 194 single users. In a subgroup analysis of 862 cases and 9017 controls, the author assessed the relative risk of bleeding for seven individual NSAIDs, ibuprofen, naproxen, diclofenac, ketoprofen, indomethacin, piroxicam and azapropazone, for multiple NSAID use, and for 'other non-steroidals' comprising a mixture of mefenamic acid, fenbufen, fenoprofen, flurbiprofen, diflunisal, sulindac, tenoxicam, tiaprofenic acid, etodolac and nabumetone (Table 5). This showed that ibuprofen had the lowest relative risk, and that the risk was significantly greater for piroxicam, azapropazone or multiple drug use. In addition a dose–response relationship could be shown for ibuprofen in doses below or above 1500 mg and indomethacin for doses below or above 75 mg.

Relative risks ibuprofen $\leq$1500 mg, 2.1 (1.1–4.1); >1500 mg, 6.5 (2.6–16.4):
Indomethacin $\leq$75 mg, 1.4 (0.3–5.8); >75 mg, 14.4 (5.7–36.4).

This GP computer-based approach is potentially the most powerful cohort technique currently available. It does, however, require an appropriate level of market penetration within the target practices. It is, nevertheless, a means of comparing directly, during the same period, the relative toxicity of different NSAIDs, and it offers the possibility of examining dose–response relationships.

Table 5 Relative risk of upper GI bleeding for individual NSAIDs (data from ref. 7)

	Cases	Controls	Adjusted relative risk
No use	615	8222	1
Ibuprofen	20	74	2.9 (1.7–5.0)
Other NSAIDs*	13	39	2.9 (1.5–5.6)
Naproxen	15	46	3.1 (1.7–5.9)
Diclofenac	25	53	3.9 (2.3–6.5)
Ketoprofen	14	20	5.4 (2.6–11.3)
Indomethacin	20	24	6.3 (3.3–12.2)
Multiple NSAID	33	43	8.9 (5.4–14.7)
Piroxicam	20	11	18.0 (8.2–39.6)
Azapropazone	11	4	23.4 (6.9–79.5)

*Mefenamic acid, fenbufen, flurbiprofen, diflunisal, sulindac, tenoxicam, tiaprofenic acid, etodolac and nabumetone

CASE-CONTROL STUDIES

The most powerful tool for examining risk is that of case-control studies. A large number of case-control studies on non-steroidals, aspirin and paracetamol have been published. In this paper I will consider data from 36 studies in which it is possible to calculate relative risk of upper GI haemorrhage or perforation, or death due to these drugs, and in which a control group was included. These data are taken from Belton et al.[8].

Nine published studies allow assessment of the relative risk of paracetamol exposure as a cause of upper GI toxicity (Figure 1). Although only two of these studies individually show a relative risk which is significantly greater than 1, a meta-analysis using a random effects model suggests a statistically significant excess risk for paracetamol of 1.42 (95% CI 1.12–1.79). Twenty-two studies allow the toxicity of aspirin to be evaluated, and all but two of these studies show a significant effect of aspirin in the doses used (Figure 2). Most older studies will, of course, involve doses higher than those generally currently used for prophylaxis of ischaemic heart disease. The meta-analysis shows an overall relative risk from aspirin exposure of 3.55 (95% CI 2.84–4.43). Eighteen case-control studies involving NSAIDs have been evaluated, and all show an excess risk (Figure 3), with relative risk, using a random effect model, of 3.94 (95% CI 2.88–5.40).

Although a large number of case-control studies have shown an increased risk of GI haemorrhage and/or perforation following exposure to NSAIDs the numbers of subjects in most studies is insufficient to allow comparison of the toxicity of single agents. Four large studies have enabled the risks associated with individual drugs to be compared (Table 6). These studies tend to confirm that ibuprofen is associated with a lower ulcer risk than other NSAIDs. Most NSAIDs

Figure 1 Meta-analysis of results of paracetamol studies. Relative risk is the risk of serious upper GI haemorrhage when taking paracetamol, compared with no use of paracetamol. Studies are listed on the vertical axis in chronological order

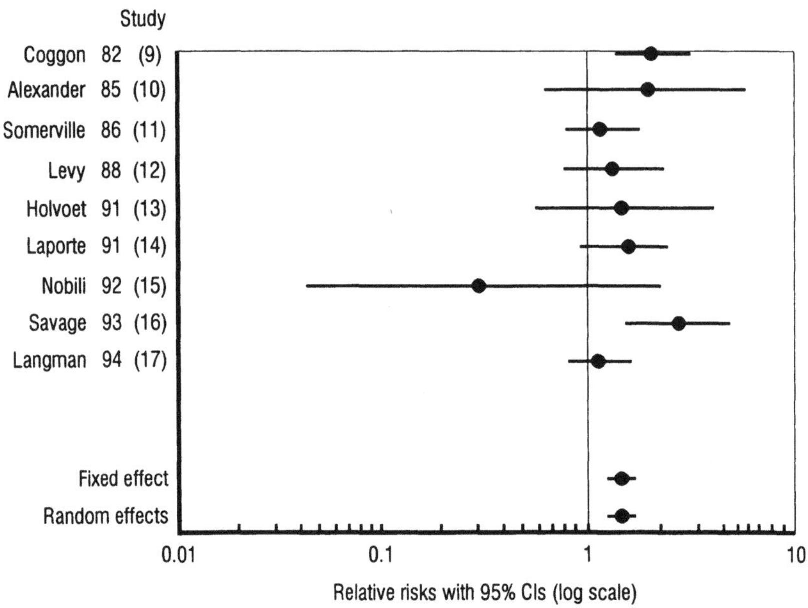

have relative risks for GI events around twice that for ibuprofen, but these studies do highlight some individual differences. Diclofenac appears more toxic in the Australian data[37] than in that from the UK[17]. Piroxicam has a high odds ratio in the Spanish study, and was towards the top of the range of other NSAIDs in the study of Savage et al.[16] from the USA and the study of Langman et al.[17] from the UK. Azapropazone and ketoprofen had very high odds ratios in the UK study[17].

These studies also suggest that the risk of GI events is greatest in the first month after starting therapy, is dose-related, where this can be evaluated, and overall the risk is greater in the elderly and in those receiving more than one NSAID. In general the rank-order in these case-control studies are in line with findings from both spontaneous reporting schemes and the large cohort study of Garcia-Rodriguez and Jick[7].

OTHER APPROACHES

The propensity of non-steroidals to cause GI toxicity can be measured in volunteers by endoscopy, or by measuring GI blood loss following administration

Figure 2 Meta-analysis of results of aspirin studies. Relative risk is the risk of serious upper GI haemorrhage when taking aspirin, compared with no use of aspirin. Studies are listed on the vertical axis in chronological order

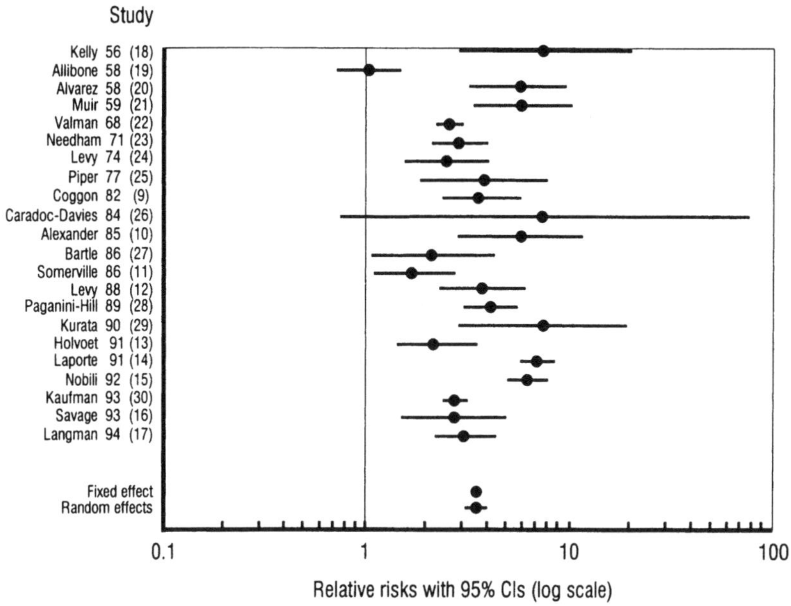

of a drug. No published comparative information compares the results of these studies, with the data that are available on the toxicity of individual drugs in clinical use. In early clinical trials most NSAIDs tend to cause dyspepsia in at least 10% of patients. A NSAID that did not cause this adverse effect might, therefore, be less likely to cause ulcer complications. Again, however, there are no published data comparing the incidence of adverse events in early clinical trials with eventual clinical toxicity. If such data could be collated, it might be a useful source for future study.

COX INHIBITION AND GI ADVERSE EVENTS

Comparison of the IC_{50} of COX-1 and COX-2 in vitro gives an indication of relative selectivity of a drug for these two enzymes[39]. The IC_{50} ratios might be expected to relate to clinical toxicity, but there is an approximate 1000-fold variation in this ratio, and while proxicam (ratio 600) has high gut toxicity, the relationship between COX selectivity and gut toxicity is far less clear for

Figure 3 Meta-analysis of results of non-acidic NSAID studies. Relative risk is the risk of serious upper GI haemorrhage when taking non-acid NSAIDs, compared to non-use. Studies are listed on the vertical axis in chronological order

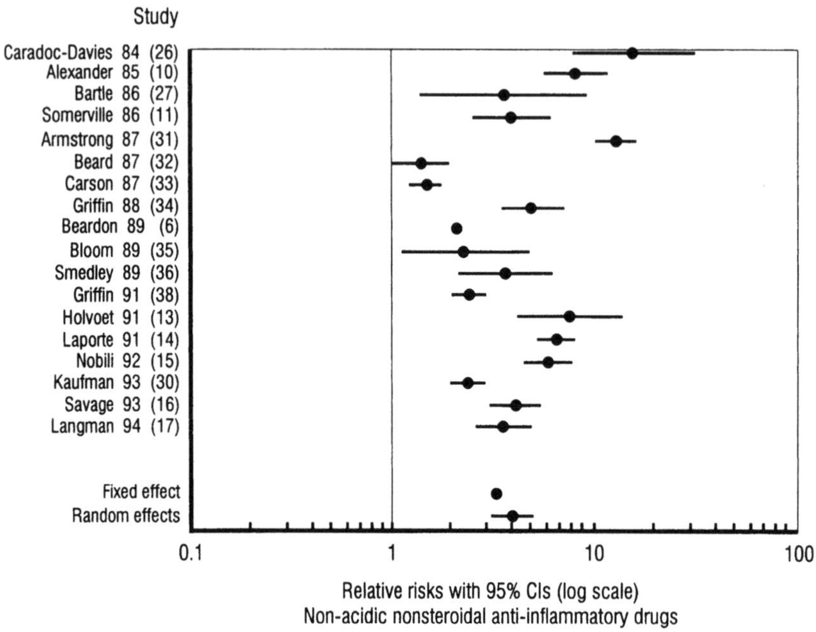

NSAIDs as a whole. For example indomethacin and diclofenac seem to have a similar clinical toxicity (Tables 2 and 6) but COX ratios of 60 and 0.7 respectively. Whether newer drugs with far greater selectivity will be a significant clinical advance remains to be seen, although preliminary data seem promising[39].

CONCLUSIONS

In this paper I have concentrated on the three principle ways in which toxicity data on NSAIDs have been collected. Of the techniques used, the most powerful is the case-control study. Such studies have been consistent in their findings, and do enable some ranking of the relative toxicity of NSAIDs on the gut. It is reassuring that these rankings are in broad agreement with those produced by the spontaneous reporting system in the UK. Cohort studies have in general been disappointing, both as methods for assessing relative risks, and for assessing magnitude of individual risk, but this is probably due to the relatively small number of subjects they recruit, which is usually insufficient to show clear differences between drugs. Computerized patient databases seem to offer a

Table 6 ***Estimated risk of upper GI haemorrhage with individual NSAIDs [odds ratio (95% CI)]. Drugs are listed alphabetically***

Drug	*Griffin et al.*[35]	*Laporte et al.*[14]	*Henry et al.*[37]	*Savage et al.*[16]	*Langman et al.*[17]	*Garcia Rodriguez and Jick*[7]
Azapropazone	–	–	–	–	16.4 (5.6–48.0)	23.4 (6.9–79.5)
Diclofenac			7.9 (4.3–14.6)	3.0 (1.8–5.4)	3.7 (2.6–5.3)	3.9 (2.3–6.5)
Ibuprofen	2.3 (1.8–3.0)	–	–	1.2 (0.4–3.2)	2.1 (1.6–2.8)	2.9 (1.7–5.0)
Indomethacin	3.8 (2.4–6.0)	4.9 (12.2)	2.4 (1.2–4.9)	7.3 (2.7–9.5)	5.9 (3.8–9.3)	6.3 (3.3–12.2)
Ketoprofen	–	–	–	2.6 (1.4–5.0)	16.7 (6.9–40.1)	5.4 (2.6–11.3)
Naproxen	4.3 (3.4–5.4)	6.5 (2.2–19.6)	5.3 (2.7–10.2)	3.6 (2.1–6.3)	6.5 (4.5–9.5)	3.1 (1.7–5.9)
Piroxicam	6.4 (4.8–8.4)	19.1 (8.2–44.3)	3.7 (2.0–6.9)	6.3 (3.3–12.0)	7.7 (4.7–12.5)	18.0 (8.2–39.6)
Sulindac	4.2 (2.8–6.3)	–	–	2.3 (1.3–4.3)	–	–

potentially powerful tool for future evaluation. The results of the single large cohort study obtained retrospectively from the UK GP database[7] agrees quite closely with the data from formal case-control studies (Table 6).

Published studies in this area show an effect of dose and age on risk. The effect of age in particular has important implications for early clinical experience with any new drug. The cautious physician will not give a new preparation to a patient perceived to be in an 'at risk' group. If, however, a marketing strategy is developed for a new NSAID which is believed from experimental data to be less likely to produce GI toxicity, there is a real risk that the initial response of prescribers to this information will be to give the drug to the higher risk groups, and hence potentially adversely affect initial adverse drug reaction reporting rates, and confound studies of GI toxicity. The design of studies which can take these factors into account is likely to be the next challenge in the search for techniques which will confirm the potentially safer adverse reaction profiles of new NSAIDs.

Acknowledgements

I am grateful for the permission of Professor M.D. Rawlins, Dr J.N.S. Matthews, Miss S.C. Lewis and Miss K.J. Belton for permission to quote data they have collected from published studies and for Figures 1, 2 and 3. I am grateful to the Medicines Control Agency for helpful discussions, for permission to publish the material in Tables 2 and 3, and for access to their database.

References

1. Douthwaite AH, Lintott GAM. Gastroscopic observation of the effect of aspirin and certain other substances on the stomach. Lancet. 1938;1222–4.
2. Committee on Safety of Medicines. Update. Br Med J. 1986;292:1191–2.
3. Committee on Safety of Medicines/Medicines Control Agency. Relative safety of oral non-aspirin NSAIDs. Curr Prob Pharmacovigilance. 1994;20:9–11.
4. Bateman DN, Chaplin S. Adverse reactions to drugs. In: Feely J, editor. New Drugs. 3rd edn. London: Br Med J. 1991:29–40.
5. Inman WHW. Comparative study of 5 NSAIDs. Prescription Event Monitoring News. 1985;3: 3–13.
6. Beardon PHG, Brown SV, McDevitt DG. Gastrointestinal events in patients prescribed non-steroidal anti-inflammatory drugs: a controlled study using record linkage in Tayside. Q J Med. 1989;266:497–505.
7. Garcia Rodriguez LA, Jick H. Risk of upper gastrointestinal bleeding and perforation associated with individual non-steroidal anti-inflammatory drugs. Lancet. 1994;343:769–72.
8. Belton KJ, Lewis SC, Matthews JNS, Rawlins MD. Systematic overview of upper gastro-intestinal haemorrhage associated with non-steroidal anti-inflammatory drugs. In: Fracchia GN, editor. European Medicines Research. Perspectives in pharmacotoxicology and pharmacovigilance. Amsterdam: IOS Press; 1994:322–330.
9. Coggon D, langman MJ, Spiegelhalter D. Aspirin, paracetamol, and haematemesis and melaena. Gut. 1982;23:340–4.
10. Alexander AM, Veitch GBA, Wood JB. Anti-rheumatic and analgesic drug usage and acute gastro-intestinal bleeding in elderly patients. J Clin Hosp Pharm. 1985;10:89–93.
11. Somerville K, Faulkner G, Langman M. Non-steroidal anti-inflammatory drugs and bleeding peptic ulcer. Lancet. 1986;1:462–4.

12. Levy M, Miller DR, Kaufman DW et al. Major upper gastrointestinal tract bleeding. Arch Intern Med. 1988;148:281–5.
13. Holvoet JL, Terriere W, Van Hee W, Verbist L, Fierens E, Hautekeete ML. Relation of upper gastrointestinal bleeding to non-steroidal and anti-inflammatory drugs and aspirin: a case-control study. Gut. 1991;32:730–4.
14. Laporte J-R, Camme X, Vidal X, Moreno V, Juan J. Upper gastrointestinal bleeding in relation to previous use of analgesics and non-steroidal anti-inflammatory drugs. Lancet. 1991;337:85–9.
15. Nobili A, Mosconi P, Franzoni MG, Tognoni G. Non-steroidal anti-inflammatory drugs and upper gastrointestinal bleeding, a post-marketing surveillance case-control study. Pharmacoepidemiol Drug Safety. 1992;1:65–72.
16. Savage RL, Moller PW, Ballantyne CL, Wells JE. Variation in the risk of peptic ulcer complications with nonsteroidal antiinflammatory drug therapy. Arthritis Rheum. 1993;36:84–90.
17. Langman MJS, Weil J, Wainwright P et al. Risks of bleeding peptic ulcer associated with individual non-steroidal anti-inflammatory drugs. Lancet. 1994;343:1075–8.
18. Kelly JJ. Salicylate ingestion: a frequent cause of gastric haemorrhage. Am J Med Sci. 1956;232: 119–27.
19. Allibone A, Flint FJ. Bronchitis, aspirin, smoking, and other factors in the aetiology of peptic ulcer. Lancet. 1958;2:179–82.
20. Alvarez AS, Summerskill WHJ. Gastrointestinal haemorrhage and salicylates. Lancet. 1958:920–5.
21. Muir A, Cossar IA. Aspirin and gastric haemorrhage. Lancet. 1959;1:539–41.
22. Valman HB, Parry DJ, Coghill NF. Lesions associated with gastroduodenal haemorrhage in relation to aspirin intake. Br Med J. 1968;4:661–3.
23. Needham CD, Kyle J, Jones PF, Johnston SJ, Kerridge DF. Aspirin and alcohol in gastrointestinal haemorrhage. Gut. 1971;12:819–21.
24. Levy M. Aspirin use in patients with major upper gastrointestinal bleeding and peptic-ulcer disease. N Engl J Med. 1974;290:1158–62.
25. Piper DW, Greig M, Landecker KD, Shinners J, Waller S, Canalese J. Analgesic intake and chronic gastric ulcer. Acute upper gastrointestinal haemorrhage, personality traits and social class. Proc RSM. 1977;70:11–15.
26. Caradoc-Davies TH. Nonsteroidal anti-inflammatory drugs, arthritis, and gastrointestinal bleeding in elderly in-patients. Age Ageing. 1984;13:295–8.
27. Bartle WR, Gupta AK, Lazor J. Nonsteroidal anti-inflammatory drugs and gastrointestinal bleeding – a case–control study. Arch Intern Med. 1986;146:2365–7.
28. Paganini-Hill A, Chao A, Ross RK. Henderson BE. Aspirin use and chronic diseases: a cohort study of the elderly. Br Med J. 1989;299:1247–50.
29. Kurata JH, Abbey DE. The effect of chronic aspirin use on duodenal and gastric ulcer hospitalizations. J Clin Gastroenterol. 1990;12:260–6.
30. Kaufman DW, Kelly JP, Sheehan JE et al. Nonsteroidal anti-inflammatory drug use in relation to major upper gastrointestinal bleeding. Clin Pharmacol Ther. 1993;53:485–94.
31. Armstrong CP, Blower AL. Non-steroidal anti-inflammatory drugs and life threatening complications of peptic ulceration. Gut. 1987;28:527–32.
32. Beard K, Walker AM, Perara DR, Jick H. Nonsteroidal anti-inflammatory drugs and hospitalization for gastroesophageal bleeding in the elderly. Arch Intern Med. 1987;47:1621–3.
33. Carson JL, Strom BL, Morse ML et al. The relative gastrointestinal toxicity of the nonsteroidal anti-inflammatory drugs. Arch Intern Med. 1987;147:1054–9.
34. Griffin MR, Ray WA, Schaffner W. Nonsteroidal anti-inflammatory drug use and death from peptic ulcer in elderly persons. Ann Intern Med. 1988;109:359–63.
35. Bloom BS. Risk and cost of gastrointestinal side effects associated with nonsteroidal anti-inflammatory drugs. Arch Intern Med. 1989;149:1019–22.
36. Smedly FH, Taube M, Leach R, Wastell C. Non-steroidal anti-inflammatory drug ingestion: retrospective study of 272 bleeding or perforated peptic ulcers. Postgrad Med J. 1989;65:892–5.
37. Henry DA, Dobson A, Turner K et al. Non-steroidal anti-inflammatory drugs and the risk of upper gastrointestinal bleeding. Lancet. 1991;337:730.
38. Griffin MR, Piper JM, Daugherty JR, Snowden M, Ray WA. Nonsteroidal anti-inflammatory drug use and increased risk for peptic ulcer disease in elderly persons. Ann Intern Med. 1991; 114:257–63.
39. Vane JR, Botting RM. This volume.

12 NSAID: can renal side effects be avoided?

J.C. FRÖLICH and D.O. STICHTENOTH

Unwanted renal effects of NSAIDs are numerous, fairly frequent and range from mild to life-threatening with a consequent life-long need for dialysis. The pursuit of drug development towards a renal-sparing NSAID is therefore a very worthy cause. This review is concerned with the physiological mechanisms which are disturbed by NSAIDs, the contribution of renal disease to this interaction (Table 1) and a comparison of NSAIDs currently used in therapy with respect to their effects on the kidney.

In this context, recent developments following the discovery of two different cyclooxygenases (COX-1 and COX-2) assume great importance. The kidney is a rich source of COX-1-produced prostaglandins (PG), which are necessary for its normal function, while COX-2-dependent PG synthesis is probably of minor importance. COX-1 inhibitors therefore cause most of the unwanted renal effects, while COX-2 inhibitors appear to be largely devoid of such effects. It has been customary to compare NSAIDs on the basis of their chemical structure, which has no discernible therapeutic relevance. It is now time to classify NSAIDs according to their relative inhibitory activity on COX-1 and COX-2, which has clinical relevance.

The incidence of renal side effects with currently used NSAIDs is not known. Because NSAIDs are widely prescribed, and also available without prescription, a large number of patients are exposed. Among the entire population exposed to NSAIDs, the incidence of renal side effects due to NSAID is probably low: for 8 million prescriptions for mefenamic acid, only 23 cases of nephropathy were reported[1]. However, NSAIDs have for many years led the list of drugs causing side effects reported to the FDA. When one looks at a selected population, the impact becomes more obvious. NSAIDs were implicated as the causative agent in approximately 6% of all patients with renal failure observed in a 2-year period[2]. In a prospective study by Kleinknecht[3] NSAIDs caused 16% of drug-induced acute renal failure and 3% of all acute renal failure. Recent observations on patients with end-stage renal failure also implicate NSAIDs[4]. The number of patients showing renal impairment may be much higher when a non-selected group of patients is carefully monitored: in a large general internal medicine practice 12% of patients treated with ibuprofen showed renal impairments[5].

Most of the unwanted renal effects of NSAIDs, including a reduction in renal blood flow (RBF), glomerular filtration rate (GFR) and papillary necrosis, sodium retention and hyperkalaemia, have been attributed to inhibition of PG

Table 1 Conditions predisposing to NSAID-induced renal failure

Dehydration	Epstein et al.[178]
Congestive heart failure	Oliver et al.[179]
Nephrotic syndrome	Arisz et al.[62]
Liver cirrhosis	Zipser[180]
Mild renal failure	Whelton et al.[68]
SLE	Patrono et al.[181]

synthesis. In addition a cytoprotective effect of PG on the kidney has been shown[6]. There may also be effects which are not related to cyclooxygenase inhibition. Interstitial nephritis is not clearly related to PG suppression. Similar considerations hold for analgesic nephropathy.

Interstitial nephritis can be caused by many drugs which are not NSAIDs, such as the β-lactam antibiotics. The frequency with which NSAIDs are involved is striking: Those implicated include fenoprofen, naproxen, piriprofen, benoxaprofen, alclofenac, piroxicam, aspirin and diflunisal (for review see Ref. 3). These drugs belong to very different chemical classes, and their only common property is their ability to act as anti-rheumatic drugs. About 2% of 398 patients presenting with drug-induced renal failure were suffering from acute interstitial nephritis. The course of the disease may be prolonged, taking up to 1 year for full recovery. About 30% of affected patients require dialysis for some time, and about 30% do not fully recover. Because the disease usually requires some months of drug exposure, it has been suggested that it is a cell-mediated immune response. Indeed, CD8 cells are the predominant species in the interstitial infiltrates. It has been suggested that COX inhibition removes an inhibitory effect of PGs on T-cells by shunting arachidonic acid away from PGs into the 5-lipoxygenase pathway[8], resulting in the production of pro-inflammatory leukotrienes. Such a shift has been shown to occur in vivo in allergic reactions[9]. However, under these conditions glucocorticoids should be very effective, yet their effect is uncertain.

Analgesic nephropathy is characterized by a slowly developing process that begins in the papilla and later involves the vasa recta. The lesions are characterized by cell death, leading to the characteristic papillary necrosis. The necrosis, however, is characterized as due to medullary ischaemia[10]. The end result is loss of concentrating ability, papillary calcification and loss of papillae. Many different factors have been alleged to participate in the damage, including concentration of the drug due to the countercurrent mechanism in the kidney (e.g. paracetamol metabolite concentration in the papilla is 10-fold higher than in the cortex; and the renal toxicity is enhanced by dehydration leading to high concentrations in the medulla); exhaustion of GSH due to the formation of reactive drug metabolites (especially paracetamol); reduction in medullary perfusion, which, due to low oxygen tension in this tissue easily leads to ischaemic damage; and loss of medullary matrix. The most important point for the present discussion is perhaps that different drugs can induce nephrotoxicity by different mechanisms. Paracetamol acts predominantly through exhaustion of GSH and only very weakly through prostaglandin inhibition[11], while other drugs, such as phenylbutazone and indomethacin, severely block cyclooxygenase, producing damage primarily through a reduction in medullary oxygen supply. The diagnosis of analgesic nephropathy does not, therefore, describe a uniform pathogenesis, and has for the most part been limited to phenacetin and paracetamol[12]. All studies of this toxicity rely on questioning patients, whose answers are often unreliable. In addition, most patients who take excessive amounts of one drug also take many other drugs. Life-long medication records are forthcoming and will shed more light on this question.

Initial investigations on the functional role of renal PG originated from studies on the role of the kidney in hypertension. Renal hypertension was thought to be due to lack of an antihypertensive medullary lipid secreted into the circulation. This was later believed to be identical with PGA_2[13] and identified in the circulation of normal volunteers and patients at a concentration of several nanograms per millilitre, an amount capable of reducing blood pressure[14,15]. Because PGE_2 can be easily dehydrated to form PGA_2 under the acidic conditions most often employed for the extraction of prostaglandins into organic solvents, we investigated the amount of PGA_2 measured in the renal medulla that might actually have arisen from this conversion. We found that all PGA_2 detected in renal medullary homogenates originated from this dehydration of PGE_2 during the extraction process[16]. In our subsequent studies on PGA_2 concentrations in the human circulation utilizing gas chromatography/mass spectrometry (GC/MS) we found that, in contrast to previous reports based on radioimmunoassay (RIA), levels were indistinguishable from zero[17].

RIA studies have detected PGE_2 in the circulation in amounts that could affect renal function. However, on the basis of measurement of the major urinary metabolite by GC/MS it was shown that these levels must be much smaller and in the range of a few picograms per millilitre[18,19]. Under conditions of shock, PGE_2 levels measured by bioassay were elevated into the range of a few nanograms per millilitre[20], and this was subsequently confirmed by GC/MS[21]. Such concentrations can exert an effect on the kidney.

PGI_2 has also been described as a prostaglandin appearing in the arterial circulation after release from the lung[22]. The metabolism of PGI_2 in humans produces 2,3-dinor-6-keto $PGF_{1\alpha}$ as the major urinary metabolite[23]. We have subsequently shown that, based upon the measurement of metabolic clearance rate and the excretion rate of the major urinary metabolite of PGI_2, the concentrations under normal conditions in man are, at most, a few picograms per millilitre[24]. These concentrations are too low to have any discernible effect on renal function.

In summary, prostaglandins affecting the kidney do not usually reach it via the circulation but are produced locally. Under certain extreme conditions such as haemorrhagic shock they can be detected in the circulation, but except for PGE_2, very little is known about their occurrence and functional role.

Great problems have arisen due to the use of RIA measurement of PG[16–18,24–26]. Quality control and comparison with the reference method GC/MS are often lacking and explain some of the discrepant results.

The interest in defining the role of PGs in the kidney has led to the application of NSAIDs as tools[27,28]. This has been a successful approach which has yielded, in addition to the information on PGs in the kidney, interesting data on the toxic effects of these drugs. It was shown that not all NSAIDs are alike with respect to their effect on renal PG synthesis and renal function. In studies on the effects of acetylsalicylic acid and its active metabolite salicylate in normal volunteers we discovered that the former reduced renal PG production, while the latter did not[29]. It is not a trivial matter to distinguish between the NSAIDs, therefore, and they should not be considered a single class of drugs. The other non-acetylated salicylates diflunisal and salsalate show a pharmacological profile similar to salicylate, i.e. they do not inhibit platelet aggregation, they lack sodium retaining properties (see page 209) and show no interactions with antihypertensive drugs and diuretics. More recently, meloxicam has been shown to be similar in the rat. It has little effect on renal PG production in a dose that shows highly effective anti-inflammatory activity[30].

ASSESSMENT OF RENAL PROSTAGLANDIN PRODUCTION

In vitro studies showed that renal cortex and medulla produce PGE_2, $PGF_{2\alpha}$ and PGI_2[13,31–33]. These studies led to the proposal that PGI_2 is primarily synthesized in cortex and PGE_2 in medulla[33–35]. While this has generally held true, there are some exceptions, presumably dependent on the experimental conditions[36]. More detailed analyses of isolated structures of the kidney have shown that the renal vasculature and glomeruli produce mainly PGI_2[37,38], while renomedullary interstitial cells synthesize predominantly PGE_2. There is also some synthesis of thromboxane A_2 (TXA_2); the functional role of this, however, is uncertain[33].

One of the substantial challenges has been to analyse renal PG production in vivo. Renal arterial and venous PG concentrations have shown a small gradient for PGE_2 and $PGF_{2\alpha}$[39,40]. However, the interpretation of blood levels of PGs is complicated by possible platelet activation and irritation of the vascular wall[41,42]. It is also technically difficult to obtain samples, particularly when repeat sampling is necessary. All of these problems are compounded when studies in humans are performed. We, therefore, considered the possibility of renal excretion of PGs and found that PGE_2, $PGF_{2\alpha}$ and 6-keto-$PGF_{1\alpha}$ appear in urine[23,43,44]. However, while 6-keto-$PGF_{1\alpha}$ is excreted in the urine after intravenous infusion of itself or PGI_2[44], PGE_2 or $PGF_{2\alpha}$ when so given do not appear in urine[18,45].

Further evidence for an intrarenal origin of PGE_2 and $PGF_{2\alpha}$ became evident, when we infused angiotensin II into one renal artery of the dog and found that only ipsilateral PG excretion increased. Contralateral PG excretion was unaffected even though GFR decreased[43]. Angiotensin must therefore have stimulated PG production in the infused kidney only, and this was shown by increased ipsilateral urinary excretion of PGs. This finding stimulated us to investigate the intrarenal origin of the PGs by stop flow experiments. With this method it was possible to identify the loop of Henle as the site of origin[46]. Further evidence for this was obtained by others using an inhibitor of the organic anion secretory pathway, probenecid. Probenecid had no effect on basal PGE_2 excretion, suggesting that it enters the tubule at a site distal to this location[45]. However, when PGE_2 reaches the kidney via the renal artery its excretion is significantly reduced by probenecid[44,45]. In contrast, 6-keto-$PGF_{1\alpha}$ is not affected by probenecid when given into the renal artery, thus showing that it does not depend on this mechanism of elimination but is simply filtered[44]. The total amount of 6-keto-$PGF_{1\alpha}$ appearing in urine under basal conditions in humans can readily be explained by filtration from plasma of the metabolite of PGI_2 formed by the whole body[24]. This might be different in renal disease.

Measurement of urinary PGE_2 thus emerges as a rather specific marker for renal PG production. There are some limitations, however. In males, seminal fluid may interfere with PGE_2 measurements as it contains about 25–50 μg/ml PGE_2 while the 24 h excretion of PGE_2 in females is only about 200 ng[41,46,47]. Furthermore, PG excretion may depend on pH as PGs are weak acids. Haylor et al.[48] showed that alkalinization of urine increased, and acidification decreased, urinary PG excretion. A further complication is the urine flow rate since there is some reabsorption of PGs, which is of course reduced when the flow rate is increased[49].

In summary, measurement of urinary PGE_2 in females provides a good index of renal PG production in humans. This parameter has been used extensively to explore the physiological and pathophysiological role of PGs and is very useful in assessing drug effects on the kidney.

REGULATION OF RENAL HAEMODYNAMICS

The first evidence for an effect of PGs on renal blood flow (RBF) was that PGE_1 infused into a renal artery of the dog produced an increase in RBF[50]. Other PGs, including PGE_2, PGD_2 and PGI_2, were also shown to increase RBF[51]. Vasoconstrictor responses to PGE_2 also exist, but these are inhibited or are converted to vasodilatation by antagonists of angiotensin II[52]. This suggests that the vasoconstriction is secondary to renin release.

Inhibition of COX by indomethacin produced a striking reduction of RBF in anaesthetized, laparotomized dogs[53,54] and led to the proposal that PGs are responsible for regulation of basal RBF. However, in later studies in conscious dogs indomethacin had no effect on RBF[55–58]. This difference points to the important role of other mediators (catecholamines, angiotensin II, vasopressin) which, when unopposed by renal PGs, cause pronounced vasoconstriction. Addressing this issue directly, Terragno studied the effect of indomethacin in conscious as opposed to laparotomized dogs. Whereas indomethacin had no effect on conscious or anaesthetized dogs, it reduced RBF >40% in the laparotomized animals[59]. The angiotensin-renin system appears to play a major role in this situation, because renin release is highly stimulated[59]. In a one clip renal hypertension model, indomethacin caused a marked reduction of RBF[60] that was abolished by an angiotensin II antagonist[61].

A wealth of information has now accumulated to suggest that PGs help to maintain RBF and GFR in pathophysiological states. This is particularly true for those disorders characterized by a low effective plasma volume: cirrhosis with ascites, heart failure and the nephrotic syndrome, where vasoconstrictor effects of renal nerve activity, catecholamines, angiotensin II and vasopressin are involved. Thus, it is not surprising that indomethacin caused a striking decrease in GFR in patients with nephrotic syndrome[62], congestive heart failure[63] and liver cirrhosis[64] (Table 1).

There are other conditions in which inhibition of PG synthesis also reduces GFR, although the underlying mechanism is not so apparent. These include Bartter's syndrome[65], chronic renal insufficiency[66], SLE with renal involvement[67] and various other conditions[68]. The inhibition of PG synthesis may have very severe effects, and may induce acute renal failure, even in patients with apparently normal renal function. Sodium depletion, of whatever cause, greatly exacerbates this effect. Thus, diuretics or dietary sodium depletion may, even in a normal kidney, decrease GFR[69,70] and obviously will have even more pronounced effects in the pathological conditions described above.

There is a further effect of renal PG inhibition which has far-reaching consequences: medullary blood flow is provided exclusively by the juxtamedullary nephrons. These nephrons are the only source of arterial blood for the medulla, which has no direct arterial blood supply. The renal medulla thus has a very low oxygen tension, and inhibition of PG synthesis will affect the distribution of blood within the kidney away from the medulla[71,72]. Thus, PGs play a critical role in protecting the renal medulla from ischaemic damage[73,74]. This may be an important factor contributing to the papillary necrosis observed in analgesic nephropathy, diabetes mellitus and after administration of currently used NSAIDs[10].

ELECTROLYTE EXCRETION

Sodium

Infusion of arachidonic acid or PGE_2 causes natriuresis[50,75]. This effect is coupled with vasodilatation, and this may be the cause of the natriuresis, presumably by an effect on proximal tubular salt and water resorption. However, there is also evidence that tubular transport is influenced by PGs directly. Indomethacin and meclofenamate enhance sodium reabsorption at a point beyond the proximal tubule[76,77]. Later studies showed that chloride was also affected and further, that during volume expansion, reabsorption of electrolytes in the thick ascending limb was inhibited by meclofenamate[78]. Direct evidence supporting a tubular action of PGE_2 on sodium reabsorption stems from microinfusions of ^{22}Na into the late proximal tubule: co-infusion of PGE_2 reduced Na reabsorption[77]. From these studies it can be deduced that PGs, most likely PGE_2, reduce sodium reabsorption in a segment beyond the proximal tubule. This could be the collecting segment or the ascending limb of the loop of Henle. In this context it should be remembered that deep nephrons are inaccessible to micropuncture. However, it is the deep nephrons which are the site of the highest PG production rate. Commonly, in addition to direct observation of electrolyte transport at the puncture site, urinary electrolytes are measured. This technique makes it impossible to determine whether a large amount of sodium in urine is due to less reabsorption at sites distal to the puncture site of the superficial nephrons, or to proportionately less reabsorption from deep nephrons. Recently, this differential handling of sodium in superficial and juxtamedullary nephrons has been described in the natriuretic response to volume expansion: the juxtamedullary nephrons reabsorbed proportionately less sodium than the superficial nephrons, and this accounted for the difference of sodium between the late puncture site and urine[78,79]. Meclofenamate has been shown, by cortical and papillary micropuncture, to enhance sodium reabsorption particularly by this mechanism of enhanced absorption in the juxtamedullary nephrons[78]. There is further evidence to support a prominent role of medulla and deep juxtamedullary nephrons for PG-dependent sodium transport. Bartelheimer and Senft reported that oxyphenbutazone, a once popular NSAID, enhanced the corticomedullary concentration gradient of sodium[80], and this was later also shown for indomethacin and meclofenamate[81,82].

Studies in isolated renal tubule segments showed that PGE_2 inhibits sodium transport out of the cortical collecting tubule, thus showing a direct inhibitory effect of PGE_2 on sodium transport[83,84]. Studies in thick ascending limb segments of medullary nephrons also showed this effect, but it was not observed in cortical segments[85]. This study confirms a pre-eminent role for juxtamedullary nephrons in PG-dependent sodium transport.

The role of antidiuretic hormone (ADH, vasopressin) on sodium transport is perhaps underestimated[86,87]. ADH enhances sodium reabsorption in the thick ascending limb and increases the corticomedullary osmolar gradient. An investigation of the interaction between ADH and PGE_2 in this segment showed that ADH-enhanced sodium transport was blocked by PGE_2 at the strikingly low K_a of 3 pM for ADH and 100 pM for PGE_2[88]. This ADH/PG antagonism probably plays a significant role in conditions such as low output congestive heart failure, liver cirrhosis and the nephrotic syndrome, because in these conditions ADH has been found to be elevated[89] and there is marked sodium and water retention.

Sodium retention following inhibition of renal PG synthesis has been observed in some experiments but not consistently (for a detailed discussion of the animal experiments see Ref. 90). However, there is firm evidence of sodium retention following PG suppression in human experiments in which the appropriate parameters have been thoroughly controlled. Of particular importance is the fact that sodium retention only occurs for a brief period in most cases, a new steady state being reached within a few days. Measurement of daily 24h urine elimination and body weight control are necessary to observe the effect. A rigorously controlled sodium intake is also a prerequisite. Under these conditions we were able to show in patients with post-malignant hypertension on a 100 mE Na^+ diet, that indomethacin (25 mg t.i.d.) readily caused inhibition of renal PG production, sodium retention and weight gain[91]. Sodium retention and weight gain are more difficult to demonstrate in normal volunteers[91]. In patients with nephrotic syndrome[62], congestive heart failure[63] and liver cirrhosis[64,92] sodium retention is easily observed after PG inhibition, and this may lead to significant clinical deterioration.

The simultaneous decrease of RBF/GFR and sodium excretion makes it difficult to localize the site of drug action. In most studies, however, sodium retention is more severe than can be explained solely by a reduction in the filtered load. Thus an increased tubular reabsorption is the only explanation. The attempt to localize the renal site of action on the basis of lithium clearance[92], which was reported to be a specific index of proximal tubular action, has been questioned because amiloride, a distally acting diuretic, enhances lithium excretion. This point is therefore unresolved.

An interaction between furosemide and indomethacin was first observed by us in 1976: indomethacin reduced simultaneously PGE_2 excretion and the diuretic response to furosemide[91]. This interaction has subsequently been observed with many other NSAIDs[93] and extends to other diuretics such as hydrochlorothiazide and piretanide[94]. The magnitude of the interaction is remarkable. A reduction in body weight of 2.2 kg produced by furosemide in patients with essential hypertension was reduced to 0.8 kg by pretreatment with indomethacin[91]. This reduction in the efficacy of a diuretic could result in clinical problems in patients with heart failure.

Potassium

Reduction of potassium excretion by inhibitors of renal COX has been observed by us in patients with Bartter's syndrome[65] and in patients with mild renal insufficiency[95]. The increase in potassium plasma concentration is associated with and probably caused by a reduction in plasma renin activity (PRA). The effect of inhibition of renal PG production on PRA has been intensively investigated and reviewed[34,91,96–100]. In essence, inhibition of renal PG production by indomethacin or ibuprofen lowers PRA together with aldosterone but increases sodium reabsorption[91]. Indomethacin also completely inhibits the increase in plasma renin activity seen within minutes after intravenous administration of furosemide to normal volunteers[91], suggesting that this renin release is due to a constitutive enzyme. The lowering of aldosterone is not due to a direct effect of PG inhibition on aldosterone secretion from the adrenal, since infusion of angiotensin II increases aldosterone to identical levels before and after indomethacin administration[91]. In sodium-depleted normal volunteers suppression of PRA by these drugs can be observed only under conditions of inhibited sympathetic drive of renin release by non-selective β-receptor blockade. When sodium retention was eliminated as a factor reducing PRA by a low sodium diet, renin release could be blocked by indomethacin[96]. Further investigations showed that the macula densa was responsible for PG-mediated renin release[97]. The prostanoid most likely involved is PGI_2 which, in contrast to PGE_2, is a potent releaser of renin from renal cortical slices[101].

Recent work has significantly enhanced our understanding of prostaglandin-mediated renin release. In studies with primary cultures of juxtaglomerular cells, PGs which stimulate cAMP production cause renin release and this is accompanied by an increase in the mRNA for renin (A. Kurtz, personal communication). Inhibition of renal PG production, leading to low PRA and aldosterone, will therefore result in decreased potassium excretion.

Hyperkalaemia is not a common problem in patients with normal renal function but it may be a severe threat to the patient with renal disease, which may itself cause potassium retention, or when drugs causing potassium retention are taken simultaneously. In particular, potassium-sparing diuretics and converting enzyme inhibitors may pose problems[102,103]. In patients with Bartter's syndrome, however, the potassium retention is advantageous[65].

Lithium

Following case reports of effects of phenylbutazone and ibuprofen on plasma levels of lithium we studied this potential drug interaction in a controlled fashion. Plasma lithium concentration increased during administration of indomethacin and diclofenac[104,105]. This effect is due to a decrease in renal lithium clearance and has now been observed with several other NSAIDs, including oxyphenbutazone and ketoprofen. Interestingly, in a cross-over study in normal volunteers, we observed a decrease in renal lithium clearance with diclofenac but no effect of aspirin despite a very similar reduction in renal PG production. The reason for this anomalous behaviour of aspirin is unknown[106]. Salicylate is also without effect on renal lithium clearance[107]. These are examples of a very pronounced difference between the NSAIDs and indicates that extrapolations between NSAIDs are not always possible.

ANTIDIURETIC HORMONE

Orloff first reported that PGE_1 inhibits increased permeability to water induced by ADH in the toad bladder, a model of the collecting duct[108]. The same phenomenon is also seen in the isolated cortical collecting tubule[109]. The question of a possible role of endogenous PGs in the modulation of ADH action was answered when PG synthesis inhibitors became available[110,111]. Studies with these drugs confirmed that endogenous PGs attenuate the hydro-osmotic effect of ADH[110,111]. This interaction obviously takes place at the medullary site, where very large amounts of PGE_2 can be synthesized[16,31,112]. COX has also been shown to be produced by the collecting duct cells[113,114].

The first in vivo study to test the hypothesis that renal PGs antagonize the action of ADH was carried out in dogs hypophysectomized to prevent endogenous ADH production. Indomethacin or meclofenamate administration produced a powerful increase in urine osmolality in response to ADH[115] and it was suggested, that PGs function as a negative feed back inhibitor of the action of ADH. Indeed, inhibition of renal PG production can cause an increase in urine osmolality produced by endogenous ADH in hydropenic conscious dogs[58] and rats[116], and can lead to a decrease in free water clearance not only in water-loaded conscious rats[116], but also in rats genetically devoid of ADH[117] and water-loaded human volunteers[118]. Similar results were obtained in other studies in which indomethacin or aspirin potentiated the action of ADH[34,119,120]. Infusion of hypertonic saline to humans also increases urine osmolality and free water reabsorption, and both effects are enhanced by indomethacin[120], showing that endogenous ADH, released in large amounts by hypertonic saline, becomes more effective, after renal PG production is suppressed.

We have studied the effect of indomethacin on free water clearance and ADH plasma levels and showed that indomethacin or ibuprofen reduced free water clearance. Surprisingly, circulating levels of ADH were suppressed simultaneously[34]. In order to study the effect of indomethacin on free water clearance during steady state ADH levels, we infused ADH. There was still a small reduction of ADH due to the unavoidable reduction of endogenous ADH secretion, but free water clearance was even more dramatically reduced, and approached zero[34]. The identity of the particular PG involved was investigated extensively after it had become clear that PGE_1 used in the primary study[108] was not found in the kidney in amounts sufficient to play such a role in vivo. Systematic studies of various PGs of the mono- and bisenoic PGs of the E, F and A series showed that PGE_2 and PGF_2 showed the greatest activity[121]. PGE_2 was found to be the most potent antagonist of ADH action in cultured canine epithelial cells[122] or in canine cortical collecting tubule cells[38].

The mechanism underlying the interaction between ADH and PGs has been studied repeatedly. No convincing evidence has been forthcoming for an interaction at the level of cAMP. Exogenous PGs have been shown to decrease the ADH-induced rise of cAMP[108,109], and blockade of PG synthesis enhanced ADH-induced cAMP[123]. However, PGs can also stimulate cAMP in renal medulla[124]. These contradictory findings have to be considered in view of the assay method for cAMP, which is performed in broken cell preparations. The entire architecture and possible compartmentalization are lost in such a crude procedure and only the sum effect is measured. Herman et al.[125] suggested that PGH_2, the precursor of PGE_2 and all other prostanoids, can reduce ADH-stimulated c-AMP. This is in agreement with a previous finding in adipocytes, where PGH_2 also inhibits adenylate cyclase[126].

ADH requires calcium from an intracellular pool for its action[127,128] and it is possible that PGs could affect this intracellular store. PGE_2 has been shown to decrease the size of this store and thus could exert its antagonistic action to ADH by this mechanism[129].

PGs are also intimately involved in water transport, affecting the solute concentration of the renal papilla. PGs enhance renal and papillary blood flow and this causes a reduction in the papillary concentration gradient; conversely, renal PG inhibition increases the solute concentration of the papilla[80]. Reduction of sodium reabsorption also reduces medullary solute levels. In the isolated medullary thick ascending limb PGE_2 inhibits sodium and chloride reabsorption[88]. This effect can only be observed in the presence of ADH, however. ADH stimulates sodium and chloride reabsorption in this segment and PGE_2 at a half maximal concentration of only 10^{-10} M will antagonize this effect. This region is also the site of the counter-current mechanism and reduced sodium and chloride in the papilla due to the action of PGE_2 render it less effective. In vivo studies support this concept as PG synthesis inhibitors enhance sodium and chloride reabsorption in the renal medulla[81,88] and increase sodium reabsorption in Henle's loop[78].

It is not certain which of the above mechanisms of the ADH/PG antagonism are operative in vivo. However, from a functional point of view it is important to recognize that under the maximal influence of ADH virtually no barrier to water reabsorption exists in the collecting duct and there is complete equilibration with the medullary interstitium. Under these conditions inhibition of PG synthesis is still effective and enhances antidiuresis, thus an influence on water permeability alone cannot explain the findings.

As suggested above, if PGs were to act as negative feedback inhibitors of ADH action there should be an increase in PG synthesis following administration of ADH that is in some way proportionate to the concentration of ADH. In vitro studies in medullary slices and in cultures of rabbit papillary collecting duct cells showed enhanced PG synthesis after ADH exposure[38,130]. We carried out experiments in vivo in rats genetically devoid of endogenous ADH production in which basal levels of urinary PGs were about 16% of those in normal rats[131]. Administration of ADH resulted in the expected restoration of urine osmolality and reduction in urine volume and urinary PGE_2 rose to the normal range[131]. This stimulatory effect of ADH on PGE_2 synthesis could also be observed in normal rats[132]. There is also a clear dose–response relationship between ADH, or its non-pressor analogue dDAVP, on urinary PG production[132]. These and numerous other studies support the concept of a negative feedback effect of PGs on ADH in the mammalian kidney.

This idea has been challenged on the basis of in vivo data obtained from humans. While some studies showed enhanced urinary PG excretion following ADH administration[133], there was no effect of dDAVP. Because angiotensin II caused the previously observed increase in urinary PG excretion[43], the authors concluded that the pressor rather than the antidiuretic effect of ADH was responsible for the stimulated PG excretion[133,134]. These findings led to the proposal that ADH leads to increased renal PG synthesis by induction of COX[135,136] and lacks an acute stimulatory effect. This has been proven wrong, because PGE_2 excretion increases within minutes following ADH and dDAVP administration[137,138]. In vitro studies also show that dDAVP acutely increases PG production in toad bladder epithelial cells[139] and in rabbit cortical collecting tubule[140]. The exact cellular source of the stimulated PG synthesis cannot be determined from these studies, but the very rapid response suggests that a constitutive COX is involved.

It is appropriate to close this discussion of the PG/ADH interaction with a case report. A 64-year-old man was admitted to the hospital twice within 4 months, disoriented and confused. His physical examination was unremarkable. He had been prescribed ibuprofen 600 mg t.i.d. for rheumatic complaints. Laboratory studies showed a slightly elevated plasma creatinine of 1.6 mg/dl and a plasma sodium of 118 mEq/l. Slow restoration of his electrolyte imbalance led to complete recovery on both occasions. On intensive questioning he described in his daily habits a water intake of one gallon because his doctor had told him that this would protect his kidney from any toxic effects of ibuprofen. While this may or may not be so, this clearly was a case of water intoxication due to decreased free water clearance caused by ibuprofen. Other similar cases have been reported[141].

DIFFERENCES BETWEEN NSAIDs ON RENAL FUNCTION

NSAIDs have been shown to induce nephrotic syndrome, acute interstitial nephritis, papillary necrosis, reduction in renal perfusion, electrolyte and water disturbances and other non-classified renal problems (for review see Refs. 8, 142). Many of these clinical problems can be related to inhibition of physiological renal PG synthesis.

The most commonly observed problem is a reduction in RBF and/or GFR and the development of oedema[5,8]. Almost all NSAIDs have been implicated, with the remarkable exception of sodium salicylate and salsalate[42]. The non-acetylated salicylate drugs have also not been reported to cause papillary necrosis in contrast to ibuprofen, indomethacin, mefenamic acid, phenylbutazone and piroxicam[10,142].

A significant problem is presented by patients with asymptomatic renal failure. In this patient group NSAIDs can rapidly and severely reduce GFR[68]. Creatinine clearance is a good predictor of risk[68]. A further high-risk group comprises patients with liver cirrhosis[92], in whom a comparison between indomethacin and diflunisal, a non-acetylated NSAID, showed remarkable differences[143]. Urinary PGE_2 was reduced by 50% by indomethacin but by only 10% by diflunisal. Indomethacin reduced GFR by about 25%, but diflunisal had no effect. The diuretic and natriuretic response to furosemide was much attenuated by indomethacin but was not affected by diflunisal.

In our own studies we observed a difference on lithium kinetics between indomethacin[104] and diclofenac[105] on the one hand and salicylate on the other[107]. This difference can be readily explained on the basis of a differential inhibitory effect of diclofenac or indomethacin and by salicylate on renal PG production in humans. Diclofenac or indomethacin, but not salicylate, given in anti-inflammatory dosage, reduced urinary PGE_2 levels in normal female volunteers by about 50%[11,29]. This inhibitory effect on renal PG production was accompanied by a similar reduction of the major urinary metabolite of PGE_2, 5,11-diketo-tetranor-prosta-1,16 dioic acid.

In animal experiments on a model of liver cirrhosis (common bile duct-ligated miniature swine) salicylate, in contrast to meclofenamate, caused natriuresis rather than sodium retention[114]. In sodium-restricted dogs, salicylate at very high dosage did decrease stimulated renal PGE_2 synthesis, but only into the range of normal sodium balance[145]. This finding[145] highlights a general problem inherent in the use of inhibitors of cyclooxygenase: their use as a tool cannot be taken as definitive proof of a PG-mediated mechanism. In human studies, when NSAIDs have to be used at doses which do not cause a threat to the health of the subject, inhibition of renal and whole body PG synthesis is always only partial. A significant amount, usually 30–50%, is left. This amount can still be regulated and thus modify renal function. In fact, a recent publication on patients suffering from overdoses of diclofenac, naproxen and sulindac very clearly makes the point that, in spite of claims to the contrary, there is an increase in the risk of renal failure with high doses of NSAID[146]. The list of causes of acute renal failure after overdose of NSAID includes other drugs such as benoxaprofen, fenprofen, ibuprofen, mefenamic acid, piroxicam and zomepirac[146]. These studies thus demonstrate that there are remarkable differences between the non-acetylated salicylates and other NSAIDs.

Another drug, sulindac, has received considerable attention because it was thought to be renal sparing, and much effort has been devoted to make this point[147]. However, experimental studies in normal volunteers which compared indomethacin and sulindac showed that sulindac blunted the natriuretic and PGE_2 response to furosemide and reduced the excretion rate of a major urinary metabolite of PGF to a similar degree[148]. In clinical trials, sulindac was also shown to reduce GFR quite as dramatically as piroxicam and ibuprofen[149]. Thus, it can no longer be claimed that sulindac is 'renal sparing'. Nabumetone has also been suggested to be renal sparing. However, the Physician's Desk Reference (Medical Economics Data, Montvale, NJ, USA, 1993) lists oedema as a known side effect, and oedema has occurred equally often with nabumetone in comparison to diclofenac and piroxicam[150]. A study on the action of nabumetone on the urinary excretion of PGE_2 in comparison to sulindac and indomethacin was reported recently[151]. Indomethacin in a dose of 100 mg/day reduced urinary PGE_2 by about 18%; sulindac in a dose of 400 mg/day caused a reduction of 25%. Nabumetone increased PGE_2 excretion by about 50% on day 7 of administration. However, 6-keto-$PGF_{1\alpha}$ was reduced by all three drugs[151]. This is surprising, since no other drug has yet been shown to decrease urinary 6-keto-$PGF_{1\alpha}$ with increasing urinary PGE_2. More reason for concern is posed by the data on baseline excretion of PGE_2: while the reference method based on GC/MS measurements indicates a 24h excretion rate of PGE_2 of 300 ng[106], the corresponding values reported in these experiments[151] are about 10-fold higher. Thus at present no statement can be made as to the effect of nabumetone on renal PG production with any degree of certainty.

RENAL CYCLOOXYGENASES AND NSAID EFFECTS

It is generally accepted that NSAIDs act by inhibiting PG production by competitive or irreversible blockade of COX. The side effects of these drugs, including damage to the gastric wall and kidney and inhibition of platelet aggregation, are also believed to result from inhibition of COX. Most interestingly, the action of steroids has also been explained on the basis of inhibition of prostaglandin synthesis. While most of the studies to support these concepts have been performed in animal experiments, the inhibition of PG production by many of these drugs, including acetylsalicylic acid, diclofenac, ibuprofen and indomethacin, has also been shown in humans and has been correlated to the inhibition of whole body or renal PGE_2 production, sodium metabolism, platelet aggregation and thromboxane production.

As has been emphasized, however, not all NSAIDs are alike. For example, paracetamol does not inhibit platelet aggregation and has a very weak effect on renal PG production in man[111]. Salicylate also shows no effect on platelet aggregation, platelet thromboxane production or renal PGE_2 synthesis at doses which are anti-inflammatory in man[29]. Furthermore, glucocorticoids, which in vitro are very effective in inhibiting PG production[152] were shown by us to have no effect on PG production in healthy animals[153] and in normal volunteers[154], even at doses that induced a Cushingoid appearance in the volunteers. The discovery of two different forms of cyclooxygenase[155–157], now known as COX-1 and COX-2, has provided an explanation of some of these discrepancies and ushered in a new generation of NSAIDs with the promise of fewer side effects on the gastrointestinal tract and kidney.

COX-1 is the constitutive enzyme serving the basic physiological functions mediated by PGs. These include regulation of peripheral vascular resistance, renal blood flow and GFR, renal sodium excretion, ADH antagonism and possibly renin release. COX-2, which shows only 60% amino acid sequence identity with COX-1, is induced by interleukins and mitogens (IL-1, transforming growth factor-β, tumour necrosis factor-α, endotoxin and fibroblast growth factors). It is induced in the uteroplacental unit and may well be the source of enhanced PG production in pregnancy[158]. COX-2 can be induced in human monocytes[159], synovial cells[160], chondrocytes[161] and many other cell types, suggesting that enhanced PG production in inflammatory reactions is due to induction of COX-2. This makes COX-2 an outstanding target for therapeutic interventions.

What are the data on COX-1 and COX-2 in the kidney? COX-1 has been found in arteries and arterioles, glomeruli and collecting ducts. Remarkably, no COX-1 has been found in the proximal or distal convoluted tubule, Henle's loop or macula densa[162]. COX-2 has been detected in low concentrations in the kidneys of accident victims, but no localization has been given[163]. In a detailed analysis of distribution of COX enzymes in the rat kidney, Harris et al.[164] reported that under control conditions, some COX-1 is observed in the cortex, papilla and in medullary interstitial cells. This showed a striking increase in the cortex during long-term sodium depletion. The major location of COX-2 was the macula densa, which is important for the control of renin release. It senses the luminal NaCl and, as we have shown previously, regulates secretion of renin by a PG-dependent mechanism[97,165]. In this context our observation that the immediate renin release caused by furosemide is completely abrogated in man by indomethacin suggests that this effect is not due to volume depletion but may be mediated by the macula densa. Further, these data suggest, that under normal basal conditions COX-2 plays a minor role in the kidney with the possible exception of renin release in the rat.

There are recent data on the occurrence and function of COX-2-mediated PG production with relevance to the kidney. Rat mesangial cells respond to IL-1 with the production of PGE_2 due to COX-2 induction, as shown by mRNA measurement[166]. This study supports the concept that the kidney is capable of producing COX-2 in inflammatory reactions and that this will lead to enhanced PG production. Radicicol, a fungal antibiotic, selectively inhibits COX-2 expression in endotoxin-stimulated macrophages and in glomerulonephritis induced by anti-basement membrane antibodies without affecting COX-1[167]. In this model of renal inflammatory disease COX-2 is typically elevated in the glomeruli[168], while it cannot be detected in glomeruli of healthy rats (an exception is described in Ref. 164). Radicicol caused a highly significant reduction of COX-2 mRNA but not of COX-1 mRNA, and simultaneously reduced PGE_2 production by the glomeruli by about 60%. Radicicol caused no significant reduction of PGE_2 production in the whole kidney, however, suggesting that the PGE_2 pool of the glomeruli is relatively small. Injection of

LPS (endotoxin) leads to the induction of COX-2 and inducible nitric oxide synthase (iNOS) and their mediators PGs and NO in the rat. The induction of these enzymes is inhibited by dexamethasone, a long acting glucocorticoid[169]. Interestingly, inhibitors of iNOS, which in vitro showed no effect on COX activity, markedly suppressed LPS-stimulated PG production, suggesting that there is a hierarchy of mediators, with iNOS regulating PG Production. The mechanism is not entirely clear, but because PGE_2 production can be immediately increased by NO donors in normal animals it may be mediated by COX-1. In renal inflammatory conditions, however, this may be different. The question of whether drugs that inhibit PG production adversely affect kidneys affected by inflammatory disease has been addressed in numerous studies. The deterioration of renal function observed with NSAIDs has been attributed to the reduction in PG synthesis. However, glucocorticoids have a pronounced effect on PG production in diseased kidneys yet they do not cause deterioration of renal function. Because glucocorticoids inhibit the induction of COX-2[159,170,171] they should have detrimental effects on renal function if COX-2-derived PGs were to support renal function normally. However, this has never been shown. The sodium retention seen after glucocorticoid administration is due to the mineralocorticoid effect and not due to PG suppression.

The effect of NSAID on COX-1 and COX-2 has been investigated repeatedly under various experimental conditions. Biochemical studies in which COX-1 and COX-2 was expressed in cells or cell membranes by transfection or in which COX-2 was induced by endotoxin showed that indomethacin and piroxicam were more effective against COX-1, while ibuprofen and the active metabolite of nabumetone, (6-MNA), were more effective against COX-2[172]. In another study, diclofenac was 10 times more powerful as an inhibitor of COX-2 relative to COX-1 than indomethacin[173]. Paracetamol was without effect on COX-2 and had only a weak effect on COX-1[174]. Interestingly, salicylate was 20 times less effective than acetylsalicylic acid against COX-1 but only half as effective against COX-2 making it a relatively selective COX-2 inhibitor. Studies on human COX-1 and 2 also showed that the two enzymes respond differently to various NSAIDs: neither was detectably affected by salicylate, COX-1 was more effectively inhibited by indomethacin and piroxicam and COX-2 was inhibited more effectively by 6-MNA, ibuprofen and diclofenac[175]. While the species and the models varied considerably, the trend that emerges is that indomethacin and piroxicam are particularly active on COX-1 while ibuprofen, diclofenac and 6-MNA are similarly active on COX-1 and COX-2.

One point needs to be stressed, however. As was observed with the β-receptor blockers, specificity is lost when high concentrations are employed. This is true for COX-1 and COX-2 selectivity of the currently used NSAIDs[172]. Thus the pharmacokinetics of the NSAID used in an individual patient become an important determinant of drug action. It is also clear that we have only marginal knowledge about COX-1 and COX-2 and know almost nothing about these two

Table 2 Difference between COX-1 and COX-2 inhibition of renal function

	COX-1 inhibition	*COX-2 inhibition*
Renal blood flow	↓	n.c.
Redistribution of RBF	+	n.c.
Reduction of GFR	+	n.c.
Reduction of Na^+ elimination	+	n.c.
Interaction with antihypertensive drugs	+	n.c.
Interaction with lithium	+	n.c.
Hyperkalaemia	+	n.c.
Reduction of free water clearance	+	n.c.

n.c. = no change

enzymes in man, particularly in the kidney in health and disease. We can, however, try to classify the NSAIDs with respect to their effects on COX-1 and COX-2 activity on the basis of known effects in man. COX-1 is present in platelets and an NSAID causing inhibition of arachidonate-induced platelet aggregation and thromboxane formation would be classified as a COX-1 inhibitor. If it is also a good analgesic, anti-inflammatory and antipyretic drug it would also qualify as a COX-2 inhibitor. Under these criteria most NSAIDs would qualify as non-selective inhibitors with minor differences. On the basis of inhibition of platelet aggregation one could assume that salicylate, salsalate and diflunisal are very weak COX-1 inhibitors. Experience with patients shows that these drugs do not cause sodium retention and oedema, reduction in renal blood flow and GFR, papillary necrosis, haematuria, water intoxication or hyperkalaemia[8,142]. They also show no interaction with β-blockers, angiotensin conversion inhibitors, diuretics or lithium. The lack of hyperkalaemia after administration of both these drugs and glucocorticoids possibly indicates that plasma renin activity is not regulated by COX-2 in humans (Table 2). These drugs have largely lost their clinical impact because they have complicated and often unpredictable pharmacokinetics: they have long elimination half-lives at antirheumatic dosage and dose-dependent pharmacokinetics with great interindividual variability.

Glucocorticoids would be expected to have unwanted gastrointestinal and renal effects similar to COX-1 inhibitors if they exerted their final effect by inhibition of PG production. However, they are devoid of these unwanted renal effects and this is probably due to their selective suppressive effect on synthesis of COX-2 mRNA[171]. Thus, selective COX-2 inhibitors promise to have significant advantages with respect to renal unwanted effects.

It is difficult to classify acetylsalicylic acid on the basis of the available data in man. Its excellent platelet inhibitory property is in part due to specific pharmacokinetic properties. Nevertheless, this would readily label it as a COX-1 inhibitor, and in accordance with this is its ulcerogenic property. However, it seems to have remarkably low renal toxicity. Even though it is the world's most popular drug, the population exposure is high and abuse frequent, it does not cause analgesic nephropathy[176]. In patients with SLE and slightly reduced renal function acetylsalicylic acid in antirrheumatic dosage has no deleterious effect. Finally, the drug does not reduce Li^+ elimination[106], in contrast to many other NSAIDs, even though it reduced urinary PGE_2 production to a similar degree.

NEW SELECTIVE COX-2 INHIBITORS

The prospect of finding new NSAIDs with selectivity for COX-2, which would eliminate the gastric and much of the renal toxicity, has led to the development of numerous new drug candidates. Of these NS 398 and CGP 28 238 showed promising selectivity but failed in early animal or clinical trials.

Meloxicam, which has recently been marketed in some European countries, showed in the rat and on human recombinant COX-2 up to 75-fold greater selectivity for COX-2 than piroxicam[30]. In a rat model of inflammation (carageenin pleurisy) it showed much greater inhibition of pleuritic PG production than renal PG production[30] and compared favourably in its selectivity in comparison to diclofenac, tenoxicam, tenidap, piroxicam and indomethacin[30]. In a double-blind, placebo-controlled clinical trial on 468 patients with rheumatoid arthritis meloxicam was found to be an effective NSAID, yet it caused no more side effects than placebo[177]. In all double-blind clinical trials meloxicam produced 60–90% fewer severe gastrointestinal side effects than diclofenac, piroxicam or naproxen.

We performed a cross-over open study of meloxicam (7.5 mg/day) in 10 normal female volunteers, comparing it with indomethacin in equi-effective anti-inflammatory doses (75 mg). We found that indomethacin but not meloxicam caused a significant inhibition of arachidonate (1 mM)-induced platelet aggregation (data not shown), indicating sparing of COX-1. Indomethacin significantly reduced urinary PGE_2 excretion by about 50% while meloxicam did not cause a significant reduction (Figure 1). Further clinical studies in patients at high risk for developing renal failure will have to be undertaken to show whether this selectivity seen in normal volunteers translates into a renal sparing effect in patients. Initial reports on a total of 3727 patients in double-blind clinical trials showed for meloxicam, 7.5 and 15 mg, a 50% reduction in renal side effects (i.e. an increase in creatinine clearance > 1.8 mg/dl) compared to piroxicam 20 mg[182]. While this shows a much reduced risk of renal problems with meloxicam, it also shows that the drug will not be completely free of renal side effects.

In summary, selective COX-2 inhibition holds the promise to provide drugs which will have significantly fewer unwanted effects on the kidney. These drugs would be expected not to cause reductions in GFR/RBF, medullary damage, sodium retention, possibly no hyperkalaemia and would show no interactions with antihypertensive drugs and lithium.

Figure 1 Effects of indomethacin and meloxicam on urinary PGE_2 excretion (mean ± SE; n = 10)

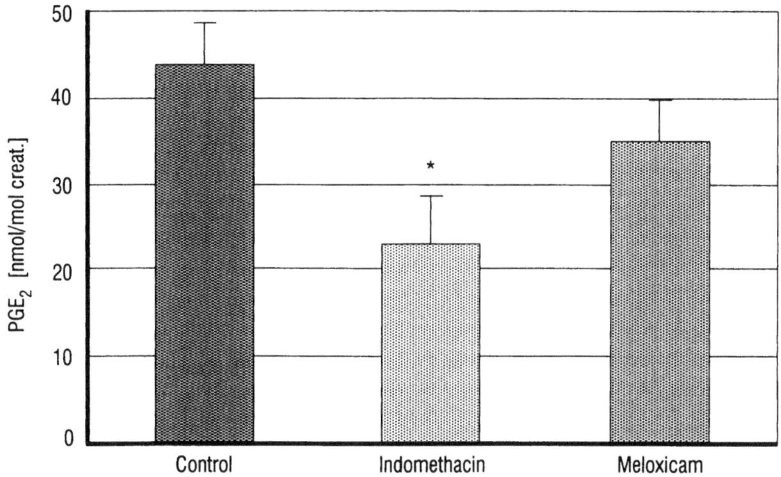

References

1. Perneger TV, Whelton PK, Klag MJ. Risk of kidney failure associated with the use of acetaminophen, aspirin, and nonsteroidal antiinflammatory drugs. N Engl J Med. 1994;331:1675–9.
2. Corwin HG, Bonventre JV. Renal insufficiency associated with non-steroidal antiinflammatory agents. Am J Kidney Dis. 1984;4:147–52.
3. Kleinknecht D. Diseases of the kidney caused by non-steroidal antiinflammatory drugs. In: Stewart JH, editor. Analgesic and NSAID-induced kidney disease. Oxford: Oxford University Press; 1993:160–79.
4. Sandler DP, Burr FR, Weinberg CR. Nonsteroidal anti-inflammatory drugs and the risk for chronic renal disease. Ann Intern Med. 1991;115:165–72.
5. Murray MD, Brater DC, Tierney WM, Jui SL, McDonald CJ. Ibuprofen-associated renal impairment in a large general internal medicine practice. Am J Med Sci. 1990;299:222–9.
6. Paller MS, Manivel JC. Prostaglandins protect kidneys against ischemic and toxic injury by a cellular effect. Kidney Int. 992;42:1345–54.
7. Finkelstein A, Fraley DS, Stachura I, Feldman HA, Gandy DR, Bourke E. Fenoprofen nephropathy. Lipid nephrosis and interstitial nephritis. A possible T lymphocyte disorder. Am J Med. 1982;72: 81–7.
8. Clive DM, Stoff JS. Renal syndromes associated with nonsteroidal antiinflammatory drugs. N Engl J Med. 1984;310:563–72.
9. Dworski R, Sheller JR, Wickersham NE et al. Allergen stimulated release of mediators into sheep bronchoalveolar lavage. Am Rev Resp Dis. 1989;139:46–51.
10. Nanra RS, Kincaid-Smith P. Experimental evidence for nephrotoxicity of analgesics. In: Stewart JH, editor. Analgesic and NSAID-induced kidney disease. Oxford: Oxford University Press; 1993:17–31.
11. Bippi H, Frölich JC. Effects of acetylsalicylic acid and paracetamol alone and in combination on prostanoid synthesis in man. Br J Pharmacol. 1990;29:305–10.
12. Spühler O, Zollinger HU. Die chronische-interstitielle Nephritis. Z Klin Med. 1953;151:1–50.
13. Lee JB, Covino BJ, Takman GH, Smith ER. Renomedullary vasodepressor substance medullin: isolation, chemical characterization, and physiological properties. Circ Res. 1965;17:57–70.

14. Zusman RM, Spector D, Caldwell BV, Speroff L, Schneider G, Mulrow PJ. The effect of chronic sodium loading and sodium restriction on plasma prostaglandin A, E, and F concentrations in normal humans. J Clin Invest. 1973;52:1093–8.
15. Zusman RM, Snider JJ, Cline A, Caldwell BV, Speroff L. Antihypertensive function of a renal-cell carcinoma: evidence for a prostaglandin-A-secreting tumor. N Engl J Med. 1974;290:843–5.
16. Frölich JC, Sweetman BJ, Carr K, Hollifield JW, Oates JA. Prostaglandin synthesis in rabbit renal medulla. Life Sci. 1975;17:1105–12.
17. Frölich JC, Sweetman BJ, Carr K, Hollifield JW, Oates JA. Assessment of the levels of PGA_2 in human plasma by gas chromatography–mass spectrometry. Prostaglandins. 1975;10:185.
18. Hamberg M, Samuelsson B. On the metabolism of PGE_1 and PGE_2 in man. J Biol Chem. 1971;246:6713–21.
19. Hamberg M, Samuelsson B. Detection and isolation of an endoperoxide intermediate in prostaglandin biosynthesis. Proc Natl Acad Sci USA. 1973;70:899–903.
20. Jakschick BA, Marshall GR, Lourik JL, Needleman P. Profile of circulating vasoactive substances in hemorrhagic shock and their pharmacologic manipulation. J Clin Invest. 1974;54:842–52.
21. Frölich JC. Gas chromatography–mass spectrometry of prostaglandins. In: Ramwell P, editor. The prostaglandins, vol. 3, New York: Plenum; 1977:1–39.
22. Gryglewski RJ. The lung as an endocrine organ. In: Vane JR, Bergström S, editors. Prostaglandins. New York: Raven; 1979:275–88.
23. Rosenkranz B, Fischer C, Weimer KE, Frölich JC. Metabolism of prostacyclin and 6-keto-prostaglandin $F_{1\alpha}$ in man. J Biol Chem. 1980;255:10194–8.
24. Rosenkranz B, Frölich JC. Problems of assessment of prostacyclin formation in vivo. Prostaglandins. 1984;27:655–7.
25. Frölich JC. Measurement of eicosanoids. Prostaglandins. 1984;27:349–50.
26. Green K, Hamberg M, Samuelsson B, Smigel M, Frölich JC. Measurement of prostaglandins, thromboxanes, prostacyclin and their metabolites by gas liquid chromatography–mass spectrometry. In: Frölich JC, editor. Advances in Prostaglandin and Thromboxane Research. V New York: Raven; 1978:1–15.
27. Smith JB, Willis AL. Aspirin selectively inhibits prostaglandin synthesis in human platelets. Nature. 1971;231:235–7.
28. Vane JR. Inhibition of prostaglandin synthesis as a mechanism of action for aspirin-like drugs. Nature. 1971;231:232–5.
29. Rosenkranz B, Fischer C, Frölich JC. Effects of salicylic and acetylsalicylic acid alone and in combination on platelet aggregation and prostanoid synthesis in man. Br J Clin Pharmacol. 1986;21:309–17.
30. Engelhard G, Pairet M. Meloxicam: A new NSAID with an improved safety profile through preferential inhibition of COX II. Eur J Clin Pharmacol. 1994;47:A98.
31. Larsson C, Anggard E. Regional differences in the formation and metabolism of prostaglandins in the rabbit kidney. Eur J Pharmacol. 1973;21:30–6.
32. Pong SS, Levine L. Biosynthesis of prostaglandins in rabbit renal cortex. Res Commun Chem Pathol Pharmacol. 1976;13:115–23.
33. Whorton AR, Smigel M, Oates JA, Frölich JC. Regional differences in prostaglandin formation by the kidney: Prostacyclin is a major prostaglandin of renal cortex. Biochim Biophys Acta. 1978;529:176–80.
34. Frölich JC, Whorton AR, Walker L et al. Renal prostaglandins regional differences in synthesis and role in renin release and ADH action. In: Proc of the VIIth International Congress of Nephrology. Montreal: University Press; 1978:107–14.
35. McGiff JC, Wong PYK. Compartmentalization of prostaglandins and prostacyclin with the kidney. Implications for renal function. Fed Proc. 1979;38:89–93.
36. Hassid A, Dunn MJ. Biosynthesis and metabolism of prostaglandins in human kidney in vitro. In: Dunn MJ, Patrono C, Cinotti GA, editors. Prostaglandins and the Kidney. New York: Plenum; 1982:3–15.
37. Grenier FC, Rollins TE, Smith WL. Kinin-induced prostaglandin synthesis by renal papillary collecting tubule cells in culture. Am J Physiol. 1981;241:94–104.
38. Garcia-Perez A, Smith WL. Apical-basolateral membrane assymetry in canine cortical collecting tubule cells: bradykinin, arginine vasopressin, prostaglandin E_2 interrelationships. J Clin Invest. 1984;74:63–74.

39. Dunn MJ, Liard JF, Dray F. Basal and stimulated rates of renal secretion and excretion of prostaglandins E_2, $F_{2\alpha}$, and 13,14-dihydro-15-keto $F_{2\alpha}$ in the dog. Kidney Int. 1978;13:136–43.
40. Zambraski EJ, Dunn MJ. Renal prostaglandin E_2 secretion and excretion in conscious dogs. Am J Physiol. 1979;236:F552–8.
41. Frölich JC. Methods in Prostaglandin Research. New York: Raven; 1979.
42. Fitzgerald GA, Pedersen AK, Patrono C. Analysis of prostaglandin and thromboxane synthesis in cardiovascular disease. Circulation. 1983;67:1174–7.
43. Frölich JC, Wilson TW, Sweetman BJ et al. Urinary prostaglandins: identification and origin. J Clin Invest. 1975;55:763–70.
44. Rosenkranz B, Kitajima W, Frölich JC. Relevance of urinary 6-keto-prostaglandin $F_{1\alpha}$ determination. Kidney Int. 1981;19:755–9.
45. Rosenblatt SG, Patak RV, Lifschitz MD. Organic acid secretory pathway and urinary excretion of prostaglandin E in the dog. Am J Physiol. 1978;235:F473–9.
46. Williams WM, Frölich JC, Nies AS, Oates JA. Urinary prostaglandins: Site of entry into renal tubular fluid. Kidney Int. 1977;11:256–60.
47. Patrono C, Wennmalm A, Ciabattoni G, Nowak J, Pugliese F, Cinotti GA. Evidence for an extra-renal origin of urinary prostaglandin E_2 in healthy men. Prostaglandins. 1979;18:623–9.
48. Haylor J, Lote CJ, Thewles A. Urinary pH as a determinant of prostaglandin E_2 excretion by the conscious rat. Clin Sci. 1984;66:675–81.
49. Frölich JC, Rosenkranz B, Fejes-Toth G, Naray-Fejes-Toth A, Frölich B. Analysis of prostanoid metabolites by gas chromatography–mass spectrometry. Adv Prostaglandin, Thromboxane Leukotriene Res. 1985;15:47–52.
50. Johnston HH, Herzog JP, Lauler DP. Effect of prostaglandin E_1 on renal hemodynamics, sodium and water excretion. Am J Physiol. 1967;213:939–46.
51. Lifschitz MD. Prostaglandins and renal blood flow. Kidney Int. 1981;19:781–5.
52. Schör N, Brenner BM. Possible mechanism of prostaglandin-induced renal vasoconstriction in the rat. Hypertension. 1981;3(suppl. II):1181–5.
53. Lonigro J, Itskovitz D, Crowshaw K, McGiff C. Dependency of renal blood flow on prostaglandin synthesis in the dog. Circ Res. 1974;32:712–7.
54. Aiken JW, Vane JR. Intrarenal prostaglandin release attenuates the renal vasoconstrictor activity of angiotensin. J Pharmacol Ther. 1973;184:678–87.
55. Swain JA, Heyndrickx CG, Borttcher DH, Vatner SF. Prostaglandin control of renal circulation in the unanesthetized dog and baboon. Am J Physiol. 1975;229:826–30.
56. Zins GR. Renal prostaglandins. Am J Med. 1975;58:14–24.
57. Kirschenbaum MA, Stein JH. Effect of inhibition of prostaglandin synthesis on urinary sodium excretion in conscious dog. J Clin Invest. 1976;57:517–21.
58. Fejes-Toth G, Fekete A, Walter J. Effect of antidiuretic hormone and indomethacin on intrarenal microsphere distribution. Pflügers Arch. 1978;376:67–72.
59. Terragno NA, Terragno DA, McGiff JC. Contribution of prostaglandins to the renal circulation in conscious, anesthetized and laparotomized dogs. Circ Res. 1977;40:590–5.
60. Nies AS, Rawl J, Cruze J, Oates JA, Frölich JC. The importance of renal prostaglandin synthesis in maintaining renal function following renal artery stenosis in the conscious dog. Invest Urology. 1978;16:72–4.
61. Satoh S, Zimmermann BG. Influence of the renin-angiotensin system on the effect of prostaglandin synthesis inhibitors on the renal vasculature. Circ Res. 1975;36:89–96.
62. Arisz L, Donker AJM, Brentjens JRH, van der Hem GK. The effect of indomethacin on proteinuria and kidney function in the nephrotic syndrome. Acta Med Scand. 1976;199:121–5.
63. Walshe JJ, Venuto RC. Acute oliguric renal failure induced by indomethacin: possible mechanism. Ann Intern Med. 1979;91:47–9.
64. Antillon M, Cominelli F, Lo S, Moran M, Somberg K, Reynolds T, Zipser RD. Effects of oral prostaglandins on indomethacin induced renal failure in patients with cirrhosis and ascites. J Rheumatol. 1990;17:46–9.
65. Gill JR, Frölich JC, Bowden RE et al. Barter's syndrome a disorder characterized by high urinary prostaglandins and a dependence of hyperreninemia on prostaglandin synthesis. Am J Med. 1976;61:43–51.
66. Berg KJ. Acute effects of acetylsalicylic acid in patients with chronic renal insufficiency. Eur J Clin Pharmacol. 1977;11:111–6.

67. Kimberley RP, Gill JR, Bowden RE, Keiser HR, Plotz PH. Elevated urinary prostaglandins and the effects of aspirin on renal function in lupus erythematosus. Ann Intern Med. 1978;89:336–41.
68. Whelton A, Stout RL, Spilman PS, Klassen DK. Renal effects of ibuprofen, piroxicam and sulindac in patients with asymptomatic renal failure. A prospective, randomized, crossover comparison. Ann Intern Med. 1990;112:568–76.
69. Frölich JC, Brill AB, Oates JA. Reduced GFR associated with decreased prostaglandin synthesis produced by indomethacin in sodium deprived humans. Clin Res. 1975;23:373A.
70. Blasingham MC, Nasjletti A. Differential renal effects of cyclooxygenase inhibition in sodium-replete and sodium-deprived dog. Am J Physiol. 1980;239:360–5.
71. Itskovitz HD, Terragno NA, McGiff JC. Effect of a renal prostaglandin on distribution of blood flow in the isolated canine kidney. Circ Res. 1974;34:770–6.
72. Kirschenbaum MA, White N, Stein JH, Ferris TG. Redistribution of renal cortical blood flow during inhibition of prostaglandin synthesis. Am J Physiol. 1974;227:801–5.
73. Roman RJ, Lianos E. Influence of prostaglandins on papillary blood flow and pressure-natriuretic response. Hypertension. 1990;15:29–35.
74. Brezis M, Rosen S. Hypoxia of the renal medulla – its implications for disease. N Engl J Med. 1995;332:647–55.
75. Tannenbaum J, Splawinski JA, Oates JA, Nies AS. Enhanced renal prostaglandin production in the dog. I. Effects on renal function. Circ Res. 1975;36:197–203.
76. Leyssac PP, Christensen P, Hill R, Skinner SL. Indomethacin blockade of renal PGE-synthesis: effect on total renal and tubular function and plasma renin concentration in hydropenic rats and on their response to isotonic saline. Acta Physiol Scand. 1975;94:484–96.
77. Kauker ML. Prostaglandin E_2 effect from the luminal side on renal tubular ^{22}Na efflux: tracer microinjection studies. Proc Soc Exp Biol Med. 1977;154:274–7.
78. Higashihara E, Stokes JB, Kokko JP, Campbell WB, Du Bose TD Jr. Cortical and papillary micropuncture examination of chloride transport in segments of the rat kidney during inhibition of prostaglandin production: a possible role of prostaglandins in the chloruresis of acute volume expansion. J Clin Invest. 1979;64:1277–87.
79. Osgood RW, Reineck HJ, Stein JH. Further studies on segmental sodium transport in the rat kidney during expansion of the extracellular fluid volume. J Clin Invest. 1978;62:311–20.
80. Bartelheimer HK, Senft G. Zur Lokalisation der tubulären Wirkung einiger antirheumatisch wirkender Substanzen. Arzneimittelforschung. 1968;18:567–70.
81. Ganguli M, Tobian L, Azar S, O'Donell M. Evidence that prostaglandin synthesis inhibitors increase the concentration of sodium and chloride in rat and renal medulla. Circ Res. 1977; 40(Suppl. I):135–9.
82. Haylor J, Lote CJ. The influence of prostaglandin E_2 and indomethacin on the renal cortico-medullary solute gradient in the rat. J Pharm Pharmacol. 1983;35:298–305.
83. Stokes JB, Kokko JP. Inhibition of sodium transport by prostaglandin E_2 across the isolated, perfused rabbit collecting tubule. J Clin Invest. 1977;59:1099–104.
84. Iino Y, Imai M. Effects of prostaglandins on Na transport in isolated collecting tubules. Pflügers Arch. 1978;373:125–32.
85. Stokes JB. Effect of prostaglandin E_2 on chloride transport across the rabbit thick ascending limb of Henle, selective inhibition of the medullary portion. J Clin Invest. 1979;64:495–502.
86. Walker LA, Valtin H. Biological importance of nephron heterogeneity. Annu Rev Physiol. 1982;44:203–19.
87. Hebert SC, Andreoli TE. Control of NaCl transport in the thick ascending limb. Am J Physiol. 1984;246:F745–56.
88. Culpepper RM, Andreoli TE. Interactions among prostaglandin E_2, antidiuretic hormone and cyclic adenosine monophosphate in modulating Cl^- absorption in single mouse medullary thick ascending limbs of Henle. J Clin Invest. 1983;71:1588–601.
89. Schrier R. Effective blood volumes revisited: pathogenesis of edematous disorders. In: Davison AM, editor. Nephrology. Proceedings of the Xth International Congress of Nephrology. London: Balliere Tindall; 1988:663–75.
90. Walker LA, Frölich JC. Renal prostaglandins and leukotrienes. Rev Physiol Biochem Pharmacol. 1987;107:1–72.
91. Frölich JC, Hollifield JW, Dormois BL et al. Suppression of plasma renin activity by indomethacin in man. Circ Res. 1976;39:447–52.

92. Wong F, Massie D, Hsu P, Dudley F. Indomethacin-induced renal dysfunction in patients with well compensated cirrhosis. Gastroenterology. 1993;104:869–76.
93. Brater DC, Anderson S, Baird C, Campbell WB. Effects of ibuprofen, naproxen and sulindac on prostaglandins in men. Kidney Int. 1985;27:66–73.
94. Dixey JJ, Noormohamed FH, Lant AF, Brewerton DA. The effect of naproxen and sulindac on renal function and their interaction with hydrochlorothiazide and piretanide in man. Br J Clin Pharmacol. 1987;25:55–63.
95. Findling J, Bedestrom D, Rawsthorne K, Kozin F, Itskovitz H. Indomethacin induced hyperkalemia in three patients with gouty arthritis. JAMA. 1980;244:1127–8.
96. Frölich JC, Hollifield JW, Michelakis AM et al. Reduction of plasma renin activity by inhibition of the fatty acid cyclooxygenase in human subjects: independence of sodium retention. Circ Res. 1979;44:781–7.
97. Data JL, Gerber JG, Crump WJ, Frölich JC, Hollifield JW, Nies AS. The prostaglandin system: A role in canine baroreceptor control of renin release. Circ Res. 1978;42:454–8.
98. Oates JA, Whorton AR, Gerkens JF, Branch RA, Hollifield JW, Frölich JC. The participation of prostaglandins in the control of renin release. Fed Proc. 1979;38:72–4.
99. Frölich JC. Prostaglandins: Role in renin regulation and mediation of antihypertensive drug effects. Arch Int Pharmacodyn Ther. 1980;Suppl:213–24.
100. Fröhlich JC. Zur Rolle der Prostaglandine bei der Reninfreisetzung. Klin Wochenschr. 1981; 59:1139–47.
101. Whorton AR, Misono K, Hollifield J, Frölich JC, Inagami T, Oates JA. Prostaglandins and renin release: I. Stimulation of renin release from rabbit renal cortical slices by PGI_2. Prostaglandins. 1977;14:1095–104.
102. Marasco WA, Gikas PW, Azizz-Baumgärtner R et al. Ibuprofen-associated renal dysfunction. Pathophysiologic mechanism of acute renal failure, hyperkalemia, tubular necrosis, and proteinuria. Arch Intern Med. 1987;147:2107–16.
103. Speirs CJ, Dollery CI, Iumqan WHW et al. Postmarketing surveillance of enalapril II. Investigation of the potential role of enalapril in deaths with renal failure. Br J Med. 1988;297:830–2.
104. Frölich JC, Leftwich R, Ragheb M, Oates JA, Reimann I, Buchanan D. Indomethacin increases plasma lithium. Br Med J. 1979;1:1115–6.
105. Reimann IW, Frölich JC. Effects of diclofenac on lithium kinetics. Clin Pharmacol Ther. 1981;30:348–52.
106. Reimann IW, Diener U, Frölich JC. Indomethacin but not aspirin increases plasma lithium levels. Arch Gen Psychiatry. 1983;40:283–7.
107. Reimann I, Golbs E, Fischer C, Frölich JC. Influence of intravenous acetylsalicylic acid and sodium salicylate on human renal function and lithium clearance. Eur J Clin Pharmacol. 1985; 29:435–41.
108. Orloff J, Handler JS, Bergstrom S. Effect of prostaglandin (PGE_1) on the permeability response of toad bladder to vasopressin, theophylline and adenosine 3′,5′-monophosphate. Nature. 1965;205:397–8.
109. Grantham JJ, Orloff J. Effect of prostaglandin E_1 on the permeability response of the isolated collecting tubule to vasopressin, adenosine 3′,5′-monophosphate and theophylline. J Clin Invest. 1968;47:1154–61.
110. Flores AGA, Sharp GWG. Endogenous prostaglandins and osmotic water flow in the toad bladder. Am J Physiol. 1972;223:1392–7.
111. Albert WC, Handler JS. Effects of PGE_1, indomethacin and polyphloretin phosphate on toad bladder response to ADH. Am J Physiol. 1974;226:1382–6.
112. Crowshaw K, Szlyk JZ. Distribution of prostaglandins in rabbit kidney. Biochem J. 1970;116: 421–4.
113. Janszen FH, Nugteren DH. Histochemical localization of prostaglandin synthetase. Histochemistry. 1971;27:159–64.
114. Smith WL, Wilkin GP. Immunochemistry of prostaglandin endoperoxide-forming cyclooxygenase: the detection of the cyclooxygenases in rat, rabbit and guinea pig kidneys by immunofluorescence. Prostaglandins. 1977;13:873–92.
115. Anderson RJ, Taber MS, Cronin RE, McDonald KM, Schrier RW. Effect of β-adrenergic blockade and inhibitors of angiotensin II and prostaglandin on renal autoregulation. Am J Physiol. 1975;229:731–6.

116. Haylor J, Lote CJ. Renal function in conscious rats after indomethacin. Evidence for a tubular action of endogenous prostaglandins. J Physiol. 1980;298:371–81.
117. Stoff JS, Rosa RM, Silva P, Eppstein FA. Indomethacin impairs diuresis in the DI rat: role of prostaglandin independent of ADH. Am J Physiol. 1982;241:231–7.
118. Walker RM, Brown RS, Stoff JS. Role of renal prostaglandins during antidiuresis and water diuresis in man. Kidney Int. 1981;21:365–70.
119. Berl T, Raz M, Wald H, Horowitz J, Czackes W. Prostaglandin synthesis inhibition and the action of vasopressin: studies in man and rat. Am J Physiol. 1977;232:529–37.
120. Kramer HJ, Backer A, Hinzen S, Dusing R. Effects of inhibition of prostaglandin-synthesis on renal electrolyte excretion and concentrating ability in healthy man. Prostaglandins Med. 1978; 1:341–9.
121. Urakabe S, Takamitsu Y, Shirai D et al. Effect of different prostaglandins on permeability of toad urinary bladder. Comp Biochem Physiol. 1975;52:1–4.
122. Martinez F, Reyes JL. Prostaglandin receptors and hormonal action on water fluxes in cultured canine renal cells (MDCK line). J Physiol. 1984;347:533–43.
123. Schlondorff D, Carvounis CP, Jacoby M, Satriano JA, Levine SD. Multiple sites for interaction of prostaglandin and vasopressin in toad urinary bladder. Am J Physiol. 1981;241:F625–31.
124. Edwards RM, Jackson BA, Dousa TP. ADH-sensitive cAMP system in papillary collecting duct: effect of osmolality and PGE_2. Am J Physiol. 1981;240:311–8.
125. Herman CA, Zenser T, Davis B. Effects of prostaglandin H_2, prostaglandin E_2 and arachidonic acid on parathyroid hormone and antidiuretic hormone activation of rat kidney adenylate cyclase. Metabolism. 1980;29:1–8.
126. Gorman RR. Prostaglandin endoperoxides: possible new regulators of cyclic nucleotide metabolism. J Cyclic Nucleotide Res. 1975;1:109.
127. Humes DM, Simmon CF, Brenner BM. Effect of verapamil in the hydroosmotic response to antidiuretic hormone in the toad urinary bladder. Am J Physiol. 1980;239:F250–1.
128. Grosse A, Cox JA, Malnoe A, deSousa RC. Evidence for a role of calmodulin in the hydroosmotic action of vasopressin in toad bladder. J Physiol. 1982;19:839–50.
129. Burch RM, Halushka PV. ^{45}Ca fluxes in isolated toad bladder epithelial cells: effects of agents which alter water or sodium transport. J Pharmacol Exp Ther. 1983;224:108–17.
130. Kalisker A, Dyer DC. In vitro release of prostaglandins from the renal medulla. Eur J Pharmacol. 1972;19:305–9.
131. Walker LA, Whorton A, Smigel M, France R, Frölich JC. Antidiuretic hormone increases renal prostaglandin synthesis in vivo. Am J Physiol. 1978;235:180–5.
132. Walker LA, Frölich JC. Dose-dependent stimulation of renal prostaglandin synthesis by deamino-8-D-arginine vasopressin in rats with hereditary diabetes insipidus. J Pharmacol Exp Ther. 1981;217:87–91.
133. Zipser RD, Little TE, Wilson W, Duke R. Dual effects of antidiuretic hormone on urinary prostaglandin E_2 excretion in man. J Clin Endocrinol Metab. 1981;53:522–6.
134. Nadler J, Zipser RD, Coleman R, Horton R. Stimulation of renal prostaglandin by pressor hormones in man: comparison of prostaglandin E_2 and prostacyclin. J Clin Endocrinol Metab. 1983;56:1260–5.
135. Beck TR, Hassid A, Dunn J. Desamino-D-arginine vasopressin induces fatty acid cyclooxygenase activity in the renal medulla of diabetes insipidus rats. J Pharmacol Exp Ther. 1982;221:269–74.
136. Bankir LR, Trinh-Trang-Tan MM, Nivez MP, Sraer J, Ardaillou R. Altered PGE_2 production by glomeruli and papillae of rats with hereditary diabetes insipidus. Prostaglandins. 1980;20: 349–65.
137. Fejes-Toth G, Filep J, Mann V. Effect of vasopressin on prostaglandin excretion in conscious dogs. J Physiol Lond. 1983;344:389–97.
138. Fejes-Toth G, Naray-Fejes-Toth A, Frölich JC. The acute effects of ADH on urinary prostaglandin excretion. J Pharmacol Exp Ther. 1983;227:215–9.
139. Burch RM, Halushka PV. Vasopressin stimulates prostaglandin and thromboxane synthesis in toad bladder epithelial cells. Am J Physiol. 1982;243:593–7.
140. Kirschenbaum MA, Lower AG, Trizna W, Fine LG. Regulation of vasopressin action by prostaglandins. J Clin Invest. 1982;70:1193–204.
141. Rault RM. Case report: hyponatremia associated with nonsteroidal antiinflammatory drugs. Am J Med Sci. 1993;305:318–20.

142. Carmichael J, Shankel S. Effects of nonsteroidal anti-inflammatory drugs on prostaglandins and renal function. Am J Med. 1985;78:992–1000.
143. Antillon M, Cominelli F, Reynolds TB, Zipser RD. Comparative acute effects of diflunisal and indomethacin on renal function in patients with cirrhosis and ascites. Am J Gastroenterol. 1989;84:153–5.
144. Zambraski EJ, Guidotti SM, Atkinson DC, Diamond J. Salicylic acid causes a diuresis and natriuresis in normal and common bile-duct-ligated cirrhotic miniature swine. J Pharmacol Exp Ther. 1988;247:983–8.
145. Zambraski EJ, Atkinson DC, Diamond J. Effects of salicylate vs. aspirin on renal prostaglandins and function in normal and sodium-depleted dogs. J Pharmacol Exp Ther. 1988;247:96–103.
146. Kulling PEJ, Beckman A, Skagius ASM. Renal impairment after acute diclofenac, naproxen and sulindac overdose. Clin Toxicol. 1995;33:173–7.
147. Patrono C, Dunn MJ. The clinical significance of inhibition of renal prostaglandin synthesis. Kidney Int. 1987;32:1–12.
148. Roberts DG, Gerber JG, Barnes JS, Zerbe GJ, Nies AS. Sulindac is not renal sparing in man. Clin Pharmacol Ther. 1985;38:258–65.
149. Murray MD, Brater DC. Renal toxicity of the nonsteroidal anti-inflammatory drugs. Annu Rev Pharmacol Toxicol. 1993;32:435–65.
150. Morgan GJ, Poland M, DeLapp RE. Efficacy and safety of nabumetone versus diclofenac, naproxen, ibuprofen, and piroxicam in the elderly. Am J Med. 1993;95(suppl 2A):19S–27S.
151. Freed MI, Audet PR, Zariffa N et al. Comparative effects of nabumetone, sulindac, and indomethacin on urinary prostaglandin excretion and platelet function in volunteers. J Clin Pharmacol. 1994;34:1098–108.
152. Flower RJ, Blackwell GJ. Anti-inflammatory steroids induce biosynthesis of a phospholipase A_2 inhibitor which prevents prostaglandin generation. Nature. 1979;278:456–9.
153. Naray-Fejes-Toth A, Fejes-Toth G, Fischer C, Frölich JC. Effect of dexamethasone on in vivo prostanoid production in the rabbit. J Clin Invest. 1984;74:120–3.
154. Rosenkranz B, Naray-Fejes-Toth A, Fejes-Toth G, Fischer C, Sawada M, Frölich JC. Dexamethasone effect on prostanoid formation in healthy man. Clin Sci. 1985;68:681–5.
155. Habenicht HJR, Goerig M, Grulich J et al. Human platelet derived growth factor stimulates prostaglandin synthesis by activation and rapid de novo synthesis of cyclooxygenase. J Clin Invest. 1986;75:1381–78.
156. Xie W, Chipman JG, Robertson DL, Erikson RL, Simmons D. Expression of a mitogen-responsive gene encoding prostaglandin synthase is regulated by mRNA splicing. Proc Natl Acad Sci USA. 1991;88:2692–5.
157. Kujubu DA, Fletcher BS, Varnum BS, Lim RW, Herschman HR. TIS10, a phorbol ester tumor promoter-inducible mRNA from Swiss 3T3 cells, encodes a novel prostaglandin synthase/ cyclooxygenase homologue. J Biol Chem. 1991;266:12866–72.
158. Slater D, Berger L, Newton R, Moore G, Bennett P. The relative abundance of type 1 to type 2 cyclooxygenase mRNA in human amnion at term. Biochem Biophys Res Commun. 1994; 198:304–8.
159. Fu J-Y, Masferrer JL, Seibert K, Raz A, Needleman P. The induction and suppression of prostaglandin H_2 synthase (cyclooxygenase) in human monocytes. J Biol Chem. 1990;265: 16737–40.
160. Angel J, Berenbaum F, Le Denmat C, Nevalainen T, Masliah J, Fournier C. Interleukin-1-induced prostaglandin E_2 biosynthesis in human synovial cells involves the activation of cytosolic phospholipase A_2 and cyclooxygenase-2. Eur J Biochem. 1994;226:125–31.
161. Knott I, Dieu M, Burton M, Houbion A, Remacle J, Raes M. Induction of cyclooxygenase by interleukin 1: Comparative study between human synovial cells and chondrocytes. J Rheumatol. 1994;21:462–6.
162. Smith WL, Bell TG. Immunohistochemical localization of the prostaglandin forming cyclooxygenase in renal cortex. Am J Physiol. 1978;235:F451–7.
163. O'Neill GP, Ford-Hutchinson AW. Expression of mRNA for cyclooxygenase-1 and 2 in human tissues. FEBS Lett. 1993;330:156–60.
164. Harris RC, McKanna JA, Akai Y, Jacobson HR, Duboid RN, Breyer MD. Cyclooxygenase-2 is associated with the macula densa of rat kidney and increases with salt restriction. J Clin Invest. 1994:94:2504–10.

165. Lorenz JN, Greenberg G, Briggs JP. The macula densa mechanism for control of renin secretion. Semin Nephrol. 1993;13:531–42.
166. Rzymkiewicz DM, DuMaine J, Morrison AR. IL-1β regulates rat mesangial cyclooxygenase II gene expression by tyrosine phosphorylation. Kidney Int. 1995;47:1354–63.
167. Chanmugam P, Feng L, Liou S et al. Radicicol, a protein tyrosine kinase inhibitor, suppresses the expression of mitogen-inducible cyclooxygenase in macrophages stimulated with lipopolysaccharide and in experimental glomerulonephritis. J Biol Chem. 1995;270:5418–26.
168. Feng L, Xia Y, Tang WW, Hwang D, Wilson C. Expression of cyclooxygenase (COX-1, COX-2) and cytosolic phospholipase A_2 (PLA-2) in anti-GBM antibody (AB) glomerulonephritis (GN). J Am Soc Nephrol. 1993;4:452.
169. Salvemini D, Settle SL, Masferrer JL, Seibert K, Currie MG, Needleman P. Regulation of prostaglandin production by nitric oxide; an in vivo analysis. Br J Pharmacol. 1995;114:1171–8.
170. Masferrer JL, Seibert K, Zweifel B, Needleman P. Endogenous glucocorticoids regulate an inducible cyclooxygenase enzyme. Proc Natl Acad Sci USA. 1992;89:3917–21.
171. Kujubu DA, Herschman HR. Dexamethasone inhibits mitogen induction of the TIS10 prostaglandin synthase/cyclooxygenase gene. J Biol Chem. 1992;267:7991–4.
172. Meade EA, Smith WL, DeWitt DL. Differential inhibition of prostaglandin endoperoxide synthase (cyclooxygenase) isozymes by aspirin and other non-steroidal antiinflammatory drugs. J Biol Chem. 1993;268:6610–4.
173. Klein T, Nüsing RM, Pfeilschifter J, Ullrich V. Selective inhibition of cyclooxygenase 2. Biochem Pharmacol. 1994;48:1605–10.
174. Mitchell JA, Akaraseenont P, Thiemermann C, Flower RJ, Vane JR. Selectivity of nonsteroidal antiinflammatory drugs as inhibitors of constitutive and inducible cyclooxygenase. Proc Natl Acad Sci USA. 1994;90:11693–7.
175. Laneuville O, Breuer DK, DeWitt DL, Hla T, Funk CD, Smith WL. Differential inhibition of human prostaglandin endoperoxide H synthases-1 and -2 by nonsteroidal anti-inflammatory drugs. J Pharmacol Exp Ther. 1994;271:927–34.
176. Dubach UC, Rosner B, Stürmer T. An epidemiologic study of abuse of analgesic drugs. Effects of phenacetin and salicylate on mortality and cardiovascular morbidity (1968–87). N Engl J Med. 1991;324:155–60.
177. Lemmel EM. A placebo controlled double blind clinical trial of 7.5 mg and 15 mg of meloxicam in short term treatment of patients with rheumatoid arthritis (RA). Eur J Clin Pharmacol. 1994;47:A105.
178. Epstein M, Lifschitz MD, Ramachandran M. Characterization of renal prostaglandin E responsiveness in decompensated cirrhosis: implications for renal sodium handling. Clin Sci. 1982;65:555–63.
179. Oliver JA, Sciacca RR, Pinto J, Cannon JA. Participation of prostaglandins in the control of renal blood flow during acute reduction of cardiac output in the dog. J Clin Invest. 1981;67: 229–37.
180. Zipser RD. Role of renal prostaglandins and the effects of non-steroidal antiinflammatory drugs in patients with liver disease. Am J Med. 1984;81(suppl. 2B):95–103.
181. Patrono C, Ciabattoni G, Remuzzi G et al. Functional significance of renal prostacyclin and thromboxane A_2 production in patients with systemic lupus erythematosus. J Clin Invest. 1985;76:1011–8.
182. Distal M, Bluhmki E. Global analysis of safety of meloxicam, a new enolic acid derived non-steroidal anti-inflammatory agent. Rheumatology in Europe. 1995;24(suppl. 3):E259.

13 Pharmacology, safety data and therapeutics of COX-2 inhibitors

P. EMERY

Non-steroid anti-inflammatory drugs (NSAIDs) are widely prescribed and effective medicines. Their use is, however, commonly associated with side effects and, despite a great deal of literature, there is still much debate as to how they should be prescribed.

The discovery by Vane[1] that both the therapeutic and the toxic effects of NSAID are produced by their action in preventing the synthesis of prostaglandins (PG) by inhibition of cyclooxygenase (COX) enzyme was undoubtedly one of the landmark discoveries of the century for the pharmaceutical industry. The elucidation of the various ways in which NSAIDs can produce inhibition – sterically, irreversibly and, in the case of certain drugs, in a time-dependent fashion, has added to the interest in the pharmacology of these compounds. These mechanisms do not explain, however, why different drugs administered at equi-active therapeutic doses exhibit side effects of differing severity, and why there is limited correlation between inhibition of PG biosynthesis and anti-inflammatory activity. The situation has now become clearer with the realization that there are isoforms of COX, a constitutive COX-1, and a form that is expressed in inflammation, COX-2. The significance of this for patients now has to be considered.

COX-1

The enzyme COX-1 has a wide tissue distribution and produces PGs with multiple physiological functions. In clinical practice the most troublesome effects associated with COX-1 inhibition are gastric ulceration, renal toxicity and a bleeding tendency.

COX-2

Role in inflammation

Under normal conditions neutrophils, macrophages, endothelial cells and fibroblasts show little or no COX activity and thus no PG production. However in response to an inflammatory stimulus COX activity is increased due to new expression of the COX-2 gene. Fibroblasts from human rheumatoid synovial tissue synthesize increased amounts of COX-2 in response to stimulation by interleukin-1 and phorbol esters (measured as mRNA for COX-2 or PGE_2 production). Glucocorticoids, and possibly some NSAIDs, can inhibit this induction of COX-2.

Role in renal function

PGs play an important role in renal homeostasis. Renal function is at least in part dependent on the ability to rapidly generate PGs from COX-1 in response to an appropriate stimulus. However, recent in vitro experimental work has suggested that COX-2 may also have an important role in this process. Stretching of rat glomerular mesangial cells stimulates the synthesis of COX-2 and PGE_2 through protein kinase C-dependent mechanisms[2]. This is thought to be important in the control of renin secretion. It is of interest that cyclosporin A, an immunosuppressant drug with renal toxicity as its major limiting factor, inhibits the synthesis of COX-2 in rat mesangial cells in response to pro-inflammatory cytokines. This may contribute to its nephrotoxicity.

Role in brain signalling

PGs have been identified as important neurotransmitters in the brain. Animal experiments have shown that COX-2 is widely distributed throughout the forebrain in discrete populations of neurones and is enriched in the cortex and hippocampus. Basal expression of COX-2 appears to be regulated by background synaptic activity. In addition it can be rapidly and transiently induced by seizures or increased synaptic activity. It has been postulated that variable COX-2 expression may be important in regulating brain PG signalling.

Role in the vascular endothelium

In vitro studies have demonstrated that the gene for COX-2 is expressed in response to vascular smooth muscle injury. Platelet derived growth factor, epidermal growth factor and thrombin have also been shown to be strong inducers of a transient increase in the production of COX-2 mRNA. In vivo, vascular injury results in an increased expression of COX-2, a response which extends over many days and may represent protracted cell activation. These results strongly suggest that COX-2 has an important pathophysiological role in vascular response to injury.

Role in skeletal muscle

Differentiated skeletal muscle in culture was reported to show a three-fold increase in COX-2 activity and anabolic myofibre growth in response to repetitive mechanical stimulation. Inhibition of COX-2 expression prevented the muscle fibre growth. The obvious conclusion was that muscle cell growth was at least part dependent on COX-2 expression.

Role in the uterus

PGs are intimately involved in normal uterine function. It has been postulated that the expression of COX-2 by uterine stromal cells in vivo may be required to support PG production necessary for the early stages of embryo implantation. In addition, COX-2 probably mediates the increase in PG synthesis in the amniotic membranes at the onset of labour.

THE CLINICAL USE OF NSAIDs

Rheumatoid arthritis

Both COX isoenzymes are present in human rheumatoid synovial explants under basal conditions, but only COX-2 is upregulated by interleukin-1 (IL-1) or phorbol ester, and only COX-2 expression is inhibited by corticosteroids. Human rheumatoid joints contain many inflammatory cytokines which will up-regulate COX-2 expression. It is probably the inhibition of this enzyme activity by NSAIDs that produces the dramatic clinical response. This is an effect on inflammation; no effect on disease progression has yet been described. There remains a possibility that PGs could influence the actual progress of the disease by an effect on the microcirculation, but this remains uncertain.

If NSAIDs are administered early in patients with RA the effect is dramatic. All signs and symptoms disappear and one may at first suspect another action of these drugs apart from simple inhibition of COX. However long-term follow-up of patients shows that NSAIDs do not affect the outcome of the disease in any detectable way. In fact one might argue that NSAIDs may be a hindrance to the management of rheumatoid (as opposed to other) patients since the symptoms are abolished when the disease is restricted in its distribution, and patients remain asymptomatic until the disease breaks through, at which time the patients believe they have become resistant to the drug. In this respect the use of selective COX-2 inhibitors will not have much impact on the treatment of RA except in the important aspect of safety. However, inhibition of COX activity is only one action of NSAIDs. If taken at higher doses, which will be possible because of reduced toxicity, then other actions, not seen with current NSAIDs used at low dosage, may be observed.

Osteoarthritis

In the case of osteoarthritis (OA) the situation is different. It is now clear that OA is not simply a degenerative disease. Clinical, histological and in vitro data have provided overwhelming evidence for an inflammatory component in the aetiology of this condition. In perimenopausal OA, circulating monocytes produce IL-6, which is probably why patients develop spinal osteoporosis at the same time. The recurrent knee effusions seen in OA can be of an inflammatory nature. They respond very well to intra-articular injections of anti-inflammatory drugs and joint biopsies show striking similarities to those from RA patients. Follow up bone scan studies in OA patients have shown that the joints that are inflamed are those that progress. Finally, it is now clear that an acute phase response is seen in OA patients: sensitive assays have shown elevated levels of C-reactive protein in OA compared with the normal population. Since there is clearly an inflammatory component in OA one would expect NSAIDs to have the same dramatic effect as they do in RA. However the major studies of the use of NSAIDs in OA have shown little beneficial effect. The major reason is that the trials exclude those patients who have symptoms of inflammatory disease (stiffness); these of course are exactly those that might benefit. It is therefore worthwhile considering the cost–benefits of the use of NSAIDs in the treatment of OA. Does the cost, in terms of the extreme toxicity of NSAIDs, outweigh the benefit? Broad patient-based surveys show that these drugs provide the most successful therapy for the symptoms of OA. These are painful conditions which inevitably result in loss of mobility, and lack of treatment produces major morbidity: the loss of mobility in elderly patients is a major cause of co-morbidity, depression and obesity for example. Early intervention with simple and effective pain relief is a priority and undoubtedly improves the long term outcome of the general condition. The problem is that physicians in general do not believe that the benefit outweighs the risk, particularly in elderly patients who are prone to develop a gastric ulcer during treatment with NSAIDs. It is this gastrointestinal toxicity that prevents their greater use. Selective inhibition of the COX-2 isoform might therefore provide an improved means of treatment of various inflammatory conditions, providing symptomatic relief with fewer side effects. However we have to consider the distribution of COX-1 and COX-2 in patients, and the data in patients is not so clear cut as in the experimental studies. It is not established for example, how widespread is the constitutive expression of COX-2 in the brain, which will be important if we have to consider the relevance of the administration of highly selective COX-2 inhibitors in humans. The distribution of COX-1 is of course widespread, and its inhibition obviously produces the familiar, undesirable side effects of NSAIDs.

Relative risks of different NSAIDs

Some relevant information is provided by examination of the side effect profile of NSAIDs in common use. Until quite recently it was believed that there was no difference between the members of this class of drug with respect to their ability to produce common toxic effects. However, recent studies have shown quite

Table 1 Comparison of the COX selectivity of NSAIDs with the reported incidence of upper gastrointestinal bleeding derived from two large case controlled studies and their toxicity index

	Odds ratio (risk)			*COX-2:COX-1 ratio*	
	Langman et al.[3]	*Garcia Rodriguez and Jick*[4]	*Toxicity index*[5]	*Mitchell et al.*[6]	*Englehardt*[7]
Azapropazone	31.5 (10.3–96.9)	23.4 (6.9–79.5)	–	–	–
Ketoprofen	23.7 (7.6–74.2)	5.4 (2.6–11.3)	4.69	–	–
Piroxicam	13.7 (7.1–26.3)	18 (8.2–39.6)	3.96	–	33
Indomethacin	11.3 (6.3–20.3)	6.3 (3.3–12.2)	5.15	60	30
Naproxen	9.1 (5.5–15.1)	3.1 (1.7–5.9)	3.01	0.6	–
Diclofenac	4.2 (2.6–6.8)	–	4.48	0.7	2.2
Ibuprofen	2.0 (1.4–2.8)	2.9 (1.7–5)	2.68	15	–
Tenoxicam	–	–	–	–	15
Meloxicam	–	–	–	–	0.33
Aspirin	–	–	1.77	166	–

conclusively that NSAIDs are not equal with regard to their toxicity. Langman et al.[3] compared the use of NSAIDs in 1144 patients aged 60 and over admitted to hospital with peptic ulcer, with age and sex-matched hospital and community controls. They found that peptic ulcer bleeding was strongly associated with the use of NSAIDs in the 3 months prior to admission. For the most commonly used NSAIDs it was possible to calculate an odds ratio for bleeding (Table 1). Those NSAIDs with the least favourable odds ratio were azapropazone and ketoprofen. An intermediate ratio was seen for indomethacin, naproxen and piroxicam, and the safest ratio was seen for ibuprofen and diclofenac. The authors noted that the risk of gastrointestinal bleeding for most drugs tended to be greatest in those who had recently started treatment. These patients were more likely to be on the full recommended dose than those who had been taking the drug for a long period.

Using a different approach to determine the risk of upper gastrointestinal bleeding with NSAID therapy, Rodriguez and Jick[4] identified 1457 cases from the records of general practitioners and calculated the odds ratios for gastrointestinal bleeding using appropriate controls (Table 1). A further measure of NSAID toxicity can be obtained from the ARAMIS (Arthritis, Rheumatism and Aging Medical Information System) database. The ARAMIS database contains detailed clinical information on more than 23000 patients with rheumatic disorders in the USA and Canada. The ARAMIS Post-Marketing Surveillance Program (PMS) has prospectively followed outcome status and drug side effects on a cohort of 2976 consecutively enrolled RA patients with 27936 patient–years of observation. Using the information obtained from this database Fries[5] has developed a 'toxicity index' to give an overall measure of the adverse effect profile of different NSAIDs (and disease modifying agents which are not considered here). The components of the index include adverse clinical symptoms, laboratory abnormalities and hospital admissions. Each side effect is weighted for severity based on the physician judgement. For each drug considered the higher the toxicity index the greater the drug toxicity (Table 1).

These three studies provide an enormous amount of information about the toxicity of NSAIDs. It is of interest to see to what extent they correlate with the known COX selectivities. The results of Langman et al. and Rodriguez and Jick show reasonable agreement, with azapropazone, piroxicam and indomethacin having the highest odds ratio for gastrointestinal bleeding. The only major difference was for ketoprofen, which had a far less favourable ratio in the study of Langman. Direct comparison of these studies with the toxicity index scores of Fries is difficult because the latter takes into account more than simply the incidence of gastrointestinal bleeding. Having said this it can be seen that indomethacin and ketoprofen (in the study of Langman) have both a high toxicity index and odds ratio for gastrointestinal bleeding. In contrast, ibuprofen has a low toxicity index and odds ratio. A further point to note is that the toxicity index is lower than might have been expected to be associated with the use of aspirin.

The variability in the ability of NSAIDs to cause gastric toxicity can now be explained on the basis of their relative ability to inhibit COX-1 rather than COX-2. COX-2 is not expressed in gastric mucosa, thus one would expect that a drug that selectively inhibited COX-2 would produce less gastrointestinal toxicity, whilst manifesting good anti-inflammatory activity. The relative effect of NSAIDs on COX-1 and COX-2 has been measured on different systems with some variability of results. Studies using whole cell preparations produce a rank order showing that selectivity against COX-2 parallels a good safety profile with regard to gastric toxicity[6,7] (Table 1). However the absolute IC_{50} values for inhibition of COX-2 and COX-1 vary and it is clear that there is as yet no experimental method that is a 'gold standard' for predicting a good clinical effect, since few drugs which purport to have a high selectivity for COX-2 have been used in patients for any length of time. Nonetheless the evidence indicates that we may have safer drugs if we use those that are highly COX-2 selective.

Renal toxicity induced by NSAIDs is also a common event. It is probably the most common reason for withdrawal of NSAIDs from hospitalized, seriously ill elderly patients. The syndrome observed with NSAIDs is fluid retention, acute renal failure, nephrotic syndrome and interstitial nephritis and, rarely these days, papillary necrosis. The kidneys of normal individuals are probably not markedly affected by NSAIDs, but patients on long term treatment are usually old and infirm and often have other conditions. For example, patients with RA have five times the incidence of hypertension and coronary artery disease and are therefore probably on multiple medication which may exacerbate the renal syndrome induced by NSAIDs. Thus highly selective COX-2 inhibitors may be of great value for these at risk patients.

NEW DEVELOPMENTS IN NSAID THERAPY

A number of new NSAIDs which demonstrate favourable side effect profiles have recently been introduced. To what extent does COX-2 selectivity account for these properties? Unfortunately there are insufficient data for this to have been included in the above studies since few of the drugs have been in long term use in patients.

Nabumetone

Nabumetone is a non-acidic NSAID established in the treatment of RA and OA. It is distinguished from other NSAIDs by its excellent side effect profile and favourable FDA labelling. Nabumetone has a number of interesting pharmacological properties which collectively may explain a reported reduced incidence of these problems. In vitro studies suggest that nabumetone is relatively COX-2 selective, since it has only a weak anti-platelet action. Consistent with this is the in vivo observation that it is relatively sparing of renal PG production. Its non-acidic nature means that it is not subject to anion trapping in the gastric mucosa, and as a prodrug, the active metabolite does not come into direct contact with the gastric mucosa.

Overall, the incidence of perforations, ulcers or bleeds observed in nabumetone-treated patients in premarketing and postmarketing studies has varied between 0.02 and 0.95%. This contrasts with the incidence of serious gastropathy associated with chronic NSAID usage of 2–4% per year. In addition, nabumetone has affected renal function in less than 1% of patients[8]. These safety data represent an improvement over the other standard, currently available NSAIDs. The lack of gastric toxicity, sparing of renal PG production and minimal anti-platelet effects may suggest a favourable COX-2 selectivity.

Meloxicam

Meloxicam is the first drug in clinical use which was specifically developed with COX-2 selectivity in mind. It is a member of the enolic class of NSAIDs, which includes piroxicam and tenoxicam. Meloxicam is administered once daily at a dose of 7.5–15 mg. At this dose it has linear pharmacokinetics and a half-life of approximately 20 h[9]. This short half-life (in contrast to piroxicam and tenoxicam with half-lives of 50 and 70 h, respectively) reduces the chance of drug accumulation and may lead to an improved side effect profile. Meloxicam has a bioavailability of 89% by the enteral route[9] and effectively penetrates the inflamed rheumatoid synovium to achieve a concentration approximately 50% of that in the plasma[10]. Studies in volunteers demonstrated almost complete metabolism, with 50% biliary and 50% renal excretion[11].

In bioassays meloxicam has demonstrated the greatest COX-2 selectivity of

***Figure 1** Selectivity of meloxicam and piroxicam against COX-2 from mouse and guinea-pig macrophages and COX-1 from bovine aortic endothelial cells (COX-2/COX-1 ratio)*

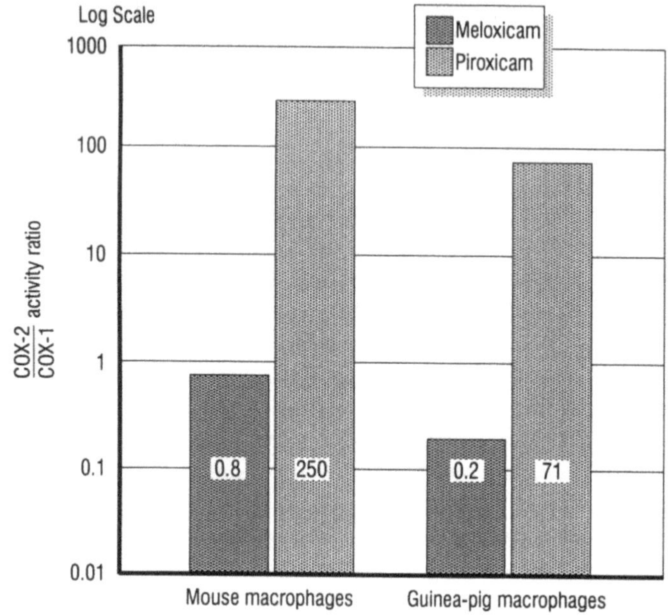

the potent inhibitors amongst the NSAIDs tested[12]. Figure 1 shows the selectivity of meloxicam against COX-2 from guinea-pig or mouse macrophages compared to COX-1 from bovine aortic endothelial cells. The COX-2/COX-1 ratios in the two systems are 0.8 and 0.2 for meloxicam compared with 250 and 71 for piroxicam (Pairet, Engelhardt, Lidbury and Vane, submitted).

Clinical trial experience

Meloxicam has now been administered to more than 5000 patients, predominantly with RA or OA. The most commonly used comparators in these trials were diclofenac 100 mg slow release, piroxicam 20 mg and naproxen 750–1000 mg. At a dose of up to 15 mg daily meloxicam has an efficacy equivalent to the other drugs with a trend in favour of improved gastrointestinal tolerability. In the early stages of use, doses of up to 60 mg were used with no gastrointestinal side effects, which suggests that the conventional dose has a reasonable safety margin.

In the treatment of OA of the hip or knee meloxicam has been used in five major double blind trials involving 1800 patients treated for 3 weeks, 6 weeks and 6 months. These studies have shown that meloxicam, at doses of 7.5 mg and 15 mg daily, is significantly superior to placebo, and comparable in efficacy to piroxicam 20 mg and diclofenac 100 mg daily[13].

In RA, approximately 2500 patients have been treated in double-blind, positive or placebo-controlled trials, of 3 weeks and 6 months duration. Open label, long-term studies of up to 18 months duration have also been undertaken. In a 3-week study comparing meloxicam 15 mg with piroxicam 20 mg in 272 patients, similar results for global efficacy, reduction in pain, Ritchie joint index, morning stiffness and withdrawals due to lack of efficacy were obtained with both drugs (Huskinson, Narjes and Bluhmki, submitted). A 6-month trial of meloxicam 7.5 mg and naproxen 750 mg also showed comparable efficacy between these two drugs[14].

Where meloxicam differed from its comparators was in its gastrointestinal safety profile. An overall analysis of data from double-blind studies in RA and OA[15] showed that total gastrointestinal side effects were significantly less frequent with meloxicam (both 7.5 mg and 15 mg) than with piroxicam 20 mg, diclofenac 100 mg and naproxen 750–1000 mg ($p<0.05$, Figure 2). Dyspepsia, abdominal pain, nausea and diarrhoea were the most common non-serious gastrointestinal side effects. Importantly, there were fewer perforations, ulcerations and bleedings, the most serious of NSAID-associated side effects, with meloxicam than with the comparators (Figure 3). This reached statistical significance compared with naproxen and piroxicam ($p<0.05$). For other body systems, meloxicam appeared to have a comparable safety profile with other NSAIDs.

In summary, meloxicam's extensive clinical trial programme has demonstrated equivalent efficacy to standard NSAIDs at equipotent doses, but with a lower incidence of gastrointestinal side effects. This improved risk/benefit ratio for meloxicam is likely to be due to its selectivity towards COX-2.

THE FUTURE

What will be the benefit of selective COX-2 inhibition in the treatment of rheumatoid disease? Will it be disease-modifying or perhaps harmful? As mentioned before it is unlikely to be disease-modifying except for the probably small, putative effect on angiogenesis. Indeed the experiment has probably already been carried out, since we have obviously had adequate COX-2 inhibition during existing treatment and we know that disease progresses despite this. It is possible, however, that high doses of selective COX-2 inhibitors may produce novel, beneficial actions. Selective COX-2 inhibitors will certainly bring symptomatic relief with less toxicity. This will allow us to differentiate clearly between symptomatic relief and a disease modifying effect, and enable us to consider how to suppress the underlying disease process. Preliminary evidence now suggests that we can do this with drugs such as anti-collagenase and anti-CD4, which previously patients would not tolerate since they do not produce symptomatic relief.

Figure 2 ***Cumulative adverse event rate. Gastrointestinal adverse events occurring in double-blind studies of RA and OA. *Significantly fewer GI side effects were observed with meloxicam 7.5 mg or 15 mg compared with diclofenac, naproxen and piroxicam (log rank test, $p < 0.05$)***

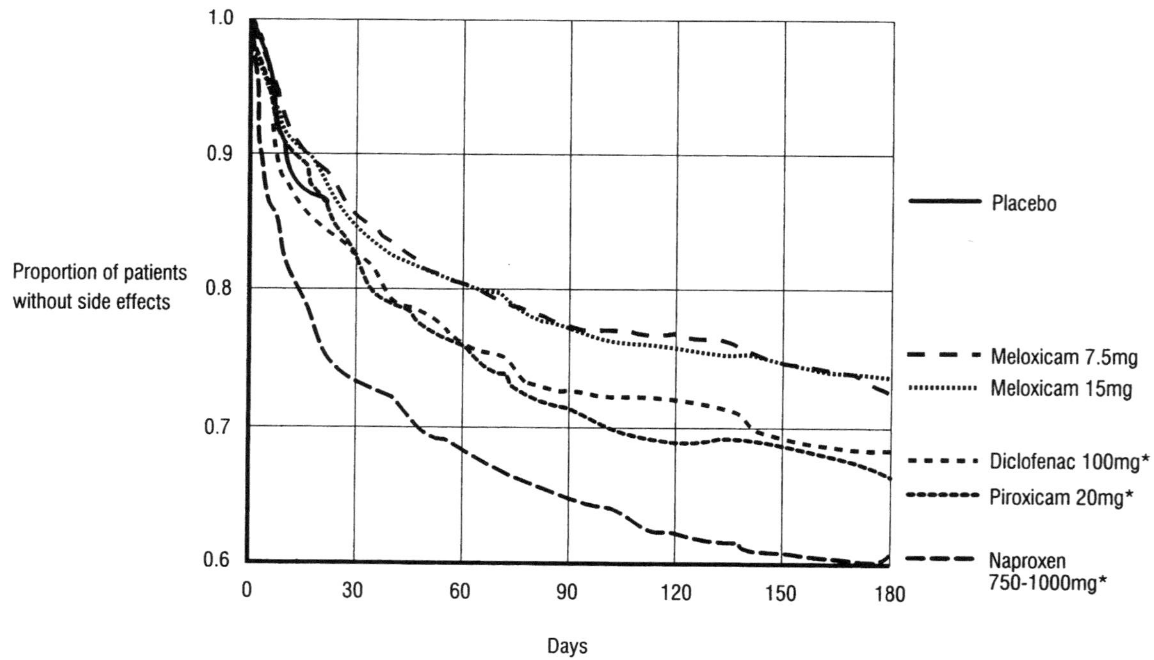

***Figure 3** Cumulative adverse event rate. Upper gastrointestinal perforations, ulcerations and bleeds (PUBs) observed occurring in double-blind studies of RA and OA. *Significantly fewer PUBs were observed with meloxicam 7.5 mg and 15 mg compared with naproxen and piroxicam (log rank test, $p < 0.05$)*

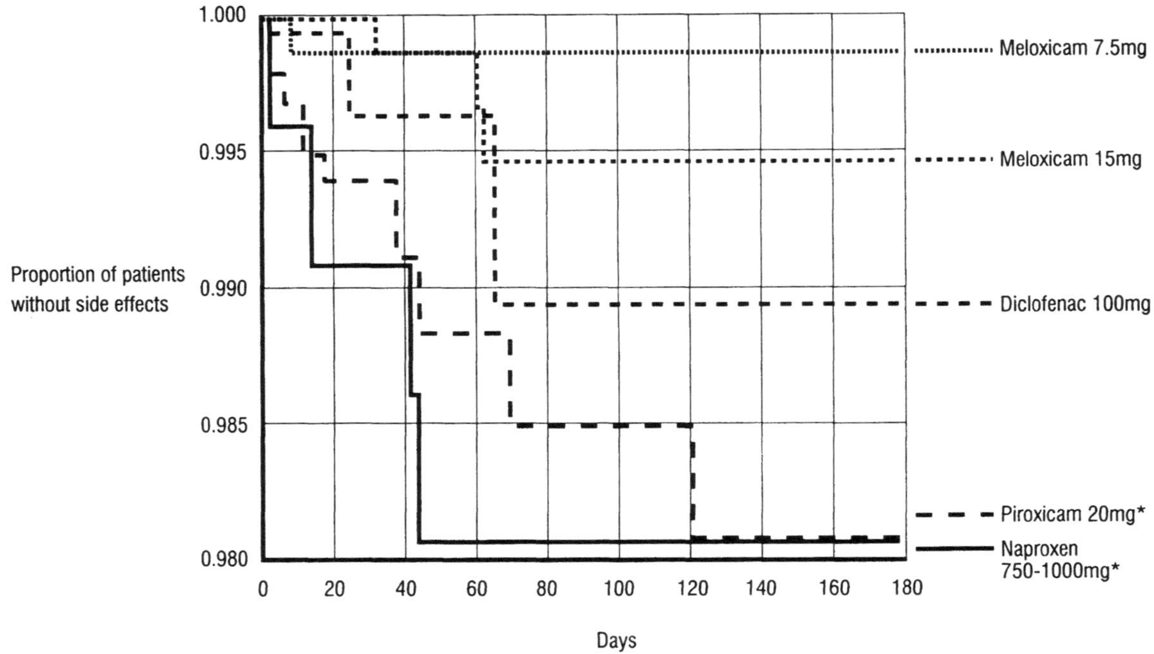

Selective COX-2 inhibitors will be of great value in ankylosing spondylitis. These patients are frequently intolerant of conventional NSAIDs. This is unfortunate since in a way the drugs are 'disease modifying', for if the patients are not kept mobile during periods of inflammation ankylosis occurs in positions of non-function. Thus less toxic, acceptable NSAIDs will be very valuable indeed. In OA, selective COX-2 inhibition will also be important: pain relief and increased mobility should result in improved quality of life. Similarly, in shoulder disease the early relief of pain is the essence of successful treatment, and non-toxic NSAIDs will achieve this with safety.

One should, however add a note of caution to our expectation of benefit from selective COX-2 inhibition. There is always the possibility that NSAIDs may have actions that are not connected with COX, uncoupling of oxidative phosphorylation for example, and there are some anomalies in the COX-2 hypothesis. Drugs that are highly selective for COX-1 can be very good in inflammatory disease. Piroxicam has a very high COX-2/COX-1 ratio yet there is no doubt it is effective in producing symptomatic relief. On the other hand flosulide is one of the most COX-2 selective drugs, with little gastric toxicity, yet it was withdrawn because of its toxic effects on the kidney. Finally, if it is definitely established that COX-2 is expressed in the central nervous system, this may have implications for therapy with selective COX-2 inhibitors. Some NSAIDs, for example diclofenac, have a mood elevating effect; others, such as indomethacin, cause the reverse. In future trials of selective COX-2 inhibitors clinicians should be alert to possible effects on the central nervous system.

References

1. Vane JR. Inhibition of prostaglandin synthesis as a mechanism of action for the aspirin-like drugs. Nature. 1971;231:232–5.
2. Akai Y, Homma T, Burns K, Yasuda T, Budr K, Harris R. Mechanical stretch/relaxation of cultured rat mesangial cells induces protooncogenes and cyclooxygenase. Am J Physiol. 1994;267: C482–90.
3. Langman MJS, Well J, Wainwright P et al. Risks of bleeding peptic ulcer associated with individual non-steroidal anti-inflammatory drugs. Lancet. 1994;343:1075–8.
4. Garcia Rodriguez LA, Jick H. Risk of upper gastrointestinal bleeding and perforation associated with individual non-steroidal anti-inflammatory drugs. Lancet. 1994;343:769–72.
5. Fries JF. NSAID-related adverse events: The view from the ARAMIS databanks. Proceedings of Symposium: New Insights into Anti-inflammatory Therapy and its Benefits. Cannes, October 1994.
6. Mitchell JA, Akarasereenont P, Thiemermann P et al. Selectivity of nonsteroidal anti-inflammatory drugs as inhibitors of constitutive and inducible cyclooxygenase. Proc Natl Acad Sci USA. 1993;90:11693–7.
7. Engelhardt G. Meloxicam. A potent inhibitor of COX-2. 9th International Conference on Prostaglandins and Related Compounds. Florence (Italy) June 6–10 1994.
8. Aronoff GR. Therapeutic implications associated with renal studies of nabumetone. J Rheumatol. 1992;19:25–31.
9. Türck D, Busch U, Heinzel G, Narjes H. Clinical pharmacokinetics of meloxicam. Eur J Rheumatol Inflam. 1996;15:23–30.
10. Degner F, Heinzel G, Busch U. Transsynovial kinetics of meloxicam. Scand J Rheumatol. 1994; Suppl 98:Abs 121.

11. Schmid J, Busch U, Heinzel G, Bozler G, Kaschke S, Kummer M. Meloxicam: pharmacokinetics and metabolic pattern after intravenous infusion and oral administration to healthy subjects. Drug Metab Dispos. 1995;23:1206–13.
12. Engelhardt G, Bögel R, Schnitzler C, Utzmann R. Meloxicam: influence on arachidonic acid metabolism. Part I. In vitro findings. Biochem Pharmacol. 1996;51:21–8.
13. Barner A, Distel M, Bluhmki E. Review of clinical trials and benefit/risk ratio of meloxicam. In: New insights into anti-inflammatory therapy and its benefits. Bollington, UK: Pennine Press; 1995:24–26.
14. Wojtulewski J, Schattenkirche M, Barceló P, Le Loet X, North N, Bluhmki E, Distel M. A six-month double-blind trial to compare the efficacy and safety of meloxicam 7.5 mg daily and naproxen 750 mg daily in patients with rheumatoid arthritis. Br J Rheumatol. (in press).
15. Distel M, Mueller C, Bluhmki F, Fries J. Global analysis of safety of a new NSAID, meloxicam. Br J Rheumatol. (in press).

Index

MIX
Papier aus verantwortungsvollen Quellen
Paper from responsible sources
FSC® C105338

If you have any concerns about our products,
you can contact us on
ProductSafety@springernature.com

In case Publisher is established outside the EU,
the EU authorized representative is:
Springer Nature Customer Service Center GmbH
Europaplatz 3, 69115 Heidelberg, Germany

Printed by Libri Plureos GmbH
in Hamburg, Germany